EUROPEAN
SOCIETY OF
CARDIOLOGY®

Sudden cardiac death

A handbook for clinical practice

EUROPEAN
SOCIETY OF
CARDIOLOGY®

THE ESC EDUCATION SERIES

Sudden cardiac death

A handbook for clinical practice

A publication based on ESC Guidelines
(www.escardio.org/knowledge/guidelines)

EDITED BY
Silvia G. Priori
Douglas P. Zipes

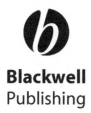

Blackwell
Publishing

Published by Blackwell Publishing
Blackwell Publishing, Inc., 350 Main Street, Malden, Massachusetts 02148-5020, USA
Blackwell Publishing Ltd, 9600 Garsington Road, Oxford OX4 2DQ, UK
Blackwell Science Asia Pty Ltd, 550 Swanston Street, Carlton, Victoria 3053, Australia

First published 2006

Library of Congress Cataloging-in-Publication Data

Sudden cardiac death: a handbook for clinical practice/edited by
Silvia G. Priori, Douglas P. Zipes.
  p. cm.
  Includes bibliographical references.
  ISBN-13: 978-1-4051-3292-3
  ISBN-10: 1-4051-3292-2
1. Cardiac arrest–Handbooks, manuals, etc. I. Priori, Silvia G.
II. Zipes, Douglas P.
  [DNLM: 1. Death, Sudden, Cardiac. WG205 S9435 2006]
RC685.C173S7713 2006
616.1'23025–dc22

                                                                    2005014112

ISBN-13: 978-1-4051-3292-3
ISBN-10: 1-4051-3292-2

A catalogue record for this title is available from the British Library

Set in 9.5/12 Meridien by Newgen Imaging Systems(P) Ltd, Chennai, India

Commissioning Editor: Gina Almond
Development Editor: Vicki Donald

For further information on Blackwell Publishing, visit our website:
www.blackwellcardiology.com

Contents

List of contributors

Editors

Silvia G. Priori, MD, PhD, Department of Cardiology, University of Pavia, Salvatore Maugeri Foundation, Pavia, Italy

Douglas P. Zipes Distinguished Professor, Professor Emeritus of Medicine, Pharmacology and Toxicology, Director Emeritus, Division of Cardiology, Indiana University, School of Medicine, Krannert Institute of Cardiology, Indianapolis, IN, USA

Contributors

Christine M. Albert, MD, Brigham and Women's Hospital, Boston, MA, USA

Elliott M. Antman, MD, Brigham and Women's Hospital, Boston, MA, USA

Charles Antzelevitch, PhD, Masonic Medical Research Laboratory, Utica, NY, USA

Cristina Basso, MD, PhD, Department of Cardiology and Pathology, University of Padua, Italy

Giuseppe Boriani, MD, PhD, Institute of Cardiology, University of Bologna, Bologna, Italy

Günter Breithardt, MD, FESC, FACC, Department of Cardiology and Angiology, Hospital of the University of Münster, Germany

Allen P Burke, MD, University of Maryland, Baltimore, MD, USA

Michael E. Cain, MD, Cardiovascular Division, Washington University School of Medicine, St Louis, MO, USA

A. John Camm, MD, Cardiological Sciences, St. George's Hospital Medical School, London, UK

D.A. Chamberlain, Wales Heart Research Institute and Prehospital Emergency Research Unit, College of Medicine, Cardiff University, Cardiff, UK

Stuart M. Cobbe, MD, FRCP, Glasgow Royal Infirmary, Glasgow, UK

Domenico Corrado, MD, PhD, Department of Cardiology and Pathology, University of Padua, Italy

Milou-Daniel Drici, MD, PhD, Department of Pharmacology, Nice-Sophia Antipolis University Medical Center, Hôpital Pasteur, Nice, Cedex, France

Helmut Drexler, MD, Cardiovascular Division, Medical University of Hannover, Hannover, Germany

K.A. Ellenbogen, MD, Department of Cardiology, Virginia Commonwealth University Health System, Richmond, VA, USA

N.A. Mark Estes III, MD, Tufts University, New England Medical Center, Boston, MA, USA

Olivier Fondard, MD, Cardiology Department, Bichat Hospital, Paris, France

Bernard J. Gersh, MD, ChB, DPhil, FACC, Division of Cardiovascular Diseases and Internal Medicine, Mayo Clinic and Mayo College of Medicine, Rochester, MN, USA

Michel Haïssaguerre, MD, Hôpital Cardiologique du Haut-Lévêque, Bordeaux, France

Mélèze Hocini, MD, Hôpital Cardiologique du Haut-Lévêque, Bordeaux, France

Stefan H. Hohnloser, MD, Division of Cardiology, J. W. Goethe University, Frankfurt, Germany

Michiel J. Janse, MD, The Experimental and Molecular Cardiology Group, Academic Medical Center, University of Amsterdam, Amsterdam, The Netherlands

Pierre Jaïs, MD, Hôpital Cardiologique du Haut-Lévêque, Bordeaux, France
Xavier Jouven, MD, PhD, Hopital Européen Georges Pompidou, University René Descartes, Paris, France
Paulus Kirchhof, MD, Department of Cardiology and Angiology, Hospital of the University of Münster, Germany
Greg Larsen, MD, Cardiology Section, Oregon VA Medical Center, Portland, USA
Mark S. Link, MD, Tufts University, New England Medical Center, Boston, MA, USA
Barry J. Maron, MD, Minneapolis Heart Institute Foundation, Minneapolis, MN, USA
William J. McKenna, BA, MD, DSc, The Heart Hospital, University College, London NHS Foundation Trust, London, UK
David Messika-Zeitoun, MD, Cardiology Department, Bichat Hospital, Paris, France
John M. Miller, MD, Indiana University School of Medicine, Indianapolis, IN, USA
Arthur J. Moss, MD, University of Rochester Medical Center, Rochester, NY, USA
Robert J. Myerburg, MD, University of Miami, Miami, FL, USA
M.A. Peberdy, MD, Department of Cardiology, Virginia Commonwealth University Health System, Richmond, VA, USA
Dan M. Roden, MD, Department of Medicine and Pharmacology, Vanderbilt University School of Medicine, Nashville, TN, USA
Prashanthan Sanders, MBBS, PhD, Hôpital Cardiologique du Haut-Lévêque, Bordeaux, France
Peter J. Schwartz, MD, University of Pavia and Policlinico S. Matteo IRCCS, Pavia, Italy
Srijita Sen-Chowdhry, MA, MBBS, MRCP, The Heart Hospital, University College, London NHS Foundation Trust, London, UK
Timothy W. Smith, MD, DPhil, Cardiovascular Division, Washington University School of Medicine, St. Louis, MO, USA
William G. Stevenson, MD, Harvard Medical School, Brigham and Women's Hospital, Boston, MA, USA
Gaetano Thiene, MD, Department of Cardiology and Pathology, University of Padua, Italy
Alec Vahanian, MD, Cardiology Department, Bichat Hospital, Paris, France
Richard L. Verrier, PhD, Harvard Medical School, Beth Israel Deaconess Medical Center, Boston, MA, USA
Renu Virmani, MD, CVPath, International Registry of Pathology, Gaithersburg, MD, USA
Hein J.J. Wellens, MD, Academic Hospital, Maastricht, The Netherlands
William Wijns, MD, Cardiovascular Centre, Aalst, Belgium
Wojciech Zareba, MD, PhD, Department of Medicine, University of Rochester, Rochester, NY, USA

Preface

Sudden cardiac death continues to present an important challenge in Europe, the United States, and other developed countries. Major difficulties exist in identifying individuals at risk prior to an episode of a ventricular tachyarrhythmia or a sudden cardiac arrest, and in responding in a timely fashion to the person suffering from the catastrophic event out of hospital. The European Society of Cardiology has established guidelines on how to address some of these issues. Another set of guidelines on evaluation and treatment of patients with ventricular arrhythmias and sudden cardiac arrest, created by joint writing committees from the American College of Cardiology, the American Heart Association, the European Society of Cardiology, and the Heart Rhythm Society, will further promote the approaches to individuals with diverse cardiac problems who are at risk of ventricular tachyarrhythmias and sudden cardiac death.

This book is part of the ESC Education Series and provides background information about the guidelines. The focus is to present an update on what we know about sudden cardiac arrest, from basic experimental studies to clinical trials. The book also serves as a compliment to the core syllabus on this topic.

Because sudden cardiac arrest is no respecter of geographic boundaries, we thought a unique contribution would be to have chapters co-authored by experts on both sides of the Atlantic to derive a truly international view on the topic. Therefore, each chapter has one or more European and American authors presenting a united view of the topic.

Chapter topics include epidemiology, genetics, arrhythmogenic mechanisms, risk stratification, autonomic nervous system, phenotypes, and there are also chapters on disease states and special populations, including coronary artery disease, cardiomyopathies, inherited diseases, valvular heart disease, heart failure, drugs, and athletes. Finally, there are chapters on drug, device and ablation treatments, and cost-effectiveness.

We plan future updates as new evidence from clinical and basic science provide substantial innovations to the field. An update of the book will parallel the publication of new sets of Guidelines.

We would like to dedicate this book to the memory of two outstanding cardiologists, Ronald Campbell and Anthony Ricketts, who have made important contributions to our understanding of sudden cardiac arrest and tragically succumbed to it.

Finally, we would like to thank our spouses, Giulio Zuanetti and Joan Zipes, for their tolerance of the time we have spent in this and other endeavors, and the support of our children, Andrea and Gabriele Zuanetti, and Debra, Jeffrey, and David Zipes.

Silvia G. Priori
Douglas P. Zipes

Section one:
Epidemiology and mechanisms

CHAPTER 1

Epidemiology of cardiac arrest

Robert J. Myerburg and Hein J.J. Wellens

Epidemiological studies related to sudden cardiac death (SCD) remain challenging for both theoretical and practical reasons. There are persisting fundamental questions about definition, inconsistencies in access to data, variations in pathophysiological mechanisms and their clinical recognition, and distinctions between population risk and individual risk. In addition, the emerging field of genetic epidemiology adds a new dimension for study, and there is need for focus on interventional epidemiology, the latter being a term coined to define the population dynamics of therapeutic outcomes. This chapter will provide an overview of each of these components of the epidemiology of SCD.

Basic definitions of SCD

A generally accepted definition of SCD is natural death due to cardiac causes, heralded by abrupt loss of consciousness within an hour of the onset of acute symptoms. Preexisting heart disease may or may not have been previously recognized, but the time and mode of death are unexpected [1]. The term "unexpected" is the hallmark of the definition because it permits inclusion of a broad range of preceding clinical states, having different levels risk.

Four time elements must be considered in the construction of a definition of SCD to satisfy clinical, scientific, legal, and social considerations: prodromes, onset, cardiac arrest, and progression to biological death. The proximate cause of SCD is an abrupt cessation of blood flow that is incompatible with maintaining life if allowed to persist. The 1-h definition is arbitrary and refers to the duration of the "terminal event," which defines the interval between the onset of symptoms signaling the pathophysiological disturbance leading to cardiac arrest and the onset of the cardiac arrest itself. A 24-h definition may be used as a SCD definition for *unwitnessed deaths* of victims known to be alive and functioning normally prior to being found, and this is appropriate within obvious limits. However, the temporal definition used affects the relative incidence of cardiac causes of sudden death and the frequency of specific cardiac disorders [1].

Biological death was viewed as an immediate consequence of cardiac arrest in the past, usually occurring within minutes. However, since the development of community-based interventions and life support systems, patients may now remain biologically alive for a long period of time after the onset of a pathophysiological process that has caused irreversible damage. In this circumstance, the causative pathophysiological and clinical event is the cardiac arrest itself, rather than the factors responsible for the delayed biological death. However, for legal, forensic, and certain social considerations, biological death is the absolute definition, in contrast to cardiac arrest, which retains survival potential.

Clinical definitions of cardiac arrest and SCD are categorized as "primary" or "secondary." These classifications are used in many clinical trials and some epidemiological surveys. "Secondary" refers to a cardiac arrest or SCD in an individual who has survived a prior cardiac arrest or its equivalent. Common use of the term "primary" is more complex, generally referring to an event in an individual who has not had a prior cardiac arrest, regardless of the clinical severity of the underlying disease. The term also refers to arrhythmic collapse as an initial or isolated feature of the disease (primary cardiac arrest – PCA), in the absence of a recognized acute state (such as acute myocardial infarction) that is an identified trigger for the event. By strict epidemiological definitions, however, none of these usages of "primary" is correct, since the term refers to the prevention of the underlying disease state, rather than of a clinical manifestation. Conversely, all cardiac arrests associated with underlying diseases are "secondary" events. Despite these differences epidemiologically, the common usage remains ingrained in clinical medicine.

General epidemiology of SCD

Overview

The worldwide incidence of SCD is difficult to estimate because it varies largely as a function of prevalence of coronary heart disease in different countries [2,3]. Estimates for the United States, largely based upon retrospective death certificate analyses [4–6] and an emergency rescue database in one study [7] range from less than 200 000 to more than 450 000 SCDs annually, with the most widely used estimates in the range of 300 000–350 000 SCDs [8]. This accounts for an incidence of 0.1–0.2% per year among the population >35 years of age. Event rates in Europe are similar to those in the United States [9]. These ranges of estimates are based, in part, on the definition of sudden death and inclusion criteria used in individual studies, and the correct number can only be defined from a carefully designed prospective epidemiological study. A recent study in a single city in the United States, using a prospective design for data collection, suggested a significantly lower national incidence when extrapolated to the entire country [10]. Because of geographic population variations [11], however, such extrapolations must be viewed with caution.

Approximately 50% of all coronary heart disease deaths are sudden and unexpected, often occurring shortly after the onset of symptoms. Because coronary heart disease is the dominant cause of both sudden and nonsudden cardiac deaths in the United States and Europe, the fraction of total cardiac deaths that are sudden is similar to the fraction of coronary heart disease deaths that are sudden. It is also of interest that the age-adjusted decline in coronary heart disease mortality in the United States during the past half-century has not changed the fraction of coronary deaths that are sudden and unexpected [12,13]. Furthermore, the decreasing age-adjusted mortality does not imply a decrease in absolute numbers of cardiac or sudden deaths because of the growth and aging of the population and the increasing prevalence of chronic heart disease [14,15].

Population subgroups and SCD

When the more than 300 000 adult SCDs that occur annually in the United States are viewed as a global incidence in an unselected adult population, the overall incidence is 1 to 2/1000 (0.1–0.2%) per year. This large population base includes those victims whose SCDs occur as a first cardiac event, as well as those whose SCDs can be predicted with greater accuracy because they are included in higher-risk subgroups. Any intervention designed for the general population must be applied to the 999/1000 who will not have an event, in order to reach and possibly influence the 1/1000 who will have. The cost and risk-to-benefit uncertainties limit the nature of broad-based interventions and demand a higher resolution of risk identification. Figure 1.1(a) highlights this problem by expressing the incidence (percent/year) of SCD among various subgroups and comparing the incidence figures to the total number of events that occur annually in each subgroup. By moving from the total adult population to a subgroup at higher risk because of the presence of selected coronary risk factors, there may be a 10-fold or greater increase in the incidence of events annually, with the magnitude of increase dependent on the number of risk factors operating in the subgroup [15]. The size of the denominator pool, however, remains very large, and implementation of interventions remains problematic, even at this heightened level of risk. Higher resolution is desirable and can be achieved by identification of more specific subgroups. However, the corresponding absolute number of deaths become progressively smaller as the subgroups become more focused, limiting the potential benefit of interventions to a much smaller fraction of the total number of patients at risk. Various estimates suggest that at least two-third of all SCDs due to coronary heart disease occur as a first clinical event or among subgroups of patients thought to be at relatively low risk for SCD [12] (Figure 1.1(b)).

Time-dependence of risk

Temporal influences on the risk of SCD have been analyzed in the context of both biological and clinical chronology. In the former, epidemiological analyses of SCD risk among populations have identified three patterns: diurnal,

6   Chapter 1

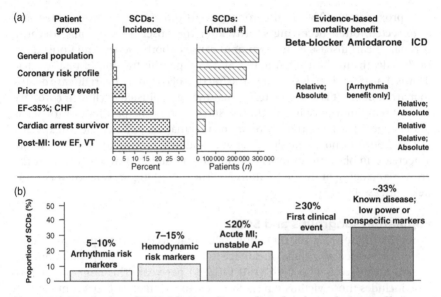

Figure 1.1 Distribution of SCD risk According to clinical and population profiles.
(a) The figure shows estimates of incidence (percent/year) and the total number of
events per year for the general adult population in the United States, and for
increasingly higher-risk subgroups. With the identification of increasingly powerful
markers of risk, the incidence increases progressively, accompanied by a progressive
decrease in the total number of events contained within each successive subgroup.
Successful interventions among larger population subgroups will require
identification of new markers, specific for high risk of a future event. Modified from
Reference 15; reproduced with permission of the American Heart Association, Inc.
(b) The figure demonstrates the distribution of clinical status of victims at the time of
SCD. Nearly two-third of cardiac arrests occur as the first clinically manifest event or
in the clinical setting of known disease in the absence of strong risk predictors.
Modified from Reference 12.

weekly, and seasonal. General patterns of heightened risk during the morning hours, on Mondays, and during the winter months have been described
[15,16]. In the clinical paradigm, risk of SCD is not linear as a function of
time after changes in cardiovascular status. Survival curves after major cardiovascular events, which identify risk for both sudden and total cardiac death,
usually demonstrate that the most rapid rate of attrition occurs during the first
6–18 months after the index event. Thus there is a time-dependence of risk
that focuses the opportunity for maximum efficacy of an intervention during
the early period after a conditioning event [15]. Curves that have these characteristics have been generated from among survivors of out-of-hospital cardiac
arrest, new onset of heart failure, and unstable angina, and from high-risk subgroups of patients having recent myocardial infarction [8,15]. Even though
attrition rates decrease over time, an effective intervention can still cause late

diversion of treated versus control risk curves, indicating continuing benefit. The patterns of early and late separation of curves reflect two different dimensions of time-dependent risk.

Age, heredity, gender, and race

Age
There are two ages of peak incidence of sudden death: between birth and 6 months of age (the sudden infant death syndrome) and between 45 and 75 years of age. Among the general adult population, the *incidence* of sudden death increases dramatically as a function of advancing age [17], in parallel with the age-related increase in incidence of total coronary heart disease deaths. For subgroups with advanced heart disease, the higher risk associated with the disease state blunts the impact of age. The incidence is 100-fold less in adolescents and adults below 30 years of age [18–20] (1 in 100 000 per year), than it is in adults above 35 years age of (1 in 1000 per year) [12].

Heredity
Among the less common causes of SCD, hereditary patterns have been reported for specific syndromes, such as the congenital long-QT-interval syndromes, hypertrophic cardiomyopathy, right ventricular cardiomyopathy, the Brugada syndrome, "idiopathic" ventricular tachycardia/fibrillation, and yet-to-be-defined patterns of familial SCD in children and young adults (see Chapter 9). Mutations and functioning polymorphisms are being mapped to genes located on many chromosomes, as the molecular bases for the entities are being defined. In addition, these observations may provide screening tools for individuals at risk for SCD due to more common causes, such as coronary heart disease [21] (see Section on Genetic Epidemiology). To the extent that SCD is an expression of underlying coronary heart disease, hereditary factors that contribute to coronary heart disease risk have been thought to operate nonspecifically for the SCD syndrome. However, recent studies have identified mutations and polymorphisms along multiple steps of the cascade from atherogenesis to plaque destabilization, thrombosis, and arrhythmogenesis, many of which are associated with altered risk of coronary events [22–25].

Gender
The risk of SCD is four to seven times greater in males compared with females during the young adult and early middle-age years because of the protection females enjoy from coronary atherosclerosis before menopause [26]. As coronary event risk increases in postmenopausal women, SCD risk increases, perhaps disproportionately, and the excess in males fades. Even though the overall risk is much lower in younger women, the classic coronary risk factors are still predictive of events among women [1,26], including cigarette smoking, diabetes, use of oral contraceptives, and hyperlipidemia.

Race

A number of early studies comparing racial differences in relative risk of SCD in whites and African Americans with coronary heart disease in the United States had yielded conflicting and inconclusive data. However, recent studies have demonstrated excess risk of cardiac arrest and SCD among African Americans compared with whites [27,28]. SCD rates among Hispanic populations were smaller. The differences were observed across all age groups.

Conventional coronary risk factors and SCD

Risk profiling for coronary atherogenesis is useful for identifying levels of population risk and individual risk [29], but cannot be used to distinguish individual patients at risk for SCD from those at risk for other manifestations of coronary heart disease. Multivariate analyses of selected risk factors (i.e. age, systolic blood pressure, heart rate, electrocardiographic abnormalities, vital capacity, relative weight, cigarette smoking, diabetes mellitus, and serum cholesterol) have determined that approximately one-half of all SCDs occur among the 10% of the population in the highest risk decile, based upon multiple risk factors. Thus, the cumulative risk derived from multiple risk factors exceeds the simple arithmetic sum of the individual risks [29]. In addition, angiographic and hemodynamic patterns discriminate SCD risk from non-SCD risk only under limited circumstances. In contrast, familial clustering of SCD as a specific manifestation of the disease may lead to identification of specific genetic abnormalities that predispose to SCD [30,31].

Hypertension is a clearly established risk factor for coronary heart disease and also emerges as a highly significant risk factor for incidence of SCD [32]. However, there is no influence of increasing systolic blood pressure levels on the ratio of sudden deaths to total coronary heart disease deaths. No relationship has been observed between cholesterol concentration and the proportion of coronary deaths that are sudden. Neither the electrocardiographic pattern of left ventricular (LV) hypertrophy nor nonspecific ST–T-wave abnormalities influence the proportion of total coronary deaths that are sudden and unexpected; only intraventricular conduction abnormalities are suggestive of a disproportionate number of SCDs [1]. The latter is an old observation that was recently reinforced by data from device trials that suggests the importance of QRS duration as a risk marker [33].

The conventional risk factors used in early studies of SCD are the risk factors for evolution of coronary artery disease. The rationale is based on two facts: (1) coronary disease is the structural basis for 80% of SCDs in the United States and Europe, and (2) the coronary risk factors are easy to identify because they tend to be present continuously over time (Figure 1.2). However, risk factors specific for fatal arrhythmias are dynamic pathophysiological events and occur transiently [13,15]. Transient pathophysiological events are being modeled epidemiologically [21], in an attempt to express and use them as clinical risk factors for both profiling and intervention.

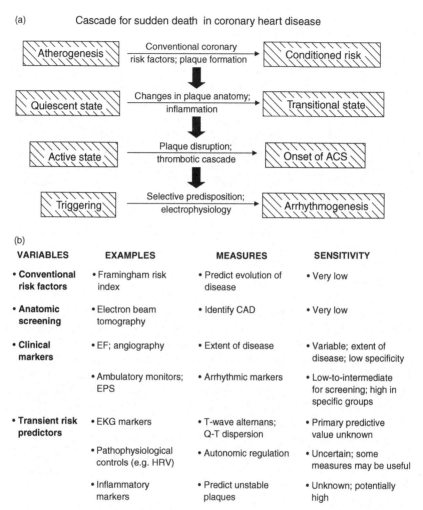

(a)   Cascade for sudden death in coronary heart disease

Atherogenesis → Conventional coronary risk factors; plaque formation → Conditioned risk

Quiescent state → Changes in plaque anatomy; inflammation → Transitional state

Active state → Plaque disruption; thrombotic cascade → Onset of ACS

Triggering → Selective predisposition; electrophysiology → Arrhythmogenesis

(b)

VARIABLES	EXAMPLES	MEASURES	SENSITIVITY
• Conventional risk factors	• Framingham risk index	• Predict evolution of disease	• Very low
• Anatomic screening	• Electron beam tomography	• Identify CAD	• Very low
• Clinical markers	• EF; angiography	• Extent of disease	• Variable; extent of disease; low specificity
	• Ambulatory monitors; EPS	• Arrhythmic markers	• Low-to-intermediate for screening; high in specific groups
• Transient risk predictors	• EKG markers	• T-wave alternans; Q-T dispersion	• Primary predictive value unknown
	• Pathophysiological controls (e.g. HRV)	• Autonomic regulation	• Uncertain; some measures may be useful
	• Inflammatory markers	• Predict unstable plaques	• Unknown; potentially high

Figure 1.2 Cascade for sudden cardiac death in coronary heart disease and levels of clinical prediction. (a) The figure demonstrates the cascade from conventional risk factors for coronary atherosclerosis to arrhythmogenesis in SCD due to coronary heart disease. The cascade identifies four levels of evolution, beginning with lesion initiation and development, progressing to the transition to an active state, then to acute coronary syndromes, and finally to the specific expression of life-threatening arrhythmias. Modified from Reference 21 with permission. (b) The figure demonstrates categories of risk factors. *Conventional risk factors* and *anatomic disease screening* have general use for predicting risk but with low sensitivity. They are not specific for arrhythmic deaths. *Clinical predictors* have variable power, some of which are useful as predictors for cardiac arrest and SCD, and have been widely used in the design of arrhythmia intervention trials. *Transient risk predictors* and *individual risk prediction* (see Figure 1.4) offer the hope for more powerful individual prediction of risk of SCD. Modified from Reference 12.

Lifestyle and psychosocial factors

Lifestyle

There is a strong association between *cigarette smoking* and all manifestations of coronary heart disease. The Framingham Study demonstrates that cigarette smokers have a two-fold to three-fold increase in sudden death risk in each decade of life at entry between 30 and 59 years, and that this is one of the few risk factors in which the proportion of coronary heart disease deaths that are sudden increases in association with the risk factor [34]. In addition, in a study of 310 survivors of out-of-hospital cardiac arrest, the recurrent cardiac arrest rate was 27% at 3 years of follow-up among those who continued to smoke after their index event, compared with 19% in those who stopped [35] ($p < .04$).

Obesity is a second factor that appears to influence the proportion of coronary deaths that occur suddenly [34]. With increasing relative weight, the percentage of coronary heart disease deaths that were sudden in the Framingham Study increased linearly from a low of 39% to a high of 70%. Total coronary heart disease deaths increased with increasing relative weight as well. Associations between levels of physical activity and SCD have been studied, with variable results. Epidemiological observations have suggested a relationship between *low levels of physical activity* and increased coronary heart disease death risk. The Framingham Study, however, showed an *insignificant* relationship between low levels of physical activity and incidence of sudden death and a high proportion of sudden to total cardiac deaths at higher levels of physical activity [34]. A case-crossover cohort study demonstrated a 17-fold relative increase in vigorous exercise-associated SCD, compared to lower-level activity or inactive states [36]. However, the absolute risk for events was very low (1 event per 1.5 million exercise sessions). Habitual vigorous exercise attenuated risk. In contrast, SCD among young athletes has a higher incidence than among young nonathletic individuals in the same age range [37]. Information about physical activity relationships in various clinical settings, such as overt and silent disease states, is still lacking.

Psychosocial factors

The magnitude of recent life changes in the realms of health, work, home and family, and personal and social factors have been related to myocardial infarction and SCD [38,39]. There is an association between significant elevations of life-change scores during the 6 months before a coronary event, and the association is particularly striking in victims of SCD. Among women, those who die suddenly are less often married, had fewer children, and had greater educational discrepancies with their spouses than did age-related controls living in the same neighborhood as the sudden death victims. A history of psychiatric treatment, cigarette smoking, and greater quantities of alcohol consumption than the controls also characterized the sudden death group. Controlling for other major prognostic factors, risk of sudden and total deaths, and other coronary events, is impacted by social and economic stresses [40]. Alteration of modifiable lifestyle factors has been proposed as a strategy for reducing risk of SCD in patients with coronary heart disease, although a study of treatment of depression following myocardial infarction failed to demonstrate an effect on event rates [1]. Acute psychosocial stressors have been associated with risk of cardiovascular events, including SCD. The risk appears to cluster around the time of the stress, and appear to occur among victims at preexisting risk, with the stressor simply advancing the time of an impending event [41].

Risk prediction and the coronary heart disease cascade

The cascade of evolution and clinical manifestations of coronary artery disease leading to risk of SCD can be viewed as a four-stage process: atherogenesis, transition, acute coronary syndromes, and arrhythmogenesis (see Figure 1.2(a)). The initial stage occurs over a long period of time and must be viewed from the perspective of population risk, rather than clinical risk, because event rates are relatively low, even among the higher-risk categories. Risk markers identified with the transitional state, those factors responsible for evolution of changes in atherosclerotic plaque anatomy and pathophysiology, are applicable to subgroups with established disease, even though it may not yet be clinically expressed. Recent interest in markers of plaque inflammation as a predictor of risk is an example of the application of pathophysiologic states in more concentrated population groups. The target is prediction of the transition of the disease to an active state over shorter time periods. The next level of the cascade is the onset of an acute coronary syndrome as the proximate trigger of SCD, or other manifestations of the underlying disease. An example is the variations in response of the thrombotic cascade to onset of the syndrome.

At the final stage of arrhythmogenesis, there is an interaction between the ischemic consequences of the earlier stages of the cascade and the generation of cardiac arrhythmias. This may be related to ion channel behavior at the single cell level and interactions between ion channel responses, or between ischemic and nonischemic regions. As one moves along the cascade of risk, there is the potential for increasing sensitivity and specificity in exchange for decreasing size of the population denominator. The challenge presently is to determine how markers of risk at each level of the cascade can be identified prospectively in order to seek subgroups at especially high risk of events prior to the onset of acute coronary syndromes. An example of such strategies is the current interest in the use of inflammatory markers as a predictor of acute coronary syndromes. The ultimate goal is to use predictors of transient risk to identify those individuals at risk for the events that trigger fatal arrhythmias [12,21] (Figure 1.2(b)). Viewed in broad perspective, these may include such pathophysiologic control mechanisms as autonomic nervous system functions (e.g. heart-rate variability, baroreceptor sensitivity, measures of alteration of repolarization, inflammatory markers, and thrombotic cascade markers).

Risk prediction in dilated cardiomyopathy

Sudden cardiac death among patients with the cardiomyopathies is even more difficult to predict. While LV ejection fraction (EF) is a strong mortality risk predictor generally among patients who have dilated cardiomyopathies, it is not as useful for specifically predicting SCD. It appears that there is a better association with functional capacity. For example, among patients with dilated cardiomyopathy who are classified as functional class I, the risk of dying is small, but the proportional probability that a death will be sudden, if it occurs, is relatively high. The fact that this category encompasses a large number of patients at relatively low risk limits the predictive power for benefit from interventions. At the other end of the spectrum, functional class III and IV patients are generally at a higher risk of mortality and a higher risk of absolute numbers of SCDs [42], although the proportional risk of sudden death is somewhat lower. This statement does not incorporate the possible impact of long-term medical therapy for heart failure on the balance between sudden and nonsudden deaths.

Interventional epidemiology

The outcomes of clinical trials, observational therapeutic data, and the results of epidemiological surveys all contribute to the management of risk for SCD [12]. However, the application of the knowledge gained from each of these sources of data may differ in terms of its population impact, compared to individual clinical impact. For example, mining of existing large databases can identify risk factors or strong associations. Observations are generally expressed in terms of relative risk statements, and often based on low absolute event rates. Low event rates with large relative differences identify effects, but usually with limited individual patient impact (Figure 1.3(a)). In contrast, randomized clinical trials with large absolute differences in outcomes are able to better define individual patient benefits. Observational studies are limited by their dependence on anticipated, rather than actual, comparison outcomes.

Studies of the benefit of the implantable cardioverter-defibrillator (ICD) for individuals at high risk of SCD are instructive. From the time of the first implant in 1980 until the publication of the first clinical trial in 1996, their use was initially prescribed on the basis of observational data and clinical judgment, and their use compared to drugs and surgery. This scientific limitation impeded their initial acceptance. With the publication of a number of randomized trials since 1996, the ICD has moved into the position of preferred therapy for specifically defined high-risk patients. The clinical trials of ICDs have included both primary and secondary prevention strategies. While the usage of the term "primary prevention" for ICD trials is technically incorrect (see above), it does serve the purpose of subgrouping patients into two general categories, the study design and outcomes of which might be interpreted and applied differently.

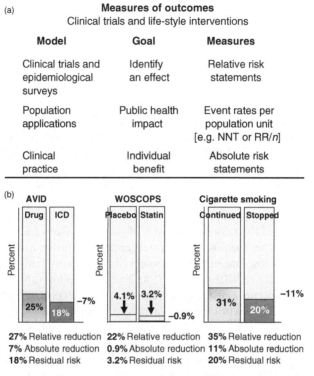

Figure 1.3 Outcomes of clinical trials can be expressed as relative risk and absolute risk improvements, as well as normalized to numbers needed to treat (NNT) or relative risk (RR) divided by the number of observations (n). (a) Here the clinical trial or epidemiological survey model, population applications, and practical clinical applications are related to the goals of identifying an effect, public health impact, or individual benefit, and the appropriate measures to express outcome in relation to those goals. (b) Here the relative and absolute risk reductions are demonstrated for three practical clinical models: the AVID trial [43] the West of Scotland Coronary Prevention Study (WOSCOPS) [44] demonstrating the effect of statins on mortality outcome, and the effect of continued cigarette smoking on outcomes after survival from an initial cardiac arrest [35]. Modified from Reference 45.

All studies of group outcomes of therapy for complex pathophysiological states must take four factors into account (Figure 1.3(b)): (1) relative risk reduction, (2) absolute risk reduction, (3) residual risk, and (4) cumulative benefits of multiple interventions. The primary endpoint reports for all clinical trials of ICD therapy, and most other large clinical trials, focus on reduction in relative risk [45,46] since this measure identifies the *effect* of the intervention. However, relative risk reduction does not quantify the benefit for the individual patient. To do so, a measure of absolute risk reduction is required, such as the absolute numerical difference in risk observed in the test and control groups, or calculations of a number of patients needed to be treated (NNT) in order to save a life [47].

Other measures of group impact that do not commonly receive attention include residual risk and cumulative benefit. The former refers to the absolute outcome among the treated group or test group in a clinical trial population, which identifies the component of total mortality risk that does not respond to the tested therapy. If residual risk is very high, the absolute and relative risk reduction benefits are correspondingly limited. Cumulative benefit refers to the increment in benefit from integration of multiple interventions. Despite its importance [45,48], this is rarely stratified in clinical trial designs because it requires larger study populations, and has not been used prospectively in any of the ICD or antiarrhythmic trials. *Post hoc* subgroup analysis can be used to suggest added benefit of a secondary strategy, but this does not replace stratifying the multiple interventions.

A comparison of the various measures of outcomes from an ICD trial, contrasted with another cardiovascular intervention, is shown in Figure 1.3(b). The relative and absolute outcomes observed in the Antiarrhythmics Versus Implantable Device (AVID) study [47] at 2 years of follow-up are compared to the West of Scotland Coronary Prevention Study (WOSCOPS) [48], a study of the impact of Pravachol versus placebo in a population of men without known preexisting coronary artery disease. While the relative risk reduction for total mortality (at 2 years of follow-up in AVID and 5 years of follow-up in WOSCOPS), was reasonably close (27% versus 22%), the absolute risk reduction and residual risks were very different. The absolute benefit in AVID was 7% over 2 years, whereas in the WOSCOPS, the absolute total mortality benefit was 0.9% over a study period of 5 years. In addition, the residual risk in AVID was considerably higher than in the WOSCOPS population, as might be expected for the populations in the two studies. The high residual risk in AVID dwarfs, to some extent, the absolute risk reduction.

In another comparison, ICD use versus amiodarone (AVID), and cessation of cigarette smoking among survivors of out-of-hospital cardiac arrest [35], both identify absolute and relative risk benefits of the same general order of magnitude. However, these two separate observations leads us to question of whether there is a positive interaction between cigarette smoking cessation and the ICD (Figure 1.3(b)). Subgroup analyses are not sufficient to answer these questions. Cessation of cigarette smoking is but one of a number of interventions that could be tested in parallel with ICD therapy, seeking positive interactions. The general principle has been suggested for amiodarone and beta-blockers in post-myocardial infarction patients.

A final consideration in the epidemiology of interventions is the comparison of entry criteria to actual enrollment. In many of the ICD trials, the range of EFs and functional classifications were unintentionally biased toward certain values, limiting the interpretation and proper application of the outcomes (see Table 1.1). EF entry criteria were largely in the range of ≤30 to ≤40%,

Table 1.1 Comparison of entry criteria to actual enrollment

	Reference	Ejection fraction		Time from qualifying event	
		Entry criterion	Actually enrolled	Entry criterion	Actually enrolled
MADIT	49	≤35%	26% (±7%) (Mean ± SD)	≥3 weeks	75% ≥6 months
MUSIT	50	≤40%	30% (21%, 35%) (Median; 25th, 75th percentile)	≥4 days	39% ≤1 year 50% ≥3 years
MADIT-2	51	≤30%	23% (±5%) (Mean ± SD)	>1 month	88% ≥6 months
SCD-HeFT	52	≤35%	25% (20%, 30%) (Median; 25th, 75th percentile)	Not specified	24 months (28, 25) (Median; 25th, 75th percentile)
COMPANION	53	≤35%	21% (±5%) (Mean ± SD)	Not specified	43 months (CHF) (Median)
DEFINITE	54	≤35%	21% (7–35%) (Mean, range)	Not specified	32 months (CHF)

but enrollment was dominated by lower ranges. Therefore, the benefit to those with the higher end of the EF range is not clear.

Genetic epidemiology of SCD

Limitations in identifying the *individual* at risk of SCD from among the general population is a major reason why SCD remains an important public health problem. The ability to identify individual-specific predisposition to expression of plaque disruption-thrombosis, and of electrophysiological responses leading to life-threatening arrhythmias, could lead to preventive actions in anticipation of the potentially fatal disturbances. New insights into specific risk at all levels of the cascade offer hope for better individual risk prediction, expressed in terms of higher orders of *single-patient probabilities*, in contrast to less specific general population risks [21].

Interest in the evolving constellation of information on genetic control of ion channel function (see Chapter 9) is reinforced by recent epidemiological studies, suggesting that SCD may be a patient-specific response in acute coronary syndromes. Two studies have demonstrated a pattern of familial clustering of SCD, with an excess risk of sudden death as the specific initial manifestation of an acute coronary syndrome when there is family history of SCD in one parent [30,31], and even higher when both sides of the family are affected [31]. While such familial clustering could be either genetic or environmental, studies on genetically-based arrhythmia syndromes provide a series of candidate

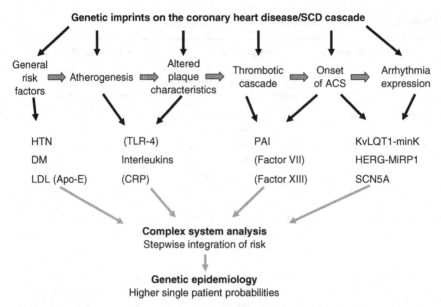

Figure 1.4 Genetic imprints on the cascade from coronary atherogenesis to sudden cardiac death. Influences of genetic variations on individual risk prediction have been identified for elements of atherogenesis, plaque evolution, the thrombotic cascade, and arrhythmia expression. Stepwise integration of these characteristics for individuals through complex system analysis methods offers the hope of a field of genetic epidemiology that may lead to higher single-patient probabilities for SCD risk prediction. Modified from Reference 21, with permission.

genes that could be the targets of studies seeking polymorphisms or mutations carried by such families. An example is a genetic variant in the cardiac sodium channel gene (*SCN5A*) observed among the African American population (carrier rate = 13.2%) that appears to predispose to arrhythmias, even though it does not express as a prototypic long-QT syndrome under control conditions [55]. Its role in predicting risk of SCD awaits clarification. Although still in its infancy, the potential impact on predicting and preventing sudden death could be huge.

A major paradigm shift in the epidemiology of coronary heart disease may emerge from new insights into the cause and expression of the multiple elements in the cascade of lesion formation, initiation of acute coronary syndromes, and triggering of cardiac arrest and SCD (Figure 1.4). Conceptually, nonexpressed variations of DNA sequences in genes encoding ion channel structure may transpose into an abnormal phenotype under pathophysiologic conditions, thus integrating with the pathophysiology of the acute coronary syndrome.

As data applicable to an expanded epidemiological approach evolves, it will call for a conceptual transformation of the sequential pathophysiologic cascade into a complex system analytic model [21,56]. The value of this approach derives from the fundamental limitation of the ability of conventional risk factors to identify specific individuals at high risk for SCD (or other manifestations of coronary artery disease) from among the *general* population. Because the majority of SCDs occur in individuals without easily identifiable high absolute risks for cardiovascular or total mortality (Figure 1.1), and risk is multifactorial, more precise predictors of *single-patient probabilities* of risk of coronary heart disease generally, and SCD in particular, must be sought. This will have to come from mathematical analyses of the interactions between multiple risks or complex system analysis.

When viewed from the perspective of a complex system, containing voluminous bioinformation, both the difficulty and the opportunity become evident. Genetic, environmental, and acquired pathophysiological states all may play roles. The value of genetically-based analysis of risk is the fact that it provides predetermined patterns far in advance of clinical events. Higher-order *single-patient probabilities*, derived from integration of properties at multiple levels of pathophysiology, will complement the power of risk expression for individual components of the SCD cascade (Figure 1.4). The ultimate goal is to profile individual risk at multiple steps in the SCD cascade, generating probability figures that are powerful enough to be useful for preventive strategies far in advance of clinical events. The degree to which analysis of genetic interactions can achieve this goal remains speculative [21,57]. However, it is clear that answering the question can be achieved only by new epidemiological models, requiring large investments into both the specialized personnel and computing power needed by a new community of science within the field of bioinformatics. Closing the gap between the numerator and denominator for SCD among the general population will offer the hope of having a far greater impact on the problem of SCD than any other approach has offered in the past, or will offer in the future, by conventional risk profiling [57].

References

1. Myerburg RJ, Castellanos A. Cardiac arrest and sudden cardiac death. In: Zipes DP, Libby P, Bonow RO, & Braunwald E, ed. *Braunwald's Heart Disease: A Textbook of Cardiovascular Medicine. 7th edn.* Elsevier Saunders Company, Philadelphia, PA, 2004: 865–908.
2. Deedwania P. Global risk assessment in the presymptomatic patient. *Am J Cardiol* 2001; **88**(7B): 17J–22J.
3. Priori SG, Aliot E, Blomstrom-Lundqvist C, *et al*. Task force on sudden cardiac death of the European Society of Cardiology. *Eur Heart J* 2001; **22**: 1374–1450.
4. Escobedo LG, Zack MM: Comparison of sudden and nonsudden coronary deaths in the United States. *Circulation* 1996; **93**: 2033–2036.
5. American Heart Association. *2001 Heart and Stroke Statistical Update.* Dallas, TX, 2000.
6. Zheng ZJ, Croft JB, Giles WH, Mensah GA. Sudden cardiac death in the United States, 1989 to 1998. *Circulation* 2001; **104**: 2158–2163.

7. Cobb LA, Fahrenbruch CE, Olsufka M, Copass MK. Changing incidence of out-of-hospital ventricular fibrillation, 1980–2000. *JAMA* 2002; **288**: 3008–3013.

8. Myerburg RJ, Kessler KM, Castellanos A. Sudden cardiac death: epidemiology, transient risk, and intervention assessment. *Ann Intern Med* 1993; **119**: 1187–1197.

9. Priori SG, Aliot E, Blomstrom-Lundqvist C, *et al.* Task force on sudden cardiac death of the European Society of Cardiology. *Eur Heart J* 2001; **22**: 1374–1450.

10. Chugh SS, Jui J, Gunson K, *et al.* Current burden of sudden cardiac death: multiple source surveillance versus retrospective death certificate-based review in a large U.S. community. *JACC* 2004; **44**: 1268–1275.

11. Gillum RF. Geographic variations in sudden coronary death. *Am Heart J* 1990; **119**: 380–389.

12. Myerburg RJ. Sudden cardiac death: exploring the limits of our knowledge. *J Cardiovasc Electrophysiol* 2001; **12**: 369–381.

13. Huikuri H, Castellanos A, Myerburg RJ. Sudden death due to cardiac arrhythmias. *N Eng J Med* 2001; **345**: 1473–1482.

14. Braunwald E. Cardiovascular medicine at the turn of the millennium: triumphs, concerns, and opportunities. *New Eng J Med* 1997; **337**: 1360–1369.

15. Myerburg RJ, Kessler KM, Castellanos A. Sudden cardiac death: structure, function, and time-dependence of risk. *Circulation* 1992; **85**(Suppl. I): I-2–I-10.

16. Arntz HR, Willich SN, Schreiber C, *et al.* Diurnal, weekly and seasonal variation of sudden death. Population-based analysis of 24,061 consecutive cases. *Eur Heart J* 2000; **21**: 315–320.

17. Holmberg M, Holmberg S, Herlitz J. Incidence, duration and survival of ventricular fibrillation in out-of-hospital cardiac arrest patients in Sweden. *Resuscitation* 2000; **44**: 7–17.

18. Wren C, O'Sullivan JJ, Wright C. Sudden death in children and adolescents. *Heart* 2000; **83**: 410–413.

19. Kuisma M, Souminen P, Korpela R. Paediatric out-of-hospital cardiac arrests: epidemiology and outcome. *Resuscitation* 1995; **30**: 141–150.

20. Steinberger J, Lucas RV Jr, Edwards JE, Titus JL. Causes of sudden, unexpected cardiac death in the first two decades of life. *Am J Cardiol* 1996; **77**: 992–995.

21. Myerburg RJ. Scientific gaps in the prediction and prevention of sudden cardiac death. *J Cardiovasc Electrophysiol* 2002; **13**: 709–723.

22. Boerwinkle E, Ellsworth DL, Hallman DM, Biddinger A. Genetic analysis of atherosclerosis: a research paradigm for the common chronic diseases. *Hum Mol Genet* 1996; **5**: 1405–1410.

23. Faber BC, Cleutjens KB, Niessen RL, *et al.* Identification of genes potentially involved in rupture of human atherosclerotic plaques. *Circ Res* 2001; **89**: 547–554.

24. Topol EJ, McCarthy J, Gabriel S, *et al.* Single nucleotide polymorphisms in multiple novel thrombospondin genes may be associated with familial premature myocardial infarction. *Circulation* 2001; **104**: 2641–2644.

25. Spooner PM, Albert C, Benjamin EJ, *et al.* Sudden cardiac death, genes, and arrhythmogenesis: consideration of new population and mechanistic approaches from a national heart, lung, and blood institute workshop. Part I. *Circulation* 2001; **103**: 2361; Part II: *Circulation* 2001; **103**: 2447–2452.

26. Albert CM, Chae CU, Grodstein F, *et al.* Prospective study of sudden cardiac death among women in the United States. *Circulation* 2003; **107**: 2096–2101.

27. Becker LB, Han BH, Meyer PM, *et al.* Racial differences in the incidence of cardiac arrest and subsequent survival. *N Engl J Med* 1993; **329**: 600–606.

28. Gillum RF. Sudden cardiac death in Hispanic Americans and African Americans. *Am J Public Health* 1997; **87**: 1461–1466.
29. Grundy SM, Balady GJ, Criqui MH, *et al.* Primary prevention of coronary heart disease: guidance from Framingham: a statement for healthcare professionals from the AHA task force on risk reduction. *Circulation* 1998; **97**: 1876–1887.
30. Friedlander Y, Siscovick DS, Weinmann S, *et al.* Family history as a risk factor for primary cardiac arrest. *Circulation* 1998; **97**: 155–160.
31. Jouven X, Desnos M, Guerot C, Ducimetiere P. Predicting sudden death in the population: the Paris prospective study I. *Circulation* 1999; **99**: 1978–1983.
32. Haider AW, Larson MG, Benjamin EJ, Levy D. Increased left ventricular mass and hypertrophy are associated with increased risk for sudden death. *J Am Coll Cardiol* 1998; **32**: 1454–1459.
33. Essebag V, Eisenberg MJ. Expanding indications for defibrillators after myocardial infarction: risk stratification and cost effectiveness. *Card Electrophysiol Rev* 2003; **7**: 43–48.
34. Grundy SM, Balady GJ, Criqui MH, *et al.* Primary prevention of coronary heart disease: guidance from Framingham: a statement for healthcare professionals from the AHA task force on risk reduction. *Circulation* 1998; **97**: 1876–1887.
35. Hallstrom AP, Cobb LA, Ray R. Smoking as a risk factor for recurrence of sudden cardiac arrest. *N Engl J Med* 1986; **314**: 271–275.
36. Albert CM, Mittleman MA, Chae CU, *et al.* Triggering of sudden death from cardiac causes by vigorous exertion. *N Engl J Med* 2000; **343**: 1355–1361.
37. Thiene G, Basso C, Corrado D. Is prevention of sudden death in young athletes feasible? *Cardiologia* 1999; **44**: 497–505.
38. Rozanski A, Blumenthal JA, Kaplan J. Impact of psychological factors on the pathogenesis of cardiovascular disease and implications for therapy. *Circulation* 1999; **99**: 2192–2217.
39. Krantz DS, Sheps DS, Carney RM, Natelson BH. Effects of mental stress in patients with coronary artery disease: evidence and clinical implications. *JAMA* 2000; **283**: 1800–1802.
40. Hemingway H, Malik M, Marmot M. Social and psychosocial influences on sudden cardiac death, ventricular arrhythmia and cardiac autonomic function. *Eur Heart J* 2001; **22**: 1082–1102.
41. Leor J, Poole WK, Kloner RA. Sudden cardiac death triggered by an earthquake. *N Engl J Med* 1996; **334**: 413–419.
42. Cleland JG, Chattopadhyay S, Khand A, *et al.* Prevalence and incidence of arrhythmias and sudden death in heart failure. *Heart Fail Rev* 2002; **7**: 229–242.
43. The Antiarrhythmics Versus Implantable Defibrillators (AVID) Investigators. A comparison of antiarrhythmic-drug therapy with implantable defibrillators in patients resuscitated from near-fatal ventricular arrhythmias. *N Engl J Med* 1997; **337**: 1576–1583.
44. Shepherd J, Cobbe SM, Ford I, *et al.* Prevention of coronary heart disease with pravastatin in men with hypercholesterolemia. West of Scotland Coronary Prevention Study Group. *N Engl J Med* 1995; **333**: 1301–1307.
45. Myerburg RJ, Mitrani R, Interian A Jr, Castellanos A. Interpretation of outcomes of antiarrhythmic clinical trials. Design features and population impact. *Circulation* 1998; **97**: 1514–1521.
46. Myerburg RJ, Mitrani RM, Interian Jr Ar, Bassett AL, Simmons J, Castellanos A. Life-threatening ventricular arrhythmias: the link between epidemiology and path

physiology. In: Zipes DP & Jalife J eds. *Cardiac Electrophysiology – From Cell to Bedside, 3rd edn*. W.B. Saunders Company, Philadelphia, PA, 2000: 521–530.

47. Laupacis A, Sackett DL, Roberts RS. An assessment of clinically useful measures of the consequences of treatment. *N Engl J Med* 1988; **318**: 1728–1733.

48. Califf RM, DeMets DL. Principles from clinical trials relevant to clinical practice: Part I. *Circulation* 2002; **106**: 1015–1021.

49. Moss AJ, Hall WJ, Cannom DS, *et al*. Improved survival with an implanted defibrillator in patients with coronary disease at high risk for ventricular arrhythmia. Multicenter Automatic Defibrillator Implantation Trial Investigators. *N Engl J Med* 1996; **335**: 1933–1940.

50. Buxton AE, Lee KL, Fisher JD, *et al*. A randomized study of the prevention of sudden death in patients with coronary artery disease. Multicenter Unsustained Tachycardia Trial Investigators. *N Engl J Med* 1999; **341**: 1882–1890.

51. Moss AJ, Zareba W, Hall WJ, *et al*. Prophylactic implantation of a defibrillator in patients with myocardial infarction and reduced ejection fraction. *N Engl J Med* 2002; **346**: 877–883.

52. Bardy GH, Lee KL, Mark DB, *et al*. Amiodarone or an implantable cardioverter-defibrillator for congestive heart failure. *N Engl J Med* 2005; **352**: 225–237.

53. Bristow MR, Saxon LA, Boehmer J, *et al*. Cardiac resynchronization therapy with or without an implantable defibrillator in advanced chronic heart failure. *N Engl J Med* 2004; **350**: 2140–2150.

54. Kadish A, Dyer A, Daubert JP, *et al*. Prophylactic defibrillator implantation in patients with nonischemic dilated cardiomyopathy. *N Engl J Med* 2004; **350**: 2151–2158

55. Splawski I, Timothy KW, Tateyama M, *et al*. Variant of SCN5A sodium channel implicated in risk of cardiac arrhythmia. *Science* 2002; **297**: 1333–1336.

56. Bonow R, Clark EB, Curfman GD, *et al*. Task force on strategic research direction: clinical science subgroup key science topics report. *Circulation* 2002; **106**: e162–e166.

57. Spooner PM, Myerburg RJ. Opportunities for sudden death prevention: directions for new clinical and basic research. *Cardiovasc Res* 2001; **50**: 177–185.

CHAPTER 2

Genetic predisposition and pathology of sudden cardiac death

Xavier Jouven, Allen P. Burke, and Renu Virmani

Introduction

The incidence of sudden cardiac death (SCD) is reported to be approximately 300 000–400 000 deaths yearly in the United States depending upon the definition used (see Chapter 1). Although the most frequent cause of death is coronary artery disease, there is a variety of underlying substrates for fatal ventricular arrhythmias, and there is a complex interaction between genetic and environmental factors regardless of the underlying cardiac disease. A precise knowledge of the morphology, risk factors, and genetic basis of a large series of SCDs is necessary to expand our understanding and therefore ability to prevent this common yet catastrophic event.

Definition of SCD and proportion of unexpected natural deaths that are cardiac in origin

Sudden cardiac death is defined as natural unexpected death due to cardiac causes that occurs within a short time after the onset of acute symptoms (usually instantaneous or within 1 h from the onset of symptoms to cardiac arrest) [1]. When the definition for sudden death includes duration of symptoms of less than 1 h between onset and death, 91% of unexpected natural deaths are due to cardiac arrhythmias. Kuller and colleagues showed that when the definition is expanded to include deaths with symptoms occurring up to 2 h before death, 12% of deaths were sudden and 88% were due to cardiac causes. However, when the duration of symptoms was increased to 24 h, 32% of deaths were sudden and cardiac cause of death declined to 75% [2,3]. Therefore, the stricter the definition of sudden instantaneous death, the smaller the proportion of natural deaths that are sudden, as would be expected, but the higher the rate that are cardiac in origin, as opposed to deaths due to internal, strokes, hemorrhages, embolic phenomena, and other noncardiac events.

Causes of SCD

Virtually any pathologic process that involves the heart may lead to SCD by virtue of a wide variety of mechanisms that may result in terminal arrhythmias. The most common cause of SCD, especially in Caucasians in developed countries, is coronary atherosclerosis, accounting for up to 80% [4]. Coronary atherosclerosis may result in sudden death by arrhythmias arising from areas of acute myocardial ischemia or healed myocardial infarction, by tamponade secondary to cardiac rupture, and by acute heart failure in cases of extensive infarcts. Other frequent causes of SCD include infiltrative diseases (mostly myocarditis and cardiomyopathies), cardiac hypertrophy, valvular heart disease (Chapter 10), and heart failure (Chapter 11), which are common substrates for arrhythmia through a variety of interrelated causes (Table 2.1).

The causes of SCD vary with the age of the patient (Tables 2.2–2.5) [6,7]. The highest incidence of sudden death is between birth and 6 months of age (sudden infant death syndrome) and between 45 and 75 years of age [1]. The incidence is 100-fold less in adolescents and young adults less than 30 years of age (one in 100 000 per year) than in adults older than 35 years (one in 1000 per year). In contrast to incidence, the proportion of deaths caused by coronary heart disease that are sudden and unexpected decreases with advancing age [1]. Men are more likely to die suddenly than women, possibly because of the protection from coronary heart disease prior to menopause [1].

The genetic basis for sudden death clearly depends on the underlying cause. In the case of atherosclerosis, there are a multitude of etiologic factors, involving inflammatory, oxidative, metabolic, and thrombotic pathways that are enhanced by a complex interplay between genetic polymorphisms and environmental factors. There are other causes of sudden death that may be traced to a single point mutation, such as channelopathies (long-QT syndrome, Brugada syndrome, catecholaminergic ventricular tachycardia and similar disorders (see Chapter 9), and hypertrophic cardiomyopathy (see Chapter 8). The genetic basis for other common causes of sudden death, such as arrhythmogenic right ventricular cardiomyopathy and anomalous coronary artery origin remain unknown [9–14]. Before genetic alterations that may be associated with sudden death are investigated, precise morphologic classification of cardiac abnormalities is required.

Pathology of common causes of SCD

Coronary heart disease

Based on autopsy studies, it has been shown that 50–60% of patients dying suddenly from coronary atherosclerosis have luminal coronary thrombi, another 20–30% have healed myocardial infarction, and approximately 10–15% of patients have stable severe coronary narrowing (>75% cross-sectional area luminal narrowing) involving one to three vessels, in the absence of any myocardial fibrosis or necrosis [15,16]. Approximately 10%

Table 2.1 Causes and mechanisms of SCD.

Immediate Cause	Underlying Causes	Mechanisms
Acute ischemia	Coronary atherosclerosis with and without thrombi Nonatherosclerotic coronary disease Aortic stenosis	Ventricular fibrillation Bradycardia EMD (usually end stage or post resuscitation)
Infiltrative diseases	Inflammatory (myocarditis) Scarring (healed infarcts, cardiomyopathy, sarcoidosis)	Ventricular fibrillation Bradyarrhythmias (uncommon)
Cardiac hypertrophy	Hypertrophic cardiomyopathy Systemic hypertension Aortic stenosis	Ventricular fibrillation Bradyarrhythmias (uncommon)[a]
Cardiac dilatation (congestive failure)	Dilated cardiomyopathy Chronic ischemia Systemic hypertension Aortic insufficiency Mitral insufficiency	Ventricular fibrillation Bradyarrhythmias (uncommon)
Tamponade	Ruptured myocardial infarct Aortic rupture	Pulseless electrical activity
Disruption of blood flow	Pulmonary embolism Mitral stenosis Left atrial myxoma	Pulseless electrical activity Ventricular fibrillation
Global myocardial hypoxia	Severe ischemic heart disease Aortic stenosis Pulmonary embolism	Baroreflex stimulation with bradyarrhythmias Ventricular tachyarrhythmias
Acute heart failure	Massive myocardial infarct Ruptured papillary muscle Chordal or leaflet rupture	Pulseless electrical activity Ventricular fibrillation
Systemic hypoxia	Pulmonary stenosis Pulmonary hypertension	Bradyarrhythmias
Vasovagal	Neuromuscular diseases	Baroreflex stimulation with bradycardia
Preexcitation	Accessory pathways	Atrial fibrillation → ventricular fibrillation
Long QT	Congenital and acquired states	Ventricular fibrillation (*torsades de pointes*)
Heart block	AV node scarring, inflammation, tumor	Bradycardia → ventricular fibrillation

Notes: EMD – electromechanical dissociation; AV – atrioventricular.
Source: Reproduced from Reference 5, with permission from Elsevier.
[a] Especially in the presence of infiltrative processes involving the conduction system.

Table 2.2 Causes of sudden death in infants and children.

Anatomic Findings	0–1 Years ($n = 20$)	1–21 Years ($n = 50$)
Coronary artery anomalies	10 (50%)	12 (24%)
Myocarditis	0	14 (28%)
No findings	7 (35%)	10 (20%)
Other findings	2 (10%)	8 (16%)
Hypertrophic cardiomyopathy	1 (5%)	6 (12%)

Source: Adapted from Reference 8, with permission from Elsevier.

Table 2.3 Causes of death, ages 14–20 years.

Cause of Death	Number (%)
No findings	18 (30)
Myocarditis	8 (13)
Hypertrophic cardiomyopathy	7 (12)
Anomalous coronary artery	5 (8)
Complex congenital heart disease	4 (7)
Atherosclerosis	3 (5)
Dilated cardiomyopathy	3 (5)
Floppy mitral valve	3 (5)
Idiopathic left ventricular hypertrophy	3 (5)
Aortic dissection	2 (3)
Kawaski disease	2 (3)
Intramyocardial coronary artery	1 (2)
Hypertensive left ventricular hypertrophy	1 (2)
Total	60

Source: Adapted from Reference 6, with permission from Elsevier.

of patients dying from noncardiac causes may have significant coronary atherosclerosis; therefore, it is essential that a complete autopsy be performed to exclude other causes of noncardiac death [17]. The terminal event in most patients with severe coronary artery disease with or without thrombosis is ventricular fibrillation. Other arrhythmias found in fatal cases of ischemic heart disease include bradyarrhythmias (20–30%), and a smaller percent of acute heart failure or pulseless electrical activity [14,18].

Before the genetic basis of sudden coronary death can be adequately explored, the heterogeneity of coronary disease needs to be understood and addressed. We have demonstrated that there are at least two forms of coronary thrombosis, each of which may precipitate sudden death, as well as contribute to plaque progression, and the formation of increased plaque burden and stable plaque. The most common cause of thrombosis is plaque

Table 2.4 Causes of death, ages 21–30 years.

Cause of Death	Number (%)
Atherosclerosis	64 (28)
No findings	49 (21)
Idiopathic left ventricular hypertrophy	27 (12)
Hypertrophic cardiomyopathy	16 (7)
Myocarditis	14 (6)
Anomalous coronary artery	9 (4)
Dilated cardiomyopathy	7 (3)
Intramyocardial coronary artery	7 (3)
Aortic dissection	7 (3)
Rheumatic mitral stenosis	6 (3)
Complex congenital heart disease	5 (2)
Hypertensive left ventricular hypertrophy	4 (2)
Endocarditis	6 (1)
Sarcoidosis	3 (1)
Aortic stenosis	3 (1)
Floppy mitral valve	2 (1)
Arrhythmogenic right ventricular dysplasia	2 (1)
Coronary aneurysm (congenital)	1 (0.4)
Amyloid	1 (0.4)
Pericarditis	1 (0.4)
Total	229

Source: Adapted from Reference 6, with permission from Elsevier.

rupture, which is uncommon prior to menopause in women, and which is highly associated with hypercholesterolemia. In contrast, plaque erosion is not associated with hypercholesterolemia or diabetes, and is proportionally quite common in premenopausal women. We have demonstrated that risk factor profiles, including diabetes mellitus and hyperhomocysteinemia, affect plaque composition in sudden coronary death victims. These data suggest that any genetic predisposition of atherosclerosis, especially if mediated by a traditional risk factor, will vary by morphologic type of coronary artery disease [19]. Although it is generally known that SCD is associated with presence of the classic risk factors, such as hypercholesterolemia, diabetes, hypertension, smoking, type A personality, and male sex [1,4,20], the contribution of multiple genetic polymorphisms to the development of coronary atherosclerotic and fatal coronary thrombosis will likely vary by type of atherothrombosis and plaque morphology.

Myocardial factors are also likely to play an important role in the susceptibility to sudden coronary death, and may be determined by an entirely different set of genetic polymorphisms. In series of individuals with sudden coronary death, the incidence of acute myocardial infarction is <20% [15,21], whereas

Table 2.5 Causes of death, ages 31–40 years.

Cause of Death	Number (%)
Atherosclerosis	258 (60)
No findings	38 (9)
Hypertensive left ventricular hypertrophy	26 (6)
Idiopathic left ventricular hypertrophy	18 (4)
Dilated cardiomyopathy	16 (4)
Hypertrophic cardiomyopathy	13 (3)
Myocarditis	12 (3)
Sarcodosis	10 (2)
Aortic stenosis	9 (2)
Aortic dissection	8 (2)
Endocarditis	6 (1)
Floppy mitral valve	6 (1)
Intramyocardial coronary artery	3 (1)
Arrhythmogenic right ventricular dysplasia	3 (1)
Rheumatic mitral stenosis	3 (1)
Anomalous coronary artery	2 (0.5)
Coronary artery dissection	2 (0.5)
Congenital heart disease	1 (0.2)
Lipomatous hypertrophy, atrial septum	1 (0.2)
Total	432

Source: Adapted from Reference 6, with permission from Elsevier.

healed myocardial infarction is 40% [15]. The rate of healed infarcts is greater in the elderly and in the diabetic population. As there is wide range of plaque burden in cases of sudden coronary death, and variation in the presence of the size of acute and healed infarcts, genetic predisposition to myocardial arrhythmias, and capacity to develop collateral circulation need to be studied in addition to those promoting atherogenesis itself.

Congenital coronary artery anomalies

The most common coronary anomaly resulting in sudden death is an aberrant left main arising from the right sinus of Valsalva with a course traveling between the pulmonary artery and aorta. The male to female ratio is 4 : 1 to 9 : 1, with majority of cases being less than 30 years of age. Sudden death is reported in up to two-thirds of individuals with this anomaly, 75% of which occur during exercise, with over 50% having symptoms prior to death [13,22]. Most patients are adolescent or young adults, although death may occur in as young as 1 month of age. The pathophysiology of sudden death may be related to the compression of the left main artery between the aorta and pulmonary trunk, diastolic compression of the vessel especially when lying within the aortic wall at its take-off from the aorta and possibly because of an ostial ridge and slit like lumen, which result in poor filling during diastole [23].

In contrast, anomalous right coronary artery from the left sinus of Valsalva is usually an incidental finding, although we have reported that up to one-third of patients may die suddenly. Again approximately 50% of these deaths are exercise related. Most deaths occur in the young and middle-aged adults younger than 35 years of age [24].

In infants less than 1 year of age, the left main coronary artery may arise from the pulmonary trunk, usually from the left sinus. Sudden death occurs in approximately 40% of cases. Typically, the artery is thin walled and vein like, and the right coronary artery, although normal in location, is tortuous and dilated.

By definition, ectopic origin of coronary arteries is a congenital condition, and therefore likely influenced by genetic factors. However, the genetic basis for these conditions is unknown. Other than reports of familial clusters of coronary artery anomalies [25], there is no knowledge of the genetic basis of this relatively common cause of exertional sudden death.

Other nonatherosclerotic coronary causes of sudden death
Spontaneous coronary dissection
Coronary artery dissection accounts for approximately 0.5% of sudden death in patients 30–40 years old (Table 2.4). Most patients are young women, and usually in the postpartum period. Most of the cases of sudden death involve the left anterior descending coronary artery (90%). Histologically, the dissection plane is the outer media, with inflammatory cell infiltrates of eosinophils, lymphocytes, neutrophils, and macrophages in the adventitia. The etiology and genetics of spontaneous coronary dissection are completely unknown.

Small vessel disease
Narrowing of small arteries supplying the sinoatrial and atrioventricular nodes has been associated with sudden death. These small vessels invariably show arterial dysplasia, which is believed to be congenital in origin. Other intramyocardial small artery dysplasias have been associated with catecholamine-induced sudden death, hypertrophic cardiomyopathy, sickle cell disease, and mitral valve prolapse. Most cases of small vessel disease and sudden death have involved the conduction system of the heart; thickened vessels within the wall of the ventricular septum have also been implicated in SCD. Although there have been reports of familial small vessel disease of the heart, and it is a component of hypertrophic cardiomyopathy, a known genetic disease, the genetic basis for isolated small vessel disease is unknown.

Cardiomyopathies
The two cardiomyopathies most frequently associated with SCD are hypertrophic cardiomyopathy and arrhythmogenic right ventricular cardiomyopathy (see Chapter 9) [5].

Hypertrophic cardiomyopathy

The morphologic features that characterize the disease are asymmetric left ventricular hypertrophy (predominantly septal), small left ventricular cavity, left atrial dilatation, and the presence of left ventricular outflow tract obstruction. Histologic features include myofiber disarray with myocyte hypertrophy with or without focal scarring and intramyocardial coronary artery thickening. The most likely cause of sudden death is ventricular fibrillation either due to ischemia from small vessel disease or due to disordered muscle bundles in the septum with or without interstitial fibrosis, altered autonomic vascular control, and ischemia secondary to subaortic stenosis [26].

Hypertensive cardiomyopathy

Other causes of left ventricular hypertrophy that may lead to sudden death include hypertensive heart disease, and concentric idiopathic left ventricular hypertrophy. Patients with hypertension and left ventricular hypertrophy have an increased risk of sudden death. In 10–40% of sudden deaths in young individuals, especially athletes, concentric left ventricular hypertrophy, as determined by body weight and height, is the only pathologic finding at autopsy.

Arrhythmogenic right ventricular cardiomyopathy

Arrhythmogenic right ventricular cardiomyopathy accounts for less than 5% of SCDs but is a relatively common cause of death from exertion [27]. Arrhythmogenic right ventricular cardiomyopathy is familial in up to 50% of cases, and the mode of inheritance is predominantly autosomal dominant with variable penetrance. Most patients are younger than 40 years at the time of death and some deaths do occur in children. Pathologic findings include dilatation of the right ventricle with focal thinning of the right ventricular wall secondary to fibrosis and fat infiltration. Left ventricular scarring, usually subepicardial is seen in at least 70% of cases, especially in individuals dying suddenly and is usually located in the lateral wall [28].

Myocarditis

Usually a sequela of viral infection, lymphocytic myocarditis is the cause of SCD in children and adolescents and less in young adults. Histologically there is lymphocytic and histiocytic infiltrate accompanied by myocyte necrosis; the degree of infiltrate is especially marked in infants and young children and it may even be predominantly neutrophilic [6]. Areas of scarring are not uncommon. Serologic and molecular studies suggest that many are caused by enteroviruses, especially Coxsackievirus B3, adenovirus, and a variety of other viruses have also been implicated in isolated cases [29,30]. Whether there is genetic predisposition to myocardial susceptibility to myocarditis viruses is unknown.

Giant cell myocarditis is a myocardial inflammation that is especially aggressive, and is characterized by chronic inflammation with numerous giant cells, myocardial necrosis with or without scarring.

Sudden death in preexcitation syndromes

The Wolff–Parkinson–White (WPW) syndrome results from preexcitation caused by an abnormal muscular connection (bypass tract) between atrium and ventricle. The most common arrhythmias observed in WPW are supraventricular arrhythmias with a favorable prognosis but sudden death may occur. The incidence of sudden death in patients with WPW syndrome is estimated to be less than 1 per 100 patient-years follow-up; 70% of patients who experience ventricular tachyarrhythmias have a previous history of symptoms [31]. Mutations in the *PRKAG2* gene encoding the gamma2 regulatory subunit of AMP-activated protein kinase have been identified in patients with familial WPW syndrome [32,33].

Genetic predisposition to SCD

The rationale to believe that there is a genetic component in SCD comes from large epidemiological studies that have addressed this topic.

Family history of CAD and/or SCD was reported as an independent risk factor for SCD in a case control study of more than 500 subjects in Seattle, WA [34]. Furthermore, a parental history of sudden death was found to be an independent risk factor for sudden death in more than 7000 men followed up for 23 years in the Paris Prospective Study I [35]. These familial aggregations of SCD cases can be related to environmental or genetic causes or interactions between both. However, three points suggest a genetic role in the Paris Prospective Study I. First, increased risk of SCD segregated independent of increased familial risk of myocardial infarction. Second, there was a positive correlation of age between parents and subjects' SCD, that is, parents and subjects die from the same cause at roughly the same age. Third, in a small subset in which there was a history of both maternal and paternal SCD, the relative risk for SCD in the offspring was 9.4 times whereas it was 1.8 times when SCD occurred in one parent only.

At present time, no single genetic mutation that can predict a higher risk for SCD in the general population has been discovered and genetic studies in this field are facing a complex scenario given the complexity of the substrate of SCD. The list of proteins that, if altered, may predispose to SCD is long and extends far beyond ion channels or other proteins directly implicated in the control of cardiac excitability. For example polymorphisms influencing levels of HDL, LDL, Apo A1, Apo B, lipoprotein A, lipoprotein receptors [36–38] may accelerate development of CAD thus increasing the risk of SCD. Similarly, polymorphisms of genes encoding critical proteins such as factor 5 Leiden, prothrombin, plasminogen activator inhibitor [39–42] may predispose to coronary thrombosis and they may also increase the risk of SCD. It is clear that it will take large studies to be able to determine the most important players among so many candidates. Furthermore it is unlikely that one or two polymorphisms will be able to account for a fraction of the global risk of SCD in an individual.

Although the difficulties are numerous, we are only at the beginning of this major challenge and genetic studies on SCD will benefit from new technological tools (including proteinomics) and from the collaboration with the other fields of research such as epidemiology, cardiac pathology, and molecular biology. These collaborations will help assemble the different pieces of the puzzle.

References

1. Myerburg RJ, Castellanos A. Cardiac arrest and sudden cardiac death. In: Braunwald E, ed. *Heart Disease. A Text Book of Cardiovascular Medicine*, 4th edn. W.B. Saunders, Philadelphia, PA, 1997: 742–779.
2. Kuller L, Lilienfeld A, Fisher R. An epidemiologic study of sudden and unexpected death in adults. *Medicine* 1967; **46:** 341–361.
3. Kuller LH. Sudden death – definition and epidemiologic considerations. *Prog Cardiovasc Dis* 1980; **23:** 1–12.
4. Myerburg RJ, Interian A, Jr, Mitrani RM *et al.* Frequency of sudden cardiac death and profiles of risk. *Am J Cardiol* 1997; **80**(5B): 10F–19F.
5. Virmani R, Burke A, Farb A, Atkinson JB, eds. *Cardiovascular Pathology*. Saunders, Philadelphia, PA, 2001: 342.
6. Burke AP, Farb A, Virmani R, Goodin J, Smialek, JE. Sports-related and non-sports-related sudden death in young adults. *Am Heart J* 1991; **121:** 568–575.
7. Burke AP, Farb A, Virmani R. Causes of sudden death in athletes. *Cardiol Clin* 1992; **10**(2): 303–318.
8. Steinberger J, Lucas R, Edwards JE, Titus JL. Causes of sudden unexpected cardiac death in the first two decades of life. *Am J Cardiol* 1996; **77:** 992–995.
9. Vincent GM. The molecular genetics of the long QT syndrome: genes causing fainting and sudden death. *Annu Rev Med* 1998; **49:** 263–274.
10. Brugada J, Brugada P. What to do in patients with no structural heart disease and sudden arrhythmic death? *Am J Cardiol* 1996; **78**(5A): 69–75.
11. Maron BJ, Roberts WC, Epstein SE. Sudden death in hypertrophic cardiomyopathy: a profile of 78 patients. *Circulation* 1982; **65**(7): 1388–1394.
12. Tada H, Aihara N, Ohe T *et al.* Arrhythmogenic right ventricular cardiomyopathy underlies syndrome of right bundle branch block, ST-segment elevation, and sudden death. *Am J Cardiol* 1998; **81**(4): 519–522.
13. Taylor AJ, Rogan KM, Virmani R. Sudden cardiac death associated with congenital coronary artery anomalies. *J Am Coll Cardiol* 1992; **20:** 640–647.
14. Zipes DP, Wellens HJ. Sudden cardiac death. *Circulation* 1998; **98**(21): 2334–2351.
15. Farb A, Tang AL, Burke AP *et al.* Sudden coronary death. Frequency of active coronary lesions, inactive coronary lesions, and myocardial infarction. *Circulation* 1995; **92**(7): 1701–1709.
16. Farb A, Burke AP, Tang AL *et al.* Coronary plaque erosion without rupture into a lipid core. A frequent cause of coronary thrombosis in sudden coronary death. *Circulation* 1996; **93**(7): 1354–1363.

17. Virmani R, Kolodgie FD, Burke AP *et al.* Lessons from sudden coronary death: a comprehensive morphological classification scheme for atherosclerotic lesions. *Arterioscler Thromb Vasc Biol* 2000; **20**(5): 1262–1275.

18. Zipes DP. Genesis of cardiac arrhythmias: electrophysiological considerations. In: Braunwald E, ed. *Heart Disease. A Textbook of Cardiovascular Medicine*, 5th edn. W.B. Saunders, Philadelphia, PA, 1997: 548–592.

19. Burke AP, Farb A, Malcom GT *et al.* Effect of risk factors on the mechanism of acute thrombosis and sudden coronary death in women. *Circulation* 1998; **97**: 2110–2116.

20. Myerburg RJ, Kessler KM, Bassett AL *et al.* A biological approach to sudden cardiac death: structure, function, and cause. *Am J Cardiol* 1989; **63**: 1512–1516.

21. Greene HL. Sudden arrhythmic cardiac death – mechanisms, resuscitation, and classification: the Seattle perspective. *Am J Cardiol* 1990; **65**: 4B–12B.

22. Virmani R, Burke AP, Farb A *et al.* Causes of sudden death in young and middle-aged competitive athletes. *Cardiol Clin* 1997; **15**(3): 439–466.

23. Taylor AJ, Byers JP, Cheitlin MD *et al.* Anomalous right or left coronary artery from the contralateral coronary sinus: "high-risk" abnormalities in the initial coronary artery course and heterogeneous clinical outcomes. *Am Heart J* 1997; **133**(4): 428–435.

24. Taylor A, Rogan KM, Virmani R. Sudden cardiac death associated with isolated congenital coronary artery anomalies. *J Am Coll Cardiol* 1992; **20**: 640–647.

25. Rowe L, Carmody TJ, Askenazi J. Anomalous origin of the left circumflex coronary artery from the right aortic sinus: a familial clustering. *Cathet Cardiovasc Diagn* 1993; **29**(4): 277–278.

26. Maron BJ, Shirani J, Poliac LC *et al.* Sudden death in young competitive athletes. Clinical, demographic, and pathological profiles. *JAMA* 1996; **276**(3): 199–204.

27. Thiene G, Nava A, Corrado D *et al.* Right ventricular cardiomyopathy and sudden death in young people. *N Engl J Med* 1988; **318**(3): 129–133.

28. Burke AP, Farb A, Tashko G *et al.* Arrhythmogenic right ventricular cardiomyopathy and fatty replacement of the right ventricular myocardium. Are they different diseases? *Circulation* 1998; **97**: 1571–1580.

29. Nicholson F, Ajetunmobi JF, Li M *et al.* Molecular detection and serotypic analysis of enterovirus RNA in archival specimens from patients with acute myocarditis. *Br Heart J* 1995; **74**(5): 522–527.

30. Towbin JA. Molecular genetic basis of sudden cardiac death. *Cardiovasc Pathol* 2001; **10**: 283–295.

31. Pappone C, Manguso F, Santinelli R *et al.* Radiofrequency ablation in children with asymptomatic Wolff–Parkinson–White syndrome. *N Engl J Med* 2004; **351**(12): 1197–1205.

32. Gollob MH, Seger JJ, Gollob TN *et al.* Novel PRKAG2 mutation responsible for the genetic syndrome of ventricular preexcitation and conduction system disease with childhood onset and absence of cardiac hypertrophy. *Circulation* 2001; **104**(25): 3030–3033.

33. Gollob MH, Green MS, Tang AS *et al.* Identification of a gene responsible for familial Wolff–Parkinson–White syndrome. *N Engl J Med* 2001; **344**(24): 1823–1831.

34. Friedlander Y, Siscovick DS, Weinmann S *et al.* Family history as a risk factor for primary cardiac arrest. *Circulation* 1998; **97**(2): 155–160.

35. Jouven X, Desnos M, Guerot C *et al.* Predicting sudden death in the population: the Paris Prospective Study I. *Circulation* 1999; **99**(15): 1978–1983.

36. Spooner PM, Albert C, Benjamin EJ *et al.* Sudden cardiac death, genes, and arrhythmogenesis: consideration of new population and mechanistic approaches from a national heart, lung, and blood institute workshop, part I. *Circulation* 2001; **103**(19): 2361–2364.

37. Spooner PM, Albert C, Benjamin EJ *et al.* Sudden cardiac death, genes, and arrhythmogenesis: consideration of new population and mechanistic approaches from a national heart, lung, and blood institute workshop, part II. *Circulation* 2001; **103**(20): 2447–2452.

38. Arking DE, Chugh SS, Chakravarti A *et al.* Genomics in sudden cardiac death. *Circ Res* 2004; **94**(6): 712–723.

39. Mikkelsson J, Perola M, Laippala P *et al.* Glycoprotein IIIa Pl(A1/A2) polymorphism and sudden cardiac death. *J Am Coll Cardiol* 2000; **36**(4): 1317–1323.

40. Reiner AP, Rosendaal FR, Reitsma PH *et al.* Factor V Leiden, prothrombin G20210A, and risk of sudden coronary death in apparently healthy persons. *Am J Cardiol* 2002; **90**(1): 66–68.

41. Snapir A, Mikkelsson J, Perola M *et al.* Variation in the alpha2B-adrenoceptor gene as a risk factor for prehospital fatal myocardial infarction and sudden cardiac death. *J Am Coll Cardiol* 2003; **41**(2): 190–194.

42. Anvari A, Schuster E, Gottsauner-Wolf M *et al.* PAI-I 4G/5G polymorphism and sudden cardiac death in patients with coronary artery disease. *Thromb Res* 2001; **103**(2): 103–107.

CHAPTER 3

Arrhythmogenic mechanisms

Michiel J. Janse and Douglas P. Zipes

Introduction

The first experimental observation linking myocardial ischemia to ventricular fibrillation was made by Erichsen in 1841, who observed that coronary artery ligation in the dog caused the action of the ventricles to cease with, "a slight tremulous motion alone continuing" [1].

McWilliam was the first to suggest that "sudden syncope from plugging or obstructing some portion of the coronary system (in patients) is very probably determined or ensured by the occurrence of fibrillar contractions in the ventricles. The cardiac pump is thrown out of gear, and the last of its vital energy is dissipated in a violent and prolonged turmoil of fruitless activity in the ventricular walls" [2]. His view was ignored for many decades, and in 1923 he wrote, "It may be permissable to recall that in the pages of this journal 34 years ago I brought forward a new view as to the causation of sudden death by a previously unrecognized form of failure of the heart's action in man (e.g. ventricular fibrillation) – a view fundamentally different from those entertained up to that time. Little attention was given to the new view for many years." ([3]; his name is now spelled MacWilliam). Hoffa and Ludwig [4] were the first to show that electrical currents could induce fibrillation. This was confirmed 49 years later by Prevost and Batelli [5], who also demonstrated that similar shocks could restore sinus rhythm.

Thus, at the turn of the twentieth century there was evidence that ventricular fibrillation could be induced by acute myocardial ischemia, that it might be responsible for sudden death in patients, and that it could be abolished by electrical shocks. It is perhaps surprising that it took more than half a century before it was realized how often ventricular fibrillation occurs in the setting of acute ischemia, and before electrical countershock became common clinical practice.

We now know that the risk of sudden death among the general population aged 35 years and older is in the order of 1–2 per 1000 per year. Between the ages of 40 and 65 years, there is a marked increase, with coronary artery disease as the most important cause. In patients with a high-risk status, the risk of sudden death may be as high as 10–25% per year. In adolescent and young adult populations, the risk is about 1% of that of the general adult population, and familial diseases, such as the congenital long QT syndrome, hypertrophic cardiomyopathy, arrhythmogenic right ventricular dysplasia, and Brugada syndrome play a dominant role [6].

Mechanisms of ventricular fibrillation

McWilliam [7] was the first to suggest that disturbances in impulse propagation could be responsible for fibrillation, and he clearly envisaged the possibility that myocardial fibers could be reexcited as soon as their refractory period had ended. Due to the inability to record simultaneously a sufficient amount of electrograms from the fibrillating heart to construct activation maps, insight into the mechanism of fibrillation during the twentieth century was initially obtained through theoretical analysis and the study of computer models. Moe *et al.* [8,9] developed the "multiple wavelet hypothesis." In their computer model, fibrillation was initiated by a rapid series of impulses and maintained by fractionation of wave fronts in partially and irregularly excitable tissue, so that independent wavelets occurred that coursed around multiple islets of refractory tissue, which continuously shifted their location, causing the pattern of conduction to shift as well. Fibrillation has been described as a random, reentrant rhythm, in which the functional reentrant circuits change size, shape, and location. When, in the 1970s, multiplexing systems became available, allowing simultaneous recording from many sites, activation maps of ventricular fibrillation in hearts with acute, regional ischemia showed activation patterns compatible with the multiple wavelet hypothesis [10,11]. In both studies, intramural reentry was documented, but non-reentrant mechanisms, especially during the ectopic ventricular impulses that initiated fibrillation, were found to be operative as well.

There is still a debate whether the functional reentrant circuits are of the "leading circle" model, or are spiral waves (or three-dimensional scroll waves). In the "leading circle" concept, the reentrant circuit is the "smallest possible pathway in which the impulse can continue to circulate ... in which the stimulating efficacy of the circulating wavefront is just enough to excite the tissue ahead, which is still in its relative refractory phase" [12]. In other words, there is no excitable gap, and maintenance of the leading circle is due to repetitive centripetal wavelets that keep the core in a constant state of refractoriness. In spiral wave reentry, there is a curving wavefront, which must not only depolarize cells in front of it in the direction of propagation, but also deliver current to cells on its sides. A curving wavefront may cease altogether when a critical curvature is reached despite the presence of excitable tissue. The essential difference between the "leading circle" and the spiral wave reentry is that in the former the core is kept permanently refractory, while in the latter the core is excitable but not excited. The slow conduction of a spiral wave is not dependent on conduction in relative refractory tissue, and therefore, there is an excitable gap [13–15]. Studies, employing isolated canine atrial preparations, demonstrated spiral wave reentry, where cells in the core sometimes were quiescent at almost normal levels of resting

(a)   (b)

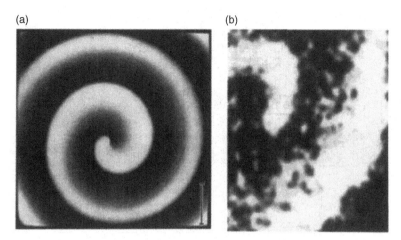

Figure 3.1 Spiral waves in a chemical Belousov–Zhabotinsky reaction (a) and in an isolated preparation of canine epicardial muscle (b). (a) Reproduced from Reference 76 with permission from AAAS and (b) from Reference 17 with permission from *Nature*.

membrane potential. The excitable gap was larger near the core of the circuit than in the periphery of the reentrant circuit, which is incompatible with the "leading circle" concept [15].

Spiral waves, also called rotors, have been described in a variety of excitable biological, physical, and/or chemical systems. The best-known example is the Belousov–Zhabotinsky reaction, where malonic acid is reversibly oxidized by bromate in the presence of ferroin. During this process, ferroin changes in color from red to blue and then back to red, allowing visualization of the reaction [16]. Figure 3.1 shows both a spiral wave in the Belousov–Zhabotinsky reaction, and a spiral wave in an isolated preparation of canine epicardial muscle, visualized by optical mapping [17].

It has been known for a long time that atrial fibrillation can be induced by application of aconitine to the atrial appendage [18]. When the appendage is clamped off, sinus rhythm is restored, while the clamped-off appendage exhibits a rapid, regular tachycardia. Thus, in this case, atrial fibrillation was caused by a focus that fired so rapidly that uniform excitation of the rest of the atria was no longer possible. The irregularity of the electrocardiogram was due to "fibrillar conduction" emerging from the focus. On the other hand, when atrial fibrillation was induced by rapid stimulation, or application of faradic shocks to the appendage, and the atrial refractory period was shortened by the administration of acetylcholine or vagal stimulation, clamping off the appendage resulted in the disappearance of fibrillation in the appendage, whereas it continued in the remainder of the atrium. In such a case, fibrillation could well be due to multiple wavelet reentry [19]. Something similar may occur in fibrillation caused by spiral wave reentry. A high frequency rotor, stabilized

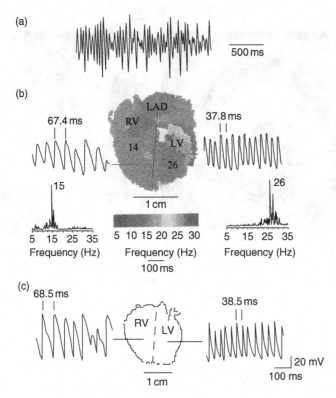

Figure 3.2 Frequency analysis of ventricular fibrillation: (a) ECG trace of ventricular fibrillation, (b) dominant frequency maps. Dominant frequencies in the right ventricle (RV) range between 10 and 16 Hz, in the left ventricle (LV) from 14 and 26 Hz. The highest frequency (26 Hz) is found in the left ventricular anterior free wall. Single pixel recordings and frequency spectra corroborate the dominant frequency findings, and (c) microelectrode recordings from the right and left ventricles during ventricular fibrillation. Reproduced from Reference 22 with permission from Lippincott, Williams and Wilkins.

somewhere in a small area of myocardium may lead to fibrillary conduction in the rest of the atria or ventricles and, in this case, the rotor causing the fibrillation is not random [20,21]. Because rotors turn around a nonexcited core, ion channels that determine the resting membrane potential in the nonexcited core, especially I_{K1}, can exert a repolarizing effect on tissue in the vicinity. Therefore, tissue with a high density of I_{K1} can produce rotors with a shorter period than tissue with lower densities. This mechanism is responsible for the observation that a single stable rotor in the anterior part of the left ventricle acts as a source for fibrillatory conduction [22] (see Figure 3.2).

Another possibility is a single rotor that drifts, and so gives rise to the typical electrocardiographic features of fibrillation [23]. Yet another mechanism is the breakup of a single spiral wave, or a pair of counter-rotating spiral waves, into a multispiral disordered state. The so-called restitution hypothesis suggests that the breakup of a single rotor into a multispiral state occurs when the oscillations in action potential duration are of sufficient amplitude to cause blockage of conduction along the wavefront [24–26]. When action potential duration is plotted against the preceding diastolic interval a restitution curve is produced. When the slope of this curve is larger than one, alternation in action potential duration may occur [27]. Alternation in action potential duration has been considered a first step in a process that leads to destabilization of wavefronts and the formation of multiple reentrant waves [28]. It has been suggested that a new type of antiarrhythmic drug would be a drug that reduces the slope of the restitution curve to values below one [28]. Whereas restitution of action potential duration certainly is a factor in determining stability of reentry, it must be remembered that spatial inhomogeneity in action potential duration, and possibly in restitution, may also play a role in breakup phenomena. Moreover, restitution of conduction velocity may also be involved in breakup of spiral waves [29]. Recent data suggest that fibrillation also can occur in situations where the restitution curve is less than one, and a hypothesis to explain fibrillation with both increased and reduced restitution curves has been offered [30]. Another factor that can increase oscillations in action potential duration and decrease stability of a spiral wave is an increased extracellular K^+ concentration. This produces a prolonged tail of refractoriness, as a consequence of the delayed recovery from inactivation of the sodium channel [31,32]. Extracellular K^+ accumulation during acute myocardial ischemia may thus destabilize reentry and lead to breakup into multiple reentrant circuits and fibrillation.

Ventricular fibrillation during acute ischemia and in hearts with a healed infarct

The arrhythmias of acute ischemia occur in two phases, the 1A phase between 2 and 10 min following coronary artery obstruction and the 1B phase between 18 and 30 min. The relative contribution of 1A and 1B arrhythmias to sudden death in humans is unknown, but animal experiments suggest that mortality in the 1B phase is larger than in the 1A phase [33–35].

For spontaneous arrhythmias to occur, both an appropriate trigger (usually a properly timed premature complex) and a substrate (a preexisting proarrhythmic condition) are required. The major causes for a substrate for reentry in the 1A phase are the depression of excitability and conduction velocity, and the marked inhomogeneity in refractoriness. These changes are due in part to extracellular K^+ accumulation, which decreases resting membrane potential. The extracellular K^+ concentration is inhomogeneous throughout the ischemic zone, accounting for inhomogeneities in refractoriness [36]. The premature ventricular complex that initiate reentry are most likely caused by reexcitation of normal cells close to the ischemic border by injury currents [10].

De Groot *et al.* [37] have defined a substrate for ventricular fibrillation during the 1B phase: a surviving epicardial layer that is depressed by electrotonic current flow from deeper, depolarized, and inexcitable layers during a time window between 14 and 35 min following coronary artery occlusion. During this time window coupling between deeper and superficial cells is mildly decreased and the electrotonic current from midmural layers partially depolarizes the subepicardium. In the depressed subepicardium, macro-reentry, predominantly due to a reduced conduction velocity, is responsible for the 1B arrhythmias. Recent optical mapping data from an isolated perfused left ventricular wedge preparation reaffirm that during ischemia, the endocardium maintains excitability long after it is lost in the epicardium. The study demonstrated that when bidirectional block occurred from the excitable endocardium to the inexcitable midmyocardium and epicardium as ischemia progressed, arrhythmias ceased (Figure 3.3) [38]. When cell-to-cell uncoupling between deep and superficial layers is complete, electrical activity in the subepicardium recovers, and reentry is no longer possible. The trigger for ventricular fibrillation during the 1B phase is most likely related to stretch of the border between ischemic and normal myocardium [39]. The clinical implication from this study is that increasing contractility or increasing afterload during this period may be arrhythmogenic. Afterload reduction in patients with acute myocardial infarction by nitroprusside resulted in abolition of severe arrhythmias [40,41]. Stimuli arising in the epicardium produce significant conduction delay because of loss of excitability during ischemia and are more effective in initiating ventricular tachycardia than endocardial stimulation (Figure 3.4) [42].

Studies in isolated, Langendorff-perfused human hearts with a healed myocardial infarction have shown that macro-reentry, utilizing a reentrant circuit made up of surviving myocardial fibers within the infarct, is the mechanism that maintains ventricular tachycardia [43]. In many hearts, however, surviving myocardial fibers and the strands of fibrous tissue were intertwined in such a complex way that reconstruction of the reentrant pathway in the whole heart was impossible. Studies on infarcted papillary muscles showed that excitation proceeded in a zig-zag way through surviving fibers embedded in a complex network of connective tissue and that very "slow" conduction was caused by the greatly prolonged pathway of the excitatory wave [44]. That electrical remodeling of the myocardium remote from the infarct also plays a role, in addition to the structural changes in the infarct itself, is shown by a study in patients with sustained ventricular tachycardia and ventricular tachycardia that rapidly degenerated into ventricular fibrillation. In the latter group, dispersion in refractoriness in the remote myocardium was several times larger than in the ventricular tachycardia group [45]. Data from optical mapping studies show that one possible reentrant pathway is between normal myocardium and that bordering the infarct area, and is related to the presence of rate-dependent slow conduction and the development of a functional line of block in the border zone [46].

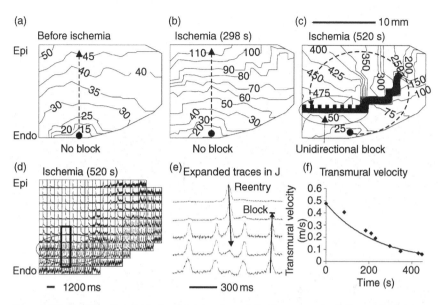

Figure 3.3 Unidirectional block of conduction at the transmural gradient of refractory period by endocardial stimulation during acute global ischemia. Activations were recorded with membrane potential sensitive fluorescence dye on a cut-exposed transmural surface of a wedge of isolated canine left ventricular free wall that was perfused through an included diagonal branch of the left anterior descending coronary artery. Acute global ischemia was created by halting perfusion. The times of ischemia are indicated in the figures. The conduction sequences (a–c) from the endocardial sites of pacing (the dots, CL: 300 ms) are shown as isochrone lines (at the times indicated by the numbers in ms) moving along the directions of the thin dashed arrow-headed lines. The thick solid line and the line with one dashed side and one solid side in (c) indicates full block and unidirectional block of conduction, respectively. Grids in the AP mosaic (d) separate the signals (1.2 s, normalized) from neighboring sensors. The framed traces in (d) are shown in (e) with an expanded time scale. The transmural velocity of conduction (f) is calculated from two recording sites with 11 mm separation along a transmural line passing through the site of pacing. Epi and Endo indicate the epicardium and endocardium. Transmural conduction from the endocardial site of pacing at the CL of 300 ms was blocked in the mid-myocardium in (c) and (d) by the longer refractory period. However, activation conducted along opposite direction (toward the endocardium) penetrated the line of unidirectional block in (c) and (d), until it collided with the refractory period of another activation initiated by the continued endocardial pacing. Reproduced from Wu and Zipes *Am J Physiol Heart Circ Physiol* 2001; **280**: H2717–2725, with permission.

Sudden death in heart failure

In patients with congestive heart failure, complex ventricular arrhythmias are often present, and sudden death is common [47,48]. It is not clear whether there is a relationship between presence of arrhythmias and subsequent

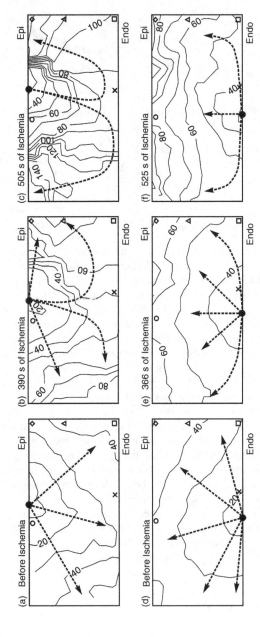

Figure 3.4 Unidirectional block of the epicardially initiated activation and transmural asymmetry in conduction during acute global ischemia. The isolated ventricular wedge and the recording area were similar to Figure 3.3. The wedge was stimulated alternately between the epicardium and endocardium at the black-dotted sites. Ischemia depressed tissue excitability more rapidly in the epicardium than in endocardium. After 505 s of ischemia (c), the epicardial-initiated activation penetrated the ventricular wall transmurally while failing to conduct laterally along the epicardium, then conducted laterally in the endocardium and mid-myocardium and reentered the epicardium. Endocardial stimulation, applied 525 s after ischemia (f), initiated activation that spread quickly along the endocardium, then transmurally to the epicardium without reentry. Therefore, ischemia-induced transmural gradient of excitability provided the substrate for reentry during epicardial stimulation. The recording area is 10 mm (transmural) by 18 mm (along the epicardium). Reproduced from Wu and Zipes *Am J Physiol Heart Circ Physiol* 2002; **283**: H2004–2011, with permission.

sudden death, because there are both reports that support such a relationship [49–51] and studies that deny it [52,53]. It has been known for a long time that the most powerful predictor for sudden death is left ventricular dysfunction [54], and one could therefore expect that sudden death would be related to the severity of heart failure. But here there is a controversy as well. Kjekshus [48] reported that in patients with New York Heart Association classes I and II heart failure, 50 to 60% of deaths were sudden, whereas in patients with class III or IV this was only 20 to 30% . In patients hospitalized for end stage heart failure, awaiting cardiac transplantation, sudden death was due to ventricular tachycardia or fibrillation in about 50%, and due to bradycardia, asystole or electromechanical dissociation in the other 50% [55,56]. These findings contrast with those of recent randomized trials on the prevention of sudden death by implantable cardioverter-defibrillator therapy, in which the device was most effective in patients with the lowest ejection fractions [57].

Three-dimensional mapping in patients with dilated cardiomyopathy, and in rabbits with heart failure caused by combined volume- and pressure-overload, showed that spontaneous and induced ventricular tachycardias arose from a focal, non-reentrant mechanism in either the endocardium or epicardium [58,59]. The non-reentrant mechanism is most likely a triggered activity based from delayed afterdepolarizations. The afterdepolarizations can be induced by rapid pacing in the presence of noradrenaline in failing myocardium [60–62]. The basis for delayed afterdepolarizations are calcium-after-transients that result from spontaneous calcium release from the sarcoplasmic reticulum [62,63]. The after-transient associated calcium is removed from the cell by the electrogenic Na/Ca exchanger [61,63] or by a calcium-activated chloride current [64], providing the transient inward current that causes the delayed afterdepolarization. The salvos of triggered activity in *in vitro* preparations are slower than the tachycardias *in vivo*. It is likely that the delayed afterdepolarizations, and the triggered activity, might initiate reentrant rhythms that lead to ventricular fibrillation.

The electrophysiological changes associated with heart failure have been the focus of intense research [65]. Heterogeneous action potential prolongation results as a function of myocardial remodeling [66], leading to an increase in the electrophysiological heterogeneity found in the normal ventricle [67]. Alterations in functional expression of ion channels and transporters, particularly those affecting potassium and calcium function, are responsible. Such changes can provide the necessary electrophysiological milieu for reentry and other mechanisms [68]. In addition, abnormal conduction due to reduced cell-to-cell coupling and sodium channel function current may play a role, along with changes caused by ventricular dilation, fibrosis, and ischemia. Gap junction remodeling from a downregulation and longitudinal redistribution of connexin43 [69] can contribute to the genesis of ventricular tachyarrhythmias. The autonomic nervous system, particularly the sympathetic limb, is important, and undergoes alterations, including sympathetic denervation and subsequent supersensitivity [70], and enhanced sympathetic regeneration called nerve sprouting [71]. While numerous studies point to the arrhythmo-genic potential of sympathetic stimulation and the benefits of beta blockade, the electrophysiologic mechanism(s) by which the sympathetic limb actually causes ventricular arrhythmias is largely unknown.

It is important to stress that drugs without direct electrophysiologic actions on the myocardium, such as aldosterone antagonists, angiotensin convert-ing enzyme inhibitors and receptor blockers, statins, magnesium, fish oil, aspirin, and beta receptor blockers, have been the only pharmacological agents shown to reduce both sudden and total mortality [72], implying that events "upstream" to the electrophysiological alterations in the myocardium, such as ischemia, fibrosis, inflammation, the renin-angiotensin system, or free radic-als are important, perhaps as triggers of the sudden ventricular event. Finally, genetics importantly program responses to stress, such as neurohumoral activ-ation, ion channel function, or prothrombic responses, that can determine susceptibility to developing a lethal ventricular arrhythmia. At least two pop-ulation based studies [73,74] provide evidence of an inherited predisposition to sudden cardiac death, with a relative risk approaching 10 for the child of two parents dying from that disorder [73]. The search for single nucleotide polymorphisms that may identify individuals at risk is intensive.

Conclusions

The mechanisms responsible for ventricular tachyarrhythmias causing sudden cardiac death are complex, multifactorial, and likely result from a conflu-ence of multiple events that portend whether a single premature ventricular complex, a run of nonsustained ventricular tachycardia, or sustained tachy-cardia/fibrillation results. Ventricular fibrillation is the final common pathway of a series of "upstream" changes that may trigger electrophysiologic altera-tions measured in milliseconds in a receptive myocardium. These relatively minor changes may determine whether an individual experiences a palpita-tion or sudden death. While we have made progress in understanding basic electrophysiologic mechanisms responsible for ventricular tachyarrhythmias, we still do not know why an apparently stable individual experiences sudden cardiac death on a Thursday at 9.15 AM, and not on Friday, or the preceding Wednesday, or 6 months before or after. Understanding the immediately pre-ceding and precipitating events, likely evanescent, remains a major challenge but may hold the clue for major progress in prediction and prevention of this calamitous event.

References

1. Erichsen JE. On the influence of the coronary circulation on the action of the heart. *London Med Gaz* 1841–1842; **2**: 561–565.
2. McWilliam JA. Cardiac failure and sudden death. *Br Med J* 1889; **1**: 6–8.

3. MacWilliam JA. Some applications of physiology to medicine: II. Ventricular fibrillation and sudden death. *Br Med J* 1923; **18**: 7–43.
4. Hoffa M, Ludwig C. Einige neue Versuche über Herzbewegung. *Z Ration Med* 1850; **9**: 107–144.
5. Prevost JL, Batelli F. Sur quelques aspets des décharges électriques sur le coeur des Mammifères. *C R Séances Acad Sci* 1899; **129**: 1267–1268.
6. Myerburg RJ, Spooner PM. Opportunities for sudden death prevention: directions for new clinical and basic research. *Cardiovasc Res* 2001; **50**: 177–185.
7. McWilliam JA. Fibrillar contraction of the heart. *J Physiol (London)* 1887; **8**: 296–310.
8. Moe GK. On the multiple wavelet hypothesis of atrial fibrillation. *Arch Int Pharmacodyn Ther* 1962; **140**: 183–188.
9. Moe GK, Rheinboldt WC, Abildskov JA. A computer model of atrial fibrillation. *Am Heart J* 1964; **67**: 200–220.
10. Janse MJ, Van Capelle FJL, Morsink H *et al.* Flow of "injury" current and patterns of excitation during early ventricular arrhythmias in acute regional myocardial ischemia in isolated porcine and canine hearts. Evidence for two different arrhythmogenic mechanisms. *Circ Res* 1980; **47**: 151–165.
11. Pogwizd SM, Corr PB. Reentrant and nonreentrant mechanisms contribute to arrhythmogenesis during early myocardial ischemia: results using three-dimensional mapping. *Circ Res* 1987; **61**: 352–371.
12. Allessie MA, Bonke FIM, Schopman FJG. Circus movement in rabbit atrial muscle as a mechanism of tachycardia: III. The "leading circle" concept: a new model of circus movement in cardiac tissue without the involvement of an anatomical obstacle. *Circ Res* 1977; **41**: 9–18.
13. Winfree AT. Electrical instability in cardiac muscle: phase singularities and rotors. *J Theor Biol* 1989; **138**: 353–405.
14. Fast VG, Kléber AG. Role of wavefront curvature in propagation of cardiac impulse. *Cardiovasc Res* 1997; **33**: 258–271.
15. Athill CA, Ikeda T, Kim Y-H *et al.* Transmembrane potential properties at the core of functional reentrant wavefronts in isolated canine right atria. *Circulation* 1998; **98**: 1556–1567.
16. Winfree AT. *When Time Breaks Down.* Princeton University Press, Princeton, NJ, 1987.
17. Davidenko JM, Pertsov AV, Salomonsz R *et al.* Stationary and drifting spiral waves of excitation in isolated cardiac muscle. *Nature* 1992; **355**: 349–351.
18. Scherf D. Studies on auricular tachycardia caused by aconitine administration. *Proc. Soc. Exp. Biol. Med.* 1947; **64**: 233–239.
19. Moe GK, Abildskov JA. Atrial fibrillation as a self-sustained arrhythmia independent of focal discharge. *Am Heart J* 1959; **58**: 59–70.
20. Jalife J, Berenfeld O, Skanes A *et al.* Mechanisms of atrial fibrillation: mother rotors or multiple daughter waves, or both? *J Cardiovasc Electrophysiol* 1998; **9**: S2–S12.
21. Samie FH, Mandapati R, Gray RA *et al.* A mechanism of transition from ventricular fibrillation to tachycardia: effect of calcium channel blockade on the dynamics of rotating waves. *Circ Res* 2000; **86**: 684–691.
22. Samie FH, Berenfeld O, Anumonwo J *et al.* Rectification of the background potassium current. A determinant of rotor dynamics in ventricular fibrillation. *Circ Res* 2001; **89**: 1216–1223.
23. Gray RA, Jalife J, Panfilov AV *et al.* Mechanisms of cardiac fibrillation. *Science* 1995; **270**: 1222–1223.

24. Panfilov AV. Spiral breakup as a model of ventricular fibrillation. *Chaos* 1998; **8**: 57–64.
25. Karma A. Electrical alternans and spiral wave breakup. *Chaos* 1994; **4**: 461–472.
26. Weiss JN, Garfinkel A, Karagueuzian HS *et al.* Chaos and the transition to ventricular fibrillation: a new approach to antiarrhythmic drug evaluation. *Circulation* 1999; **99**: 2819–2826.
27. Gilmour RF Jr, Otani NF, Watanabe MA. Memory and complex dynamics in cardiac Purkinje fibers. *Am J Physiol* 1997; **272**: H1826–H1832.
28. Riccio ML, Koller ML, Gilmour RF Jr. Electrical restitution and spatiotemporal organization during ventricular fibrillation. *Circ Res* 1999; **84**: 955–963.
29. Fenton F, Cherry E, Hastings H *et al.* Multiple mechanisms of spiral wave breakup in a model of cardiac activity. *Chaos* 2002; **12**: 852–892.
30. Chen P-S, Wu T-J, Ting C-T *et al.* A tale of two fibrillations. *Circulation* 2003; **108**: 2298–2309.
31. Gettes LN, Reuter H. Slow recovery from inactivation of inward currents in mammalian myocardial fibers. *J Physiol (London)* 1974; **240**: 703–724.
32. Shaw RM, Rudy Y. Electrophysiologic effects of acute myocardial ischemia: a theoretical study of altered cell excitability and action potential duration. *Cardiovasc Res* 1997; **35**: 256–272.
33. Kaplinsky E, Ogawa S, Balke CW *et al.* Two periods of early ventricular arrhythmias in the canine acute myocardial infarction model. *Circulation* 1979; **60**: 397–403.
34. Smith WT, Fleet WF, Johnson TA *et al.* The 1B phase of ventricular arrhythmias in ischemic *in situ* porcine heart is related to changes in cell-to-cell coupling. *Circulation* 1995; **92**: 3051 3060.
35. Cinca J, Warren M, Carreno A *et al.* Changes in myocardial electrical impedance induced by coronary artery occlusion in pigs with and without preconditioning: correlation with local ST-segment potential and ventricular arrhythmias. *Circulation* 1997; **96**: 3079–3086.
36. Coronel R, Fiolet JWT, Wilms-Schopman FJG *et al.* Distribution of extracellular potassium and its relation to electrophysiologic changes during acute myocardial ischemia in the isolated perfused porcine heart. *Circulation* 1988; **77**: 1125–1138.
37. De Groot JR, Wilms-Schopman FJG, Opthof T *et al.* Late ventricular arrhythmias during acute regional ischemia in the isolated blood perfused pig heart. Role of electrical cellular coupling. *Cardiovasc Res* 2001; **50**: 362–372.
38. Wu J, Zipes DP. Transmural reentry during global acute ischemia and reperfusion in canine ventricular muscle. *Am J Physiol* 2001; **280**: H2717–H2725.
39. Coronel R, Wilms-Schopman FJG, de Groot JR. Origin of ischemia-induced 1b arrythmias in pig hearts. *J Am Coll Cardiol* 2002; **39**: 166–176.
40. Mukherjee D, Feldman MS, Helfant RH. Nitroprusside therapy: treatment of hypertensive patients with recurrent chest pain, ST-segment elevation, and ventricular arrhythmias. *J Am Med Assoc* 1976; **235**: 2406–2409.
41. Durrer JD, Lie KI, van Capelle FJL *et al.* Effect of sodiumnitroprusside on mortality in acute myocardial infarction. *New Engl J Med* 1982; **306**: 1121–1128.
42. Wu J, Zipes DP. Transmural reentry triggered by epicardial and not endocardial stimulation during acute ischemia in canine ventricular muscle. *Am J Physiol* 2002; **283**: H2004–H2011.
43. De Bakker JMT, Coronel R, Tasseron S, *et al.* Ventricular tachycardia in the infarcted, Langendorff-perfused human heart: role of the arrangement of surviving cardiac fibers. *J Am Coll Cardiol* 1990; **15**: 1594–1607.

44. De Bakker JMT, van Capelle FJL, Janse MJ *et al.* Slow conduction in the infarcted human heart. "Zigzag" course of activation. *Circulation* 1993; **88**: 915–926.
45. Ramdat Misier A, Opthof T, van Hemel NM *et al.* Dispersion in "refractoriness" in noninfarcted myocardium of patients with ventricular tachycardia or fibrillation after myocardial infarction. *Circulation* 1995; **91**: 2566–2572.
46. Takahashi T, van Dessel P, Lopshire J *et al.* Optical mapping of the functional reentrant circuit of ventricular tachycardia in acute myocardial infarction. *Heart Rhythm*, 2004; **4**: 451–459.
47. Chakko S, de Marchena E, Kessler KM *et al.* Ventricular arrhythmias in congestive heart failure. *Clin Cardiol* 1989; **12**: 525–530.
48. Kjekshus J. Arrhythmias and mortality in congestive heart failure. *Am J Cardiol* 1990; **65**: 42–48.
49. De Maria R, Gavazzi A, Caroli A *et al.* Ventricular arrhythmia in dilated cardiomyopathy as an independent prognostic hallmark. *Am J Cardiol* 1992; **69**: 1451–1457.
50. Romeo F, Pellicia F, Cianfrocca C *et al.* Predictors of sudden death in idiopathic dilated cardiomyopathy. *Am J Cardiol* 1996; **63**: 138–140.
51. Doval HC, Nul DR, Grancelli HO *et al.* Non-sustained ventricular tachycardia in severe heart failure: independent marker of increased mortality due to sudden death. *Circulation* 1996; **94**: 3189–3203.
52. Packer M. Lack of relation between ventricular arrhythmias and sudden death in patients with chronic heart failure. *Circulation* 1992; **85**: 50–56.
53. Teerlink JR, Jaladuddin M, Anderson S *et al.* Ambulatory ventricular arrhythmias in patients with heart failure do not specifically predict an increased risk of sudden death. *Circulation* 2000; **101**: 40–46.
54. Bigger JT Jr, Flaiss JL, Kleiger J *et al.* The relationship among ventricular arrhythmias, left ventricular dysfunction, and mortality two years after myocardial infarction. *Circulation* 1984; **69**: 250–258.
55. Luu M, Stevenson WG, Stevenson LW *et al.* Diverse mechanisms of unexpected cardiac arrest in advanced heart failure. *Circulation* 1989; **80**: 1675–1680.
56. Stevenson WG, Stevenson LW, Middlekauf HR *et al.* Sudden death prevention in patients with advanced ventricular dysfunction. *Circulation* 1993; **88**: 2953–2961.
57. Moss AJ. Implantable cardioverter-defibrillator therapy. The sickest patients benefit most. *Circulation* 2000; **101**: 1638–1640.
58. Pogwizd SM. Nonreentrant mechanisms underlying spontaneous ventricular arrhythmias in a model of nonischemic heart failure in rabbits. *Circulation* 1995; **92**: 1034–1048.
59. Pogwizd SM, McKenzie JP, Cain ME. Mechanisms underlying spontaneous and induced ventricular arrhythmias in patients with idiopathic dilated cardiomyopathy. *Circulation* 1998; **98**: 2404–2414.
60. Vermeulen JT, McGuire MA, Opthof T *et al.* Triggered activity and automaticity in ventricular trabeculae of failing human and rabbit hearts. *Cardiovasc Res* 1994; **28**: 1547–1554.
61. Pogwizd SM, Schlotthauer K, Li L *et al.* Arrhythmogenesis and contractile dysfunction in heart failure. Roles of sodium–calcium exchange, inward rectifier potassium current, and residual beta-adrenergic responsiveness. *Circ Res* 2001; **88**: 1159–1167.
62. Baartscheer A, Schumacher CA, Belterman C *et al.* SR calcium handling and calcium after-transients in a rabbit model of heart failure. *Cardiovasc Res* 2003; **58**: 99–108.

63. Pogwizd SM, Qi M, Yuan W *et al.* Upregulation of Na/Ca-exchanger expression in an arrhythmogenic model of heart failure. *Circ Res* 1999; **85**: 1015–1024.

64. Verkerk AO, Veldkamp MW, Bouman LN *et al.* Calcium-activated Cl-current contributes to delayed afterdepolarizations in single Purkinje and ventricular myocytes. *Circulation* 2000; **101**: 2639–2644.

65. Tomaselli GF, Zipes DP. What causes sudden death in heart failure? *Circ Res*, 2004; **95**: 754–763.

66. Tomaselli GF, Marban E. Electrophysiological remodeling in hypertrophy and heart failure. *Cardiovasc Res* 1999; **42**: 270–283.

67. Antzelevitch C, Sicouri S, Litkovsky SH *et al.* Heterogeneity within the ventricular wall. Electrophysiology of epicardial, endocardial, and M cells. *Circ Res* 1991; **69**: 1427–1449.

68. Ueda N, Zipes DP, Wu J. Prior ischemia enhances arrhythmogenicity in isolated canine ventricular wedge model of long QT3. *Cardiovasc Res* 2004; **63**: 69–76.

69. Peters NS, Green CR, Poole-Wilson PA *et al.* Reduced content of connexin43 gap junctions in ventricular myocardium from hypertrophied and ischemic human hearts. *Circulation* 1993; **88**: 864–875.

70. Inoue H, Zipes DP. Results of sympathetic denervation in the canine heart: supersensitivity that may be arrhythmogenic. *Circulation* 1987; **75**: 877–887.

71. Cao JM, Chen LS, KenKnight BH *et al.* Nerve sprouting and sudden cardiac death. *Circulation* 2000; **101**: 1960–1969.

72. Alberte C, Zipes DP. Use of nonantiarrhythmic drugs for prevention of sudden cardiac death. *J Cardiovasc Electrophysiol* 2003; **14**: S87–SS95.

73. Jouven X, Desnos M, Guerot C *et al.* Predicting sudden death in the population of the Paris Prospective Study. *Circulation* 1999; **99**: 1978–1983.

74. Friedlander Y, Siscovick DS, Weinmann S *et al.* Family history as a risk factor for primary cardiac arrest. *Circulation* 1998; **97**: 155–160.

75. Müller SC, Plesser T, Hess B. The structure of the core of the spiral waves in the Belousov–Zhabotinskii reaction. *Science* 1985; **230**: 661–663.

CHAPTER 4

Risk stratification for SCD

Stefan H. Hohnloser and Wojciech Zareba

Sudden cardiac death (SCD) is defined as the unexpected natural death, from cardiac causes, within a short time period of a person without a cardiac condition that would appear fatal [1]. SCD is responsible for approximately 300 000 fatalities in the United States alone [2,3]. It is estimated that 50% of all cardiac deaths are sudden, and this proportion has remained constant despite the overall decline in cardiovascular mortality during the last decades [3]. In approximately three quarter of cases, SCD is due to ventricular tachycardia (VT) and fibrillation [4–6] although in patients with underlying congestive heart failure, a significant proportion of SCD is the consequence of bradycardic events or electromechanical dissociation [7]. The majority of patients with a cardiac arrest suffer from coronary artery disease [8,9], but acute myocardial infarction is seen in less than half [9,10]. In a series of observations on 151 hearts from men dying from SCD, the presence of acute thrombus/ plaque rupture or erosion was noted in 67% of patients aged 30–39 years, but this declined with age and was present in only 31%, aged 60–69 years [11]. In another series of patients surviving a cardiac arrest who underwent angiography, recent coronary occlusions were noted in 48% [12].

The magnitude of the problem in specific subgroups of patients with SCD was addressed by Myerburg *et al.* [13], in a review of the population impact of emerging implantable cardioverter-defibrillator (ICD) trials (see Chapter 1). The highest incidence of SCD occurred in survivors of out-of-hospital cardiac death and high-risk postinfarction subgroups, but the greatest absolute number of SCD events (population attributable risk) occurred in larger subgroups of patients at somewhat lower risk including patients with left ventricular dysfunction, congestive heart failure, or any prior coronary events. The challenge, therefore, is to identify risk factors for SCD among the large group of patients at relatively low risk, and this applies directly to survivors of myocardial infarction, in an era when the prognosis has improved substantially in comparison with prior series antedating the widespread use of reperfusion therapy.

Risk stratification aims at the identification of quantitative and qualitative measurements that can serve as sensitive and specific predictors of cardiac, and in particular, arrhythmogenic mortality in patients with coronary disease or other cardiovascular diseases [14]. Although risk stratification is always a topic of interest from an intellectual perspective, its clinical relevance is dependent upon the availability of a therapeutic intervention that reduces the risk of arrhythmogenic death. With the advent of the ICD, particularly in the light of the modifications and refinements to this technology during the last decade, such an intervention is now in our hands [15–19].

This chapter will discuss the issue of risk stratification in patients with structural heart disease as it applies to contemporary cardiology.

Epidemiological impact of risk stratification

There are a number of potentially useful modalities that can be used to stratify postinfarction patients according to their risk of an arrhythmogenic death. In order to exert an impact on SCD from an epidemiologically meaningful point of view, prognostic tests need to achieve a high positive predictive accuracy together with a reasonable degree of sensitivity. Otherwise, the test or the combination of tests would be too specific to have any significant impact on the epidemiological problem of SCD simply because these yield positive findings only in a small minority of the postinfarction population. The first step towards this goal requires knowledge of the total number of sudden deaths within a specific patient population expressed as a fraction of total mortality within this group. For example, in patients with congestive heart failure, Kjekshus demonstrated that in studies in which the mean functional NYHA class was between I and II, the overall death rate was relatively low but 67% of death were sudden [20]. In contrast, among studies with a mean functional class of IV, there was a high total mortality but the fraction of sudden death was only 29%. Thus, for an intervention specific for the problem of SCD, it is important not only to identify infarct survivors at high risk of death, but also to predict the most likely mode of death, that is, arrhythmic or nonarrhythmic death since such a distinction would have a major influence upon the treatment strategy. Patients with a high propensity for arrhythmic death may benefit from preventive antiarrhythmic interventions whereas such treatment may provide no advantage or even increase the risk of mortality in patients more likely to die from nonarrhythmic death. Similarly the likelihood of a significant benefit from an ICD would only be present in the former group. Accordingly, the various risk stratifiers currently in clinical use need to be examined in regard to their ability not only to predict total mortality but also with respect to their potential to predict specific causes of death.

A pivotal aspect of the clinical impact of risk stratification is that the methodology be applicable not only to specialized referral centers, but also in the community hospital setting in which the majority of patients with acute myocardial infarction will receive care. For these reasons, invasive procedures are unlikely to gain widespread acceptance. Accordingly, current investigations focus upon the development of newer methods of noninvasive risk stratification. Another prerequisite for the process of risk stratification for arrhythmic death is that this be initiated in the predischarge period. The highest risk for SCD is within the first 12 months following the index infarction, and the majority of events occur within the first few months [21,22].

The Bayesian approach to the impact of the changing prognosis upon tests used for risk stratification

Bayesian principles are commonly employed in the evaluation of the incremental value of a new test in the diagnosis of coronary artery disease [23,24], but these basic concepts can be extended to the utilization of a variety of tests in which the endpoint is prognostic. Bayes' theorem can facilitate an understanding of the impact of a lower event rate upon the utility of tests used for risk stratification as is the case of myocardial infarction survivors in the contemporary era. Bayes' theorem suggests that the likelihood of disease or an event following testing (post-test probability) can be calculated from the characteristics (sensitivity and specificity) of the test and the pretest probability, and this can be plotted graphically (Figure 4.1) [25].

In the context of death or arrhythmic events post-myocardial infarction, line B in the figure would represent a patient with an intermediate probability of event, and lines A and C, patients with low or high probability of an event. In the case of the latter, the event rate (e.g. SCD or late ventricular arrhythmias) is high irrespective of the results of the test, and in the case of the latter (A), the converse is the case. Irrespective of whether the test is positive or negative, the event rate is low. In clinical situations corresponding to patients with a high

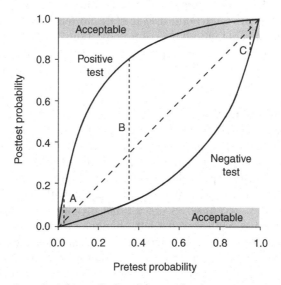

Figure 4.1 Bayesian principles applied to risk stratification (see text for details). Reproduced with permission from Reference 26.

or low probability of an event, the test does not provide a significant amount of incremental value over the pretest knowledge of the likelihood of an event. In contrast, however, among patients with an intermediate probability of an event (line B), the difference in outcomes between a positive and negative test is substantial. The crux of the issue in the modern era of myocardial and post-myocardial therapy and risk stratification, is to what extent, tests that had a strong predictive value in the reperfusion era (in which the late event rate ranged from 20% to 50%) still apply to a population in the reperfusion era with a much lower event rate.

Risk stratification in postinfarction patients

Clinical and demographic data

The GISSI-II Trial of 10 219 hospital survivors following thrombolytic therapy, identified a number of clinical variables, which were independently predictive of 6-month mortality. In order of importance, those were the ineligibility for an exercise test (for cardiac or noncardiac reasons), early left ventricular failure, left ventricular dysfunction in the recovery phase, age greater than 70 years, electrical instability, late left ventricular failure, prior myocardial infarction, and a history of hypertension [27]. For example, in a recent study of 103 164 patients with myocardial infarction who were 65 years or older, a single-risk model [including older age, comorbidity, heart failure, reduced left ventricular ejection fraction (LVEF), and peripheral vascular disease] effectively stratified patients according to their risk of death 1 year after discharge [28].

Numerous other series have confirmed the adverse prognostic impact of older age and diabetes upon both early and late mortality [29]. Other high-risk groups include patients who have contraindications to reperfusion therapy, patients who receive such therapy late, and patients who, for whatever reason, fail to be treated with reperfusion therapy, even in the absence of contraindications [30,31].

Left ventricular function

Ventricular function as defined by the predischarge ejection fraction has been recognized as a major determinant of late mortality for decades [14,22,32,33]. Although the proportion of patients with impaired left ventricular function has declined following reperfusion therapy, the correlation between impaired ejection fraction and late mortality persists [32]. Nonetheless, in comparison with earlier studies, recent series suggest that the curve relating mortality to ejection fraction has "shifted to the left," implying that for a given degree of left ventricular dysfunction, the increase in mortality is somewhat less than previously reported. A recent study of 313 patients, all of whom had a patent infarct-related artery at the time of discharge, identified that an ejection fraction of ≤35% still had a positive predictive value of 28% for cardiac death or sustained ventricular arrhythmias during follow-up [34].

In another series of patients with an anterior myocardial infarction, all of whom underwent primary percutaneous transluminal coronary angioplasty (PTCA), the presence of restrictive diastolic filling as defined by deceleration time on echocardiography of less than 130 ms was associated with a 2-year mortality over a mean of 32 months of 21% versus only 3% in patients without restrictive features [35]. Data such as these point to the presence of smaller patient subgroups (30% of the total in this series) who may well benefit from further risk stratification. On the other hand, these data also suggest that the remaining 70% of patients with an excellent prognosis might not require any additional risk stratification, given a mortality rate of only 3% at 2 years. What is important in this study is that the predictive power of diastolic dysfunction was independent of ejection fraction.

Ambulatory ECG monitoring

Ambulatory Holter monitoring is a comprehensive tool for identifying and quantifying factors that might contribute to the mechanism of SCD (Figure 4.2). Historically, detecting and quantifying Holter-recorded ventricular arrhythmias was the first ECG-based approach to determine the risk of patients and to implement antiarrhythmic therapy [1]. There is clear association between increased frequency and complexity of ventricular arrhythmias with cardiac and SCD. However, diminishing these arrhythmias with pharmacological agents was not leading to improved survival, and in case of several drugs such therapy was associated with worse outcome [1]. Primary prevention of sudden death with ICD therapy was introduced by Multicenter Automatic Defibrillator Implantation Trial (MADIT) and MUSTT in patients

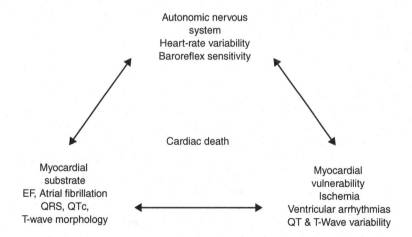

Figure 4.2 Factors contributing to cardiac death and respective Holter-derived ECG parameters. Reproduced with permission from Reference 36.

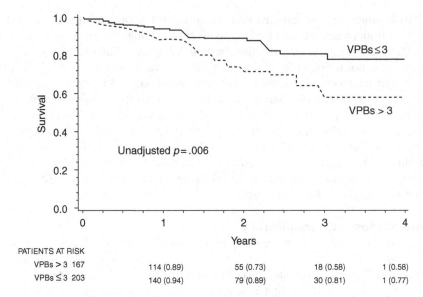

Figure 4.3 Cumulative probability of survival in MADIT II patients randomized to conventional therapy in relationship to presence or absence of frequent VPBs. Reproduced with permission from Reference 38.

with documented nonsustained VT and inducibility of ventricular tachyar-rhythmias [15,16]. After the MADIT II [18] and Sudden Cardiac Death in Heart Failure Trial SCD-HeFT [37] trials, EF ≤30% is considered a sufficient risk stratifier without the need for documenting Holter-detected ventricu-lar arrhythmias or inducible VT. Nevertheless, as shown in a secondary MADIT II analysis (Figure 4.3) frequent premature ventricular beats identify significantly increased risk of mortality and arrhythmic events even in patients with such low ejection fractions. Therefore, tracking frequency and severity of ventricular arrhythmias might still assist clinicians in prioritization of patients to ICD therapy.

The effects of the autonomic nervous system on the heart could be evalu-ated by quantifying heart-rate variability (HRV) illustrating the relationship between parasympathetic and sympathetic components of this system. Heart-rate turbulence (HRT) complements HRV analysis by providing insight into a baroreflex sensitivity component of central regulation of the cardiovascular system. Abnormalities of central regulation of the heart are very unlikely to cause SCD without altered myocardial substrate and additional factors increasing vulnerability of myocardium to VT. Holter technology provides clinicians with several parameters illustrating changes in myocardial substrate and vulnerability. As discussed above, ejection fraction and other meas-ures of left ventricular dysfunction are the most acceptable measures of the changes in myocardial substrate. However, complementary information about substrate could be obtained from electrocardiology (including ambulatory ECG monitoring). The parameters of interest include QRS duration and morphology (conduction disturbances and hypertrophy), late potentials, and changes in repolarization duration or morphology. Vulnerability of myocardium could be evaluated using Holter monitoring in which one could determine presence or absence of ischemic ST-segment changes, frequency and complexity of ventricular arrhythmias, and abnormal dynamics of repolarization as reflected by QT–RR relationship and QT or T-wave variability. T-wave alternans, usually analyzed in exercise testing, is yet another measure of myocardial vulnerability to arrhythmias.

Signal-averaged ECG

A broad QRS complex is associated with an increased risk of mortality and patients with conduction disturbances do not benefit much from signal-averaged ECG (SAECG) analyses. However, presence of late potentials and/or prolonged filtered QRS duration in SAECG in patients with normal QRS duration on standard ECG indicates increased risk of cardiac events. Data from MUSTT trial [39] in 1925, patients demonstrated that filtered QRS duration >114 ms was significantly associated with the primary study endpoint (arrhythmic death or cardiac arrest) after adjustment for clinical covariates. Patients with an abnormal SAECG had a 28% incidence of primary endpoints in comparison to 17% in those with normal SAECG ($p < .001$) during 5-year follow-up. Cardiac death and total mortality also were significantly higher. In this study, combination of prolonged filtered QRS duration >114 ms and EF <30% identified a very high-risk subset of patients (Figure 4.4). This finding was of particular importance since the clinical usefulness of inducible VT was found to be limited in this study. Recent, as yet unpublished data from the MADIT II trial also indicate that abnormal SAECG in patients with normal QRS duration identifies high-risk individuals or lack of SAECG abnormalities identifies group of patients with a low mortality who are unlikely to benefit from ICD therapy. Results from these two large clinical trials support the notion that normal SAECG with its high negative predictive value could be used to identify postinfarction patients with depressed left ventricular function who might not benefit from ICD therapy. Remaining patients, that is, those with abnormal SAECG while having normal QRS duration on standard ECG, and patients with wide QRS on standard ECG constitute a group with a risk high enough (>20% mortality in 2-year period) to warrant ICD therapy without hesitation. There is growing evidence for rebirth of interest in SAECG as a useful risk stratification tool in high-risk postinfarction patients with left ventricular dysfunction. Abnormal SAECG recorded in the early postinfarction period, however, has insufficient predictive power, which seems to be overwhelmed by better predictive value of other ECG parameters (including HRT and T-wave alternans). However, there is data indicating that the combination of abnormalities in SAECG with positive results of T-wave alternans test might be useful in identifying high-risk individuals in the early postinfarction period [40,41]. Bailey *et al.* [42] suggested the use of SAECG together with

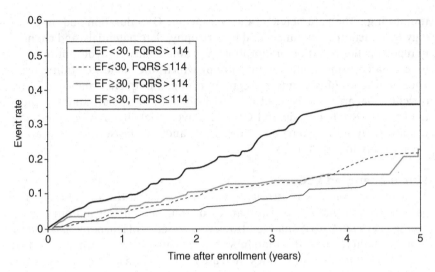

Figure 4.4 Kaplan–Meier estimates of arrhythmic death or cardiac arrest by SAECG result and EF. Two-year and five-year event rates for patients with EF <30% and FQRS >114 ms were 17% and 36%, respectively; for patients with EF <30% and FQRS ≤114 ms, they were 10% and 23%, respectively; for patients with EF ≥ 30% and FQRS >114 ms, they were 11% and 22% respectively; and for patients with EF ≥30% and FQRS ≤114 ms, they were 6% and 13%, respectively. Differences between those with EF <30% and FQRS >114 ms compared with those with FQRS ≤114 ms was highly significant ($p = .0001$). Difference between those with EF ≥30% and FQRS >114 ms compared with those with FQRS ≤114 ms was also significant ($p = .01$). Reproduced with permission from Reference 39. FQRS = filtered QRS duration.

ejection fraction as first steps of risk stratification process in postinfarction patients. Patients with normal SAECG and preserved left ventricular function have a very low risk of arrhythmic events (about 2% over 5-year period), whereas those with abnormal SAECG and depressed LVEF have very high risk of such events (about 38%). Intermediate groups, with either test abnormal, require further stratification using Holter-based HRV and ventricular arrhythmia analysis or programmed ventricular stimulation. Ultimately, this strategy is likely to identify the majority of patients eligible for ICD therapy as well as those who may not need this treatment.

Microvolt T-wave alternans
The presence of subtle beat-to-beat changes in the amplitude of the T-wave in the surface ECG, which is termed microvolt T-wave alternans (MTWA), has been shown to be associated with an increased risk of SCD or other serious ventricular tachyarrhythmic events [40,41,43]. Particularly in patients with ischemic and nonischemic cardiomyopathy, assessment of MTWA has been shown to be useful for prediction of arrhythmic complications during the

subsequent course of treatment of these patients. For instance, a recent report on 129 patients with ischemic cardiomyopathy found that over a 24 months follow-up no major arrhythmic event or SCD occurred in those patients who tested negative; on the other hand, in MTWA positive patients or in those with an indeterminate test result, the event rate was 15.6% [44]. Bloomfield *et al.* recently reported their findings in 177 MADIT II-like patients in whom they assessed MTWA and whom they followed for 2 years [45]. They found that a positive MTWA was associated with a higher mortality rate than that associated with a prolonged QRS duration of >120 ms. In fact, the actual mortality was 17.8% in patients with a positive MTWA compared to only 3.8% in those patients who tested negative for MTWA (hazard ratio 4.8, 95% confidence interval 1.1–20.7, $p = .02$). It is of particular note that in all studies, evaluating MTWA for arrhythmic risk stratification MTWA carried a high negative predictive value of between 96% and 100%. This indicates that analysis of MTWA may be particularly helpful to avoid unnecessary ICD implantations in patients with depressed LV function who test negative for MTWA.

Measures of autonomic control

Numerous studies explored the prognostic value of HRV parameters for predicting outcomes in postinfarction patients [47–50]. They consistently showed that depressed HRV is associated with increased mortality. However, there is limited data regarding the prognostic significance of HRV parameters for predicting sudden or arrhythmic death. The limited evidence for the association between depressed HRV parameters and SCD might be due to the difficulty in categorizing sudden or arrhythmic nature of death, but also could be because of lack of strong evidence for this association. HRV also operates differently in different patient population depending not only on the disease but also on advancement of the disease process. HRV parameters predict well CHF worsening and total mortality in congestive heart failure patients whereas the predictive value of HRV for SCD is limited. Similarly, there are no studies linking HRV with electrophysiology (EP) inducibility, further indicating that HRV might not be the right approach to identify susceptibility to arrhythmias. Reported associations with arrhythmic events are most likely driven by congestive heart failure which predisposes to SCD itself [51].

A new method for evaluating the response of sinus beats to single ventricular premature beats is HRT [52]. Normal response to VPBs consists of immediate acceleration with subsequent deceleration of heart rate whereas blunted response, which does not show such reaction, is considered as a noninvasive sign of impaired baroreflex sensitivity. Schmidt *et al.* [52] demonstrated that HRT quantified using two parameters describing turbulence onset and turbulence slope is an independent predictor of total or cardiovascular mortality in MPIP and EMIAT postinfarction populations. This observation was further substantiated by recent analysis of data in postinfarction patients from ATRAMI study [53] and ISAR study [54] with majority of patients treated with primary coronary interventions. However, again like for HRV parameters there is no support for direct association between HRT parameters and sudden death.

The last few years saw an increased clinical interest in nonlinear dynamic methods for risk stratification purposes. There are few studies suggesting that low levels of alfa1, short-term scaling component of heart-rate dynamics, is associated with increased mortality in postinfarction patients [55,56]. The limitation of both HRT and nonlinear dynamic is their limited accessibility.

Therefore, there is strong evidence linking depressed HRV and abnormal HRT with cardiac mortality and these methods should be used in the risk stratification process, however, with full realization that their predictive value might not be directly related to sudden death or arrhythmic events.

Invasive electrophysiologic testing

Testing inducibility of VT in postinfarction patients became a standard modality for identifying high-risk individuals prone to sudden death. MADIT and MUSTT were designed to enroll postinfarction patients with depressed LVEF who presented with nonsustained VT and inducibility of ventricular tachyarrhythmias during invasive electrophysiologic testing [15,16]. Both these primary prevention trials with the use of ICDs demonstrated that the above risk stratification algorithm was able to select a subset of postinfarction patients with very high mortality risk. However, secondary analysis from MUSTT [57] published in 1999, revealed that despite significant difference in outcome between inducible patients enrolled in the trial and noninducible patients enrolled in a registry, EP inducibility was found of limited use since 5-year mortality in inducible patients was 48% compared to 44% in noninducible. In 1997, MADIT II was launched to determine whether primary prevention with ICD therapy is justified in postinfarction patients with EF ≤30% but without additional risk stratifiers [18]. This trial demonstrated a significant 31% reduction in the risk of mortality in patients treated with ICDs when compared to conventionally treated patients. MADIT II also showed that there is no need for additional risk stratifiers (including EP testing) when ejection fraction is so low. In fact, in over 80% randomized to ICD arm of MADIT II, invasive EP testing with an attempt to induce tachyarrhythmias was performed at the time of ICD placement. VT inducibility, observed in 40% of studied patients, was not effective in identifying patients with cardiac events defined as VT, ventricular fibrillation, or death (MADIT II – personal communication). These observations from both MUSTT and MADIT II subanalyses suggest that in patients with substantially depressed left ventricular function, EP inducibility should not be considered as useful predictor of outcome. It is, however, possible that inducibility might have much better predictive value in postinfarction patients with EF >30% or >35%. Cappato *et al.* [58] investigated usefulness of EP inducibility in 285 survivors of cardiac arrest enrolled in the Cardiac Arrest Study Hamburg (CASH) and found that EP inducibility was predictive for sudden death in patients with EF >35% (HR = 3.0; $p = .006$)

whereas it was not useful in patients with lower ejection fraction (HR = 1.1; $p = .81$).

Risk stratification in nonischemic cardiomyopathy

The above sections focused on postinfarction patients, whereas a growing number of CHF patients with nonischemic cardiomyopathy is being seen by cardiologists and are considered for prophylactic ICD therapy. DEFINITE [19] was a recent trial evaluating the effects of ICD therapy on mortality in patients with nonischemic cardiomyopathy. About half of patients enrolled in SCD-HeFT [37] had nonischemic cardiomyopathy. Both these studies indicated that ICD therapy reduces mortality in nonischemic cardiomyopathy patients and following these findings new indications for ICD in the United States include nonischemic cardiomyopathy with EF ≤30% [59].

The question remains how to identify patients with nonischemic cardiomyopathy who might benefit from ICD therapy more than other individuals. Invasive EP testing with inducibility of ventricular arrhythmias is not useful as a risk stratification method. Several noninvasive techniques were explored including presence of nonsustained VT, abnormal signal-averaged ECG, HRV, and recently T-wave alternans. Among these noninvasive modalities, T-wave alternans seems to be of increasing interest in dilated cardiomyopathy patients. Hohnloser *et al.* [60] studied 137 dilated cardiomyopathy patients followed for a mean 14 months and they found that decreased baroreflex sensitivity and presence of MTWA were the only two significant predictors of arrhythmic events outperforming other tested parameters including NSVT, SAECG, LVEF, and HRV. However, in a larger Marburg Cardiomyopathy Study of 343 cardiomyopathy patients with mean 52-month follow-up, Grimm *et al.* [61] found that ejection fraction was the only effective predictor of arrhythmia-free survival. Nonsustained VT added to ejection fraction was further refining the risk stratification model. In Marburg Cardiomyopathy Study, other tests including SAECG, HRV, baroreflex sensitivity, and T-wave alternans were not useful in predicting arrhythmia-free survival. Secondary analyses from DEFINITE and SCD-HeFT trials will bring more data to further clarify this controversy. Nevertheless, since the above ICD trials gave basis for ICD indications in dilated cardiomyopathy patients with EF ≤30%, future research is needed to determine optimal risk stratification algorithms in patients with EF >30% and in this group NSVT and T-wave alternans might be of major value.

Summary

Ejection fraction remains the number one risk stratifier in both ischemic and nonischemic cardiomyopathy patients. Patients with EF ≤30% should undergo primary prevention therapy by device implantation. Predictive value of various noninvasive parameters in patients with such profound left ventricular dysfunction is limited, although the high negative predictive values of SAECG and T-wave alternans might help prioritizing postinfarction patients. In patients with EF >30%, T-wave alternans especially in combination with other parameters reflecting abnormalities in myocardial substrate (prolonged QRS, abnormal SAECG) or increased vulnerability (NSVT) might be considered as useful noninvasive measures of risk stratification competing with invasive EP induction of ventricular tachyarrhythmias.

References

1. Zipes DP, Wellens HJJ. Sudden cardiac death. *Circulation* 1998; **98**: 2334–2351.
2. Gillum RF. Sudden coronary deaths in the United States 1980–1985. *Circulation* 1989; **79**: 756–765.
3. Myerburg RJ, Kessler KM, Catellanos A. Sudden cardiac death: structure, function, and time-dependence of risk. *Circulation* 1992; **85**(Suppl. I): 2–10.
4. Schaffer WA, Cobb LA. Recurrent ventricular fibrillation and modes of death in survivors of out-of-hospital ventricular fibrillation. *N Engl J Med* 1975; **293**: 259–262.
5. Wilber DJ, Garan H, Finkelstein D, *et al*. Out-of-hospital cardiac arrest. Use of electrophysiologic testing in the prediction of long-term outcome. *N Engl J Med* 1988; **318**: 19–24.
6. Meissner AD, Akhtar M, Lehman MH. Nonischemic sudden tachyarrhythmic death in artherosclerotic heart disease. *Circulation* 1991; **84**: 905–912.
7. Liu M, Stevenson WG, Stevenson LW, Baron K, Walden J. Diverse mechanisms of unexpected cardiac arrest in advanced heart failure. *Circulation* 1989; **80**: 1675–1680.
8. Liberthson RR, Nagel EL, Hirschman JC, *et al*. Pathophysiologic observations in prehospital ventricular fibrillation and sudden cardiac death. *Circulation* 1974; **49**: 790–797.
9. Reichenbach DD; Moss NS, Meyer E. Pathology of the heart in sudden cardiac death. *Am J Cardiol* 1977; **39**: 865–869.
10. Kannel WB, Thomas HE. Sudden coronary death: the Framingham study. *Ann NY Acad Sci* 1982; **382**: 3–21.
11. Farb A, Burke AP, Kolodgie FD, Virmani R. Risk profiles are more abnormal and acute thrombi more frequent in young men with sudden death. *J Am Coll Cardiol* 1999; **33**: 324A (abstract).
12. Spaulding CM, Joly LM, Rosenberg A, *et al*. Immediate coronary angiography in survivors of out-of-hospital cardiac arrest. *N Engl J Med* 1997; **336**: 1629–1633.
13. Myerburg RJ, Mitrani R, Interian A, Castellanos A. Interpretation of outcomes of antiarrhythmic clinical trials. Design features and population impact. *Circulation* 1998; **97**: 1514–1521.
14. Camm AJ, Katrisis DG. Risk stratification of patients with ventricular arrhythmias. In: Zipes DP & Jalife J, eds. *Cardiac Electrophysiology: From Cell to Bedside*. W.B. Saunders Co, Philadelphia, PA, 2000: 808–828.
15. Moss AJ, Hall WJ, Cannom DS, *et al*. Improved survival with an implanted defibrillator in patients with coronary disease at high risk for ventricular arrhythmias. *N Engl J Med* 1996; **335**: 1933–1940.

16. Buxton AE, Lee KL, Fischer JD, Josephson ME, Prystowski EN, Hafley G (for the Multicenter Unsustained Tachycardia Trial Investigators). A randomized study of the prevention of sudden death in patients with coronary artery disease. *N Eng J Med* 1999; **341**: 1882–1890.

17. The Antiarrhythmics Versus Implantable Defibrillators (AVID) Investigators. A comparison of antiarrhythmic-drug therapy with implantable defibrillators in patients resuscitated from near-fatal ventricular arrhythmias. *N Eng J Med* 1997; **337**: 1576–1583.

18. Moss AJ, Zareba W, Hall WJ, *et al.* (for the Multicenter Automatic Defibrillator Implantation Trial II Investigators). Prophylactic implantation of a defibrillator in patients with myocardial infarction and reduced ejection fraction. *N Engl J Med* 2002; **346**: 877–883.

19. Kadish A, Dyer A, Daubert JP, *et al.* Prophylactic defibrillator implantation in patients with nonischemic dilated cardiomyopathy. *N Engl J Med* 2004; **350**: 2151–2158.

20. Kjekshus J. Arrhythmias and mortality in congestive heart failure. *Am J Cardiol* 1990; **65**: 421–428.

21. Myerburg Kessler M, Castellanos A. Sudden cardiac death: epidemiology, transient risk, and intervention assessment. *Ann Int Med* 1993; **119**: 1187–1197.

22. Hohnloser SH, Klingenheben T, Zabel M. Identification of patients after myocardial infarction at risk of life-threatening arrhythmias. *Eur Heart J* 1999; 1(Suppl C): C11–C20.

23. Epstein SE. Implications of probability analysis on the strategy used for noninvasive detection of coronary artery disease. *Am J Cardiol* 1980; **46**: 491–499.

24. Gibbons RG. Obtaining incremental information from diagnostic tests. In: Yusuf S, Cairns JA, Camm AJ, Fallen EL, & Gersh BJ, eds. *Evidence-Based Cardiology*. BMJ Books, London, 1998.

25. Berman BS, Garcia EV, Maddahi J. Thallium-201 scintigraphy in the detection and evaluation of coronary artery disease. In: Berman DS & Mason DT, eds. *Clinical Nuclear Cardiology*. Grune and Stratton, New York, 1981.

26. Hohnloser SH, Gersh BJ. Changing late prognosis of acute myocardial infarction. *Circulation* 2003; **107**: 941–946.

27. Tavazzi L, Volpi A. Remarks about postinfarction prognosis in light of the experience with the Gruppo Italiano per lo Studio della Sopravivenza nell' Infarto Miocardico (GISSI) Trials. *Circulation* 1997; **95**: 1341–1345.

28. Krumholz HM, Chen J, Chen YT, Wang Y, Radford MJ. Predicting one-year mortality among elderly survivors of hospitalization for an acute myocardial infarction: results from the cooperative cardiovascular project. *J Am Coll Cardiol* 2001; **38**: 453–459.

29. Berger AK, Breall JA, Gersh BJ, *et al.* Effect of diabetes mellitus and insulin use on survival after acute myocardial infarction in the elderly (The Cooperative Cardiovascular Project). *Am J Cardiol* 2001; **87**: 272–277.

30. Gottlieb S, Boyko V, Harpaz D, *et al.* Long-term (three-year) prognosis of patients treated with reperfusion or conservatively after acute myocardial infarction. *J Am Coll Cardiol* 1999; **34**: 70–82.

31. Canto JG, Shlipak MG, Rogers WJ, *et al.* Prevalence, clinical characteristics, and mortality among patients with myocardial infarction presenting without chest pain. *JAMA* 2000; **283**: 3223–3229.

32. Rouleau JL, Talajic M, Sussex B, *et al.* Myocardial infarction patients in the 1990s. Their risk factors, stratification and survival in Canada: the Canadian

Assessment of Myocardial Infarction (CAMI) Study. *J Am Coll Cardiol* 1996; **27**: 1119–1127.

33. Gomes JA, Winters SL, Martison M, Machac J, Steward D, Targonski A. The prognostic significance of quantitative signal-averaged variables related to clinical variables, site of myocardial infarction, ejection fraction and ventricular arrhythmias. A prospective study. *J Am Coll Cardiol* 1988; **1**: 377–384.

34. Klingenheben T, Sporis S, Mauss O, Hohnloser SH. Value of autonomic markers for noninvasive risk stratification in post infarction patients with a patent infarct-related artery. *PACE* 2000; **23**(II): 733 (abstract).

35. Cerisano G, Bolognese L, Buonamici P, *et al*. Prognostic implications of restrictive left ventricular filling in reperfused anterior acute myocardial infarction. *J Am Coll Cardiol* 2001; **37**: 793–799.

36. Zareba W, Moss AJ. Noninvasive risk stratification in postinfarction patients with severe left ventricular dysfunction and methodology of the MADIT II noninvasive electrocardiology substudy. *J Electrocardiol* 2003: **36**(Suppl.): 101–108.

37. Bardy GH, Lee KL, Mark DB, *et al*. Sudden Cardiac Death in Heart Failure Trial (SCD-HeFT) Investigators. Related articles, links amiodarone or an implantable cardioverter-defibrillator for congestive heart failure. *N Engl J Med* 2005; **352**: 225–237.

38. Berkowitsch A, Zareba W, Neumann T, *et al*. Risk stratification using heart rate turbulence and ventricular arrhythmia in MADIT II: usefulness and limitations of a 10-minute Holter recording. *Ann Noninvasive Electrocardiol* 2004; **9**: 270–279.

39. Gomes JA, Caine ME, Buxton AE. Prediction of long-term outcomes by signal-averaged electrocardiography in patients with unsustained ventricular tachycardia, coronary artery disease, and left ventricular dysfunction. *Circulation* 2001; **104**: 436–441.

40. Ikeda T, Sakata T, Takami M, *et al*. Combined assessment of T-wave alternans and late potentials used to predict arrhythmic events after myocardial infarction. A prospective study. *J Am Coll Cardiol* 2000; **35**: 722–730.

41. Gold MR, Bloomfield DM, Anderson KP, *et al*. Comparison of T-wave alternans, signal averaged electrocardiography and programmed ventricular stimulation for arrhythmia risk stratification. *J Am Coll Cardiol* 2000; **36**: 2247–2253.

42. Bailey JJ, Berson AS, Handelsman H, Hodges M. Utility of current risk stratification tests for predicting major arrhythmic events after myocardial infarction. *J Am Coll Cardiol* 2001; **38**: 1902–1911.

43. Hohnloser SH. T wave alternans. In: Zipes DP & Jalife J, eds. *Cardiac Electrophysiology: From Cell to Bedside*, 4th edn. W.B. Saunders Co, Philadelphia, PA, 2004: 839–847.

44. Hohnloser SH, Ikeda T, Bloomfield DM, *et al*. T-wave alternans negative coronary patients with low ejection fraction and benefit from defibrillator implantation. *Lancet* 2003; **362**: 126–127.

45. Bloomfield DM, Steinman RC, Namerow PB, *et al*. Microvolt T-wave alternans distinguishes between patients likely and patients not likely to benefit from implanted cardiac defibrillator therapy. *Circulation* 2004; **110**: 1885–1889.

46. Kleiger RE, Miller JP, Bigger JT Jr, Moss AJ. Decreased heart rate variability and its association with increased mortality after acute myocardial infarction. *Am J Cardiol* 1987; **59**: 256–262.

47. Bigger JT Jr, Fleiss JL, Kleiger R, Miller JP, Rolnitzky LM. The relationships among ventricular arrhythmias, left ventricular dysfunction, and mortality in the 2 years after myocardial infarction. *Circulation* 1984; **69**: 250–258.
48. Bilchick KC, Fetics B, Doukeng R, *et al*. Prognostic value of heart rate variability in chronic congestive heart failure (Veterans Affairs' Survival Trial of Antiarrhythmic Therapy in Congestive Heart Failure). *Am J Cardiol* 2002; **90**: 24–28.
49. Nolan J, Batin PD, Andrews R, *et al*. Prospective study of heart rate variability and mortality in chronic heart failure: results of the United Kingdom heart failure evaluation and assessment of risk trial (UK Heart). *Circulation* 1998; **98**: 1510–1516.
50. Fauchier L, Babuty D, Cosnay P, Fauchier JP. Prognostic value of heart rate variability for sudden death and major arrhythmic events in patients with idiopathic dilated cardiomyopathy. *J Am Coll Cardiol* 1999; **33**: 1203–1207.
51. La Rovere MT, Pinna GD, Maestri R, *et al*. Short-term heart rate variability strongly predicts sudden cardiac death in chronic heart failure patients. *Circulation* 2003; **107**: 565–570.
52. Schmidt G, Malik M, Barthel P, *et al*. Heart-rate turbulence after ventricular premature beats as a predictor of mortality after acute myocardial infarction. *Lancet* 1999; **353**: 1390–1396.
53. Ghuran A, Reid F, La Rovere MT, *et al*. The ATRAMI Investigators. Heart rate turbulence-based predictors of fatal and nonfatal cardiac arrest (The Autonomic Tone and Reflexes After Myocardial Infarction substudy). *Am J Cardiol* 2002; **89**: 184–190.
54. Barthel P, Schneider R, Bauer A, *et al*. Risk stratification after acute myocardial infarction by heart rate turbulence. *Circulation* 2003; **108**: 1221–1226.
55. Makikallio TH, Huikuri HV, Hintze U, *et al*. Fractal analysis and time- and frequency-domain measures of heart rate variability as predictors of mortality in patients with heart failure. *Am J Cardiol* 2001; **87**: 178–182.
56. Perkiomaki JS, Zareba W, Daubert JP, Couderc JP, Corsello A, Kremer K. Fractal correlation properties of heart rate dynamics and adverse events in patients with implantable cardioverter-defibrillators. *Am J Cardiol* 2001; **88**: 17–22.
57. Buxton AE, Lee KL, DiCarlo L, *et al*. Electrophysiologic testing to identify patients with coronary artery disease who are at risk for sudden death. *N Engl J Med* 2000; **342**: 1937–1945.
58. Cappato R, Boczor S, Kuck KH. Response to programmed ventricular stimulation and clinical outcome in cardiac arrest survivors receiving randomized assignment to implantable cardioverter defibrillator or antiarrhythmic drug therapy. *Eur Heart J* 2004; **25**: 642–649.
59. Draft Decision Memo for Implantable Cardioverter Defibrillators (CAG-00157R2). Accessed on October 9, 2004 at https://www.cms.hhs.gov/mcd/viewdraftdecision memo.asp?id=139.
60. Hohnloser SH, Klingenheben T, Bloomfield D, *et al*. Usefulness of microvolt T-wave alternans for prediction of ventricular tachyarrhythmic events in patients with dilated cardiomyopathy: results from a prospective observational study. *J Am Col Cardiol* 2003; **41**: 2220–2224.
61. Grimm W, Christ M, Bach J, Muller HH, Maisch B. Noninvasive arrhythmia risk stratification in idiopathic dilated cardiomyopathy. Results of the Marburg Cardiomyopathy Study. *Circulation* 2003; **108**: 2883–2891.

CHAPTER 5

Autonomic nervous system: Emerging concepts and clinical applications

Peter J. Schwartz and Richard L. Verrier

Introduction

The concept that neural activity exerts a potent influence on arrhythmogenesis, which gained credence in the 1970s [1,2], has received strong affirmation in ensuing literature. In recent years, fascinating new insights have been gained regarding the mechanisms of neurocardiac interactions and important practical tools have been developed for human studies of neural influences on heart rhythm in health and disease. This chapter provides a succinct update of progress in both the basic science and clinical literature with special focus on risk stratification and implications for therapy.

Integration of neural control of cardiac electrical activity

Regulation of cardiac neural activity is highly integrated and is achieved by circuitry at multiple levels [3]. Higher brain centers operate through elaborate pathways within the hypothalamus and medullary cardiovascular regulatory sites. Baroreceptor mechanisms have long been recognized as integral to autonomic control of the cardiovascular system. The intrinsic cardiac nerves provide local neural coordination, partly independent of higher brain centers. The entire neural control of the heart is enriched by afferent information, relayed centrally through vagal and sympathetic cardiac afferents [4–6]. This sensory system, besides signaling hemodynamic changes through cardiac mechanoreceptors provides the basis for reflex changes in sympathetic [7] and vagal activity [8] which contribute significantly to the cardiac arrhythmias associated with acute myocardial ischemia [9]. At the level of the myocardial cell, autonomic receptors interact with G proteins to control ionic channels, pumps, and exchangers.

Autonomic nervous system tone and reflexes

Heart-rate variability

Autonomic nervous system tone has been studied in human subjects primarily by employing the tool of heart-rate variability (HRV), which reflects the fact that the pattern of beat-to-beat control of the sinoatrial (SA) node provides a reflection of cardiac-bound autonomic activity [10]. Parasympathetic influences exert a unique imprimatur of rapid, dynamic control, as acetylcholine affects muscarinic receptors, and are therefore reflected in the high-frequency (HF) component. Sympathetic nerve activity, through the influence of norepinephrine on beta-adrenergic receptors, has a considerably slower influence and is evident in the lower frequency (LF) components. Thus, while HRV is only an indirect measure of cardiac autonomic function as it reflects influences on the SA node and not on the ventricular myocardium, nevertheless, HRV studies underscore the universal influence of the autonomic nervous system in cardiovascular disease and arrhythmic events. The parameter is capable of stratifying risk for mortality after myocardial infarction (MI) [10,11,12] and noncardiac surgery [13] and in patients with chronic congestive heart failure [14] or cardiomyopathy [15]. In patients with cardiovascular disease, HRV provides evidence of vagal withdrawal immediately prior to onset of ischemia [16] and ventricular arrhythmias [17], a mechanism suggested by experimental laboratory studies.

Baroreceptor sensitivity

The early studies by Billman, Schwartz, and Stone [18] drew attention to the importance of baroreceptor function in susceptibility to life-threatening arrhythmias associated with myocardial ischemia and infarction. In the initial investigations in canines, it was demonstrated that more powerful the baroreflex response, the less vulnerable were animals to ventricular fibrillation during myocardial ischemia superimposed on prior MI. The protective effect of the baroreceptor mechanism has been linked primarily to the antifibrillatory influence of vagus nerve activity, which presynaptically inhibits norepinephrine release [19] and maintains heart-rate low during myocardial ischemia [20]. The latter effect improves diastolic coronary perfusion, minimizing the ischemic insult from coronary artery occlusion. The experimental findings were soon matched by clinical studies and the importance of baroreflex sensitivity (BRS) was subsequently documented in human subjects in whom baroreceptor function was evaluated with the pressor agent phenylephrine [21–23]. It was indeed demonstrated that post-MI patients were less likely to experience sudden cardiac death (SCD), and total cardiac mortality, if their baroreceptor function was not depressed. Overall, it appears that BRS and HRV, which reflect disturbances in autonomic reflexes and tone, respectively, provide complementary information pertaining to autonomic factors in the precipitation of life-threatening arrhythmias. From the clinical standpoint, the most important finding probably is the evidence that, among patients

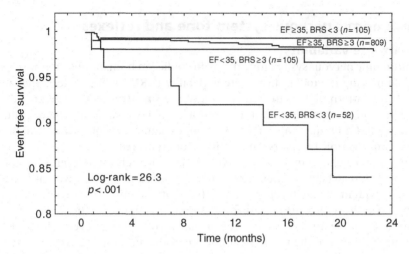

Figure 5.1 Kaplan–Meier event-free survival curves for arrhythmic events according to the combination of EF with BRS. The total population has been divided in four groups after dichotomization of EF according to <35% and ≥35%. The total population has been divided in four groups after dichotomization of BRS according to the ATRAMI cut-off values of <3 ms/mm Hg and ≥3 ms/mm Hg. The probability value refers to differences in events rate between subgroups. Reprinted from Reference 23, with permission.

with depressed (35%) left ventricular ejection fraction (LVEF), the presence of either preserved or depressed BRS allow identification of two subgroups at significantly different risk (Figure 5.1). As the Multicenter Automatic Defibrillator Implantation Trial (MADIT II) results have led to the suggestion of implanting Cardioverter-defibrillators (ICDs) in all post-MI patients with LVEF <30%, the evidence that the use of appropriate autonomic markers can help to identify a significant subgroup at much lower risk among patients with LVEF <35% [23] and even <30% [24] has important practical implications for national health policies.

Recently, BRS testing has also been performed by measuring heart-rate turbulence (HRT), a term that refers to fluctuations of sinus-rhythm cycle length after a single ventricular premature beat (VPB), which appears to be mechanistically linked with BRS [25]. The basic principle, introduced by Schmidt et al. [26], is that the reaction of the cardiovascular system to a VPB and subsequent decrease in arterial blood pressure is a direct function of baroreceptor responsiveness, as reflex activation of the vagus nerve controls the pattern of sinus rhythm. Several retrospective studies confirm that in low-risk patients, after a VPB, sinus rhythm exhibits a characteristic pattern of early acceleration and subsequent deceleration. By contrast, patients at high risk exhibit essentially a flat, nonvarying response to the VPB, indicating their inability to activate vagal nerves and access their cardioprotective effect. HRT appears to be a promising independent predictor of total mortality in patients with ischemic heart disease or heart failure [26,27].

Heart-rate turbulence is an inexpensive, simple method that can be analyzed from routine ambulatory ECGs (AECGs). Its main limitation is its requirement of spontaneous, single VPBs, without which the analysis cannot be performed from AECG recordings.

Intrinsic cardiac innervation

Armour [28] introduced and investigated the elaborate intrinsic neural network within the heart that provides local, independent heart rhythm control. This important advance is in line with the findings by Randall and Ardell [29] and Zipes and coworkers [30], who drew attention to the fact that components of this innervation system reside within discrete fat pads. The cardiac fat pads and local cardiac regulatory systems, although somewhat enigmatic in their regulatory function, are of considerable clinical significance. For example, myocardial ischemia can compromise the functional capacity of cardiac intrinsic neurons residing in the fat pad and thus has the potential to increase electrical inhomogeneity and susceptibility to arrhythmias [31]. Intrinsic innervation is also vulnerable to diabetic neuropathy, which accordingly could exacerbate vulnerability to arrhythmias [32].

Nerve growth and degeneration

Whereas the concept of remodeling has been well established with respect to the myocardium, the importance of restructuring of cardiac innervation has not received due attention until the past few years. Infarction of either the right of left ventricle results in heterogeneous autonomic denervation in the viable peri-infarct territory, which establishes a substrate for enhanced susceptibility to arrhythmias. Fundamental contributions in this regard have emerged from the laboratories of Elvan and Zipes [33] and Chen and coworkers [34–38], who provided evidence implicating "nerve sprouting" in ventricular arrhythmogenesis and potentially SCD. Chen and colleagues reported a significant correlation between increased sympathetic nerve density as reflected in immunocytochemical markers with history of arrhythmias including ventricular tachycardia and SCD in native hearts of human transplant recipients with severe heart failure [34]. Their observations suggested an association between post-injury sympathetic nerve density and susceptibility to life-threatening ventricular arrhythmias in these patients. In a canine post-MI model, they demonstrated that induction of nerve sprouting by infusion of nerve growth factor (NGF) into the left stellate ganglion (LSG) resulted in increased incidence of ventricular tachycardia and fibrillation [35], thus providing novel support for the prior multiple evidence of the unique arrhythmogenic potential associated with activation of left sided cardiac nerves [39,40]. Significantly, the predisposition to arrhythmias was again linked to immunocytochemical evidence of a heterogeneous pattern of sympathetic reinnervation. In a similar ambulatory canine model, the group reported the frequent occurrence prior to VT of visible T-wave alternans (TWA) [36], a noninvasive marker of risk for ventricular arrhythmias in the post-MI population [41]. Recently, Liu *et al.* [37] demonstrated in rabbits that hypercholesterolemia can produce proarrhythmic neural and electrophysiological remodeling that is highly arrhythmogenic and is associated with important changes in ionic currents including I_{Ca}. Collectively, this evidence points to the lability of autonomic innervation and the intricate changes that may be responsible for derangements in neural activity and predisposition to arrhythmias. This adverse effect of heterogeneous remodeling of sympathetic innervation to the heart is likely to play a role in the increased risk for life-threatening arrhythmias and strengthens the rationale for the use of autonomic interventions in the prevention of sudden cardiac death.

Behavioral state
The view that behavioral factors may predispose to malignant arrhythmias has gained strong support in recent years because of batteries of psychometric tests for behavioral testing and indicators of cardiac electrical instability including ICD discharge frequency and TWA.

Lampert *et al.* [42] systematically examined the potential of emotional and physical stressors to provoke spontaneous ventricular arrhythmias in patients with ICDs. Detailed diaries of mood states and physical activity were obtained during two periods preceding spontaneous, appropriate ICD shocks and during control periods 1 week later. A total of 107 documented ICD shocks were reported by 42 patients, the majority of whom had coronary artery disease. In the 15-min period preceding shocks, there was a significant incidence of high levels of anger, with odds ratios of 1.83 ($p < .04$). Other mood states, notably anxiety, worry, sadness, and happiness, did not trigger ICD discharge. Physical activity was also associated with increased incidence of shocks. These observations are consistent with recent experimental [43] and clinical [44] (Figure 5.2) studies demonstrating that mental stress is capable of significantly increasing cardiac electrical instability as assessed by TWA.

The dynamic influence of mental and physical activity on cardiac electrical function finds further support in a recent study of ambulatory ECG-based TWA analysis in post-MI patients [41]. Modified moving average (MMA) analysis was used to measure TWA from 24-h AECGs from patients enrolled in the autonomic tone and reflexes after myocardial infarction (ATRAMI) study obtained at an average of 15 days following the index event. The patients were followed for 21 ± 8 months and were matched for gender, age, site of MI, LVEF, thrombolysis, and beta-adrenergic blockade therapy. A four-to-seven-fold higher odds of cardiac arrest or arrhythmic death was predicted by TWA levels at the 75th percentile of controls, that is, approximately 50 μV. Individuals at risk for arrhythmic death showed increased TWA levels at maximum heart rate and at 8:00 AM, suggesting that daily mental and physical stress can disclose clinically significant levels of electrical instability. Although the increase in TWA may be associated with maximum daily heart-rate, elevated

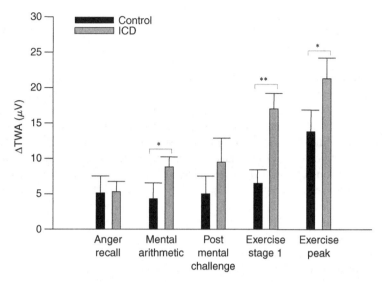

Figure 5.2 Comparison of ICD patients with controls in TWA responses to mental stress and exercise (Δ = change from baseline). Increases in TWA were higher in ICD patients than in controls during mental arithmetic ($p = .043$), exercise stage 1 ($p = .0004$), and peak exercise ($p = .038$). $^*p < .05,^{**}p < .01$ (ICD versus control). Reprinted from Reference 16, with permission from Lippincott, Williams, and Wilkins.

heart-rate *per se* does not appear to be the sole factor, as TWA measured at peak heart rate did not correlate with the magnitude of the heart-rate change nor did the maximum heart rates differ between patients with and without events. These increases in TWA in such cases are likely to reflect the influence of enhanced sympathetic nerve activity, since beta-adrenergic receptor blockade reduces TWA magnitude [45], an effect shown to be independent of heart rate, when this variable was controlled by pacing [43].

An important evolving literature addresses the profound changes in autonomic nervous system activity and respiration during sleep and their provocation of increased risk for sudden death, particularly in individuals with apnea and/or heart failure [46].

Autonomically based antiarrhythmic therapy
The evidence that life-threatening arrhythmias are enhanced either by increases in sympathetic activity or by inability to increase vagal activity appropriately has provided the rationale for preventive strategies aimed at counteracting these two conditions.

Antiadrenergic interventions
This approach is specifically useful for patients with ischemic heart disease and with congenital disorders that decrease cardiac electrical stability such

as the congenital long QT syndrome (LQTS). The realization that acute myocardial ischemia elicits a reflex increase in cardiac sympathetic activity [7] contributed to the rationale for the use of beta-blockers in patients with acute MI. The unquestionable success of this therapy [47] attests the clinical impact of the autonomic nervous system and of its manipulation.

The recognition that left-sided cardiac nerves have a higher arrhythmogenic potential, probably because they are quantitatively dominant at ventricular level [48], has contributed to the exploration of its clinical use. In the only randomized clinical trial performed, post-MI patients at high risk for sudden death were allocated to either placebo, beta-blockade, or left cardiac sympathetic denervation (LCSD)[49]. Both pharmacologic and surgical antiadrenergic interventions reduced significantly sudden cardiac death from 22% to 3%. This trial provided the "proof of concept" for the antifibrillatory effect of LCSD in man. In clinical practice, however, the main current use of LCSD is for patients affected by LQTS. The most recent worldwide data on 147 high-risk patients demonstrate that when beta-blockade is unable to prevent syncope, LCSD is a valid alternative to the ICD [50]. The 5-year mortality in this group was 3%, thus showing that protection by sympathectomy is not 100% effective. On the other hand, the reduction >90% in the number of episodes of syncope and cardiac arrest, also in the unfortunate patients with multiple ICD shocks (average 30/year), indicates a major improvement in quality of life. Reduction of QTc below 500 ms after LCSD identifies patients at minimal risk for subsequent events (Figure 5.3). Thus, LQTS patients who have syncope despite beta-blockade should be informed of the pros and cons of the next therapeutic steps, the ICD and LCSD.

The clinical impact of removing specific cardiac sympathetic nerves is a good example of the tight relationship between cardiovascular physiology and therapy.

Vagal interventions

Several lines of evidence suggest that whenever autonomic markers indicate the presence of reduced vagal activity, tonic but especially reflex, there is an increase in risk for cardiac mortality and sudden death and this provides a strong rationale to develop means to increase vagal activity in selected groups of patients. Of the three main possibilities (pharmacologic activation, exercise training, and direct vagal stimulation) the first seems the most distant from clinical applicability because selective and safe pharmacologic activation of cardiac M2 receptors is not yet available.

The experimental evidence that increasing vagal activity by exercise training, increased depressed BRS in high-risk post-MI dogs and prevented VF during acute myocardial ischemia [51] and that it also provided antifibrillatory protection in high-risk dogs with a normal heart [52] paved the way for clinical studies aimed at assessing its impact on cardiac mortality. Ninety-five post-MI patients, matched for all major variables, were randomized to a 4-week endurance training period or to no training [53]. During a 10-year

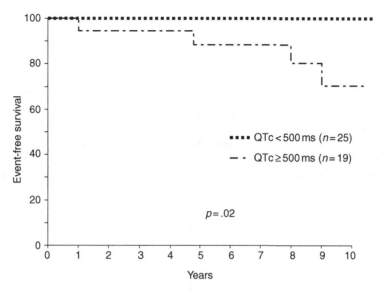

Figure 5.3 Kaplan–Meier curves of event-free survival and survival according to post-LCSD QTc in patients with only syncope or aborted cardiac arrest pre-LCSD. Reprinted from Reference 50, with permission.

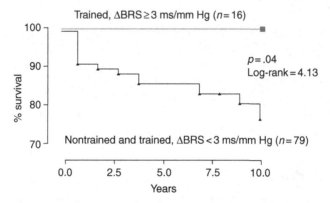

Figure 5.4 Cardiac mortality estimated by the Kaplan–Meier method among the patients with a training-induced increase in BRS ≥3 ms/mm Hg and the group including patients who trained without the same BRS increase and nontrained patients. Reprinted from Reference 53, with permission.

follow-up, cardiac mortality among the trained patients who had an exercise-induced increase in BRS >3 ms/mm Hg was strikingly lower compared to that of the trained patients without such a baroreflex response and to that of the non-trained patients (0 of 16 versus 18 of 79, $p = .04$) (Figure 5.4). These data demonstrate that when exercise training shifts the autonomic balance toward a quantitatively sufficient increase in vagal activity, it can significantly improve long-term prognosis.

Classic studies in anesthetized animals indicating the potential of vagal stimulation to reduce the prevalence of ventricular fibrillation induced by coronary artery occlusion [54] were followed by a study in a conscious canine model for sudden death recognized for its clinical relevance [55]. Vanoli *et al.* [56] demonstrated that direct stimulation of the right cervical vagus, initiated through a chronically implanted electrode, at 15 s after onset of acute myocardial ischemia in dogs with a healed MI, performing an exercise stress test, was able to reduce the incidence of ventricular fibrillation by 92%. Furthermore, this effect was only partly due to the attendant heart-rate reduction, as in half of the animals, the efficacy of vagal stimulation persisted despite maintenance of constant heart rate by atrial pacing, thus proving that the protective effect was also mediated by direct sympathetic–parasympathetic interactions.

This important evidence has represented the springboard for the current interest in the use of chronically implanted vagal electrodes for the prevention of ventricular fibrillation in man and also for the evaluation of value of neurally mediated heart-rate control in patients with heart failure. Preliminary clinical investigations related to feasibility and safety are currently ongoing in Italy.

Conclusions

Our understanding of the role of the autonomic nervous system has continued to evolve in a fascinating and productive manner.

The findings as discussed in this chapter provide cogent evidence that the progressive unraveling of our understanding of the physiology underlying neural control of the heart is allowing a fine-tuning of the autonomic nervous system, which has already resulted in an improved risk stratification and in a greater array of therapeutic tools.

Acknowledgments

Supported by Grants R01 HL63968 (RLV) and HL66394 (PJS) from the National Heart, Lung, and Blood Institute of the National Institutes of Health.

References

1. Lown B, Verrier RL. Neural activity and ventricular fibrillation. *N Engl J Med* 1976; **294**: 1165–1170.
2. Schwartz PJ, Brown AM, Malliani A *et al. Neural Mechanisms in Cardiac Arrhythmias.* New York: Raven Press, 1978.
3. Lathrop DA, Spooner PM. On the neural connection. *J Cardiovasc Electrophysiol* 2001; **12**: 841–844.

4. Malliani A, Recordati G, Schwartz PJ. Nervous activity of afferent cardiac sympathetic fibres with atrial and ventricular endings. *J Physiol (London)* 1973; **229**: 457–469.
5. Malliani A. Cardiovascular sympathetic afferent fibers. *Rev Physiol Biochem Pharmacol* 1982; **94**: 11–74.
6. Levy MN, Schwartz PJ (eds.). *Vagal Control of the Heart: Experimental Basis and Clinical Implications*. Futura Publishing Co, Armonk, NY, 1994: 644.
7. Malliani A, Schwartz PJ, Zanchetti A. A sympathetic reflex elicited by experimental coronary occlusion. *Am J Physiol* 1969; **217**: 703–709.
8. Schwartz PJ, Pagani M, Lombardi F, Malliani A, Brown AM. A cardio–cardiac sympatho-vagal reflex in the cat. *Circ Res* 1973; **32**: 215–220.
9. Schwartz PJ, Foreman RD, Stone HL, Brown AM. Effect of dorsal root section on the arrhythmias associated with coronary occlusion. *Am J Physiol* 1976; **231**: 923–928.
10. Lombardi F. Clinical implications of present physiological understanding of HRV components. *Card Electrophysiol Rev* 2002; **6**: 245–249.
11. Camm AJ, Pratt CM, Schwartz PJ, *et al.* Mortality in patients after a recent myocardial infarction: a randomized, placebo-controlled trial of azimilide using heart rate variability for risk stratification. *Circulation* 2004; **109**: 990–996.
12. Carney RM, Blumenthal JA, Stein PK, *et al.* Depression, heart rate variability, and acute myocardial infarction. *Circulation* 2001; **104**: 2024–2028.
13. Filipovic M, Jeger R, Probst C, *et al.* Heart rate variability and cardiac troponin I are incremental and independent predictors of one-year all-cause mortality after major noncardiac surgery in patients at risk of coronary artery disease. *J Am Coll Cardiol* 2003; **42**: 1767–1776.
14. La Rovere MT, Pinna GD, Maestri R, *et al.* Short-term heart rate variability strongly predicts sudden cardiac death in chronic heart failure patients. *Circulation* 2003; **107**: 565–570.
15. Fauchier L, Babuty D, Cosnay P, Fauchier JP. Prognostic value of heart rate variability for sudden death and major arrhythmic events in patients with idiopathic dilated cardiomyopathy. *J Am Coll Cardiol* 1999; **33**: 1203–1207.
16. Kop WJ, Verdino RJ, Gottdiener JS, O'Leary ST, Bairey Merz CN, Krantz DS. Changes in heart rate and heart rate variability before ambulatory ischemic events. *J Am Coll Cardiol* 2001; **38**: 742–749.
17. Pruvot E, Thonet G, Vesin JM, *et al.* Heart rate dynamics at the onset of ventricular tachyarrhythmias as retrieved from implantable cardioverter-defibrillators in patients with coronary artery disease. *Circulation* 2000; **101**: 2398–2404.
18. Billman GE, Schwartz PJ, Stone HL. Baroreceptor reflex control of heart rate: a predictor of sudden cardiac death. *Circulation* 1982; **66**: 874–880.
19. Levy MN, Blattberg B. Effect of vagal stimulation on the overflow of norepinephrine into the coronary sinus during cardiac sympathetic nerve stimulation in the dog. *Circ Res* 1976; **38**: 81–84.
20. Kolman BS, Verrier RL, Lown B. The effect of vagus nerve stimulation upon vulnerability of the canine ventricle. Role of sympathetic–parasympathetic interactions. *Circulation* 1975; **52**: 578–585.
21. La Rovere MT, Specchia G, Mortara A, Schwartz PJ. Baroreflex sensitivity, clinical correlates and cardiovascular mortality among patients with a first myocardial infarction. A prospective study. *Circulation* 1988; **78**: 816–824.
22. La Rovere MT, Bigger JT Jr, Marcus FI, *et al.* Baroreflex sensitivity and heart-rate variability in prediction of total cardiac mortality after myocardial infarction.

ATRAMI (Autonomic Tone and Reflexes After Myocardial Infarction) Investigators. *Lancet* 1998; **351**: 478–484.

23. La Rovere MT, Pinna GD, Hohnloser SH, *et al*. Baroreflex sensitivity and heart rate variability in the identification of patients at risk for life-threatening arrhythmias: implications for clinical trials. *Circulation* 2001; **103**: 2072–2077.

24. La Rovere MT, Camm AJ, Malik M, Hohnloser SH, Mortara A, Schwartz PJ on behalf of the ATRAMI Investigators. A preserved autonomic balance identifies among MADIT II patients a subgroup at low risk for implantable cardioverter-defibrillator discharge. *Eur Heart J* 2004; **25**(Abstr Suppl.): 168.

25. Lin LY, Lai LP, Lin JL, *et al*. Tight mechanism correlation between heart rate turbulence and baroreflex sensitivity: sequential autonomic blockade analysis. *J Cardiovasc Electrophysiol* 2002; **13**: 427–431.

26. Schmidt G, Malik M, Barthel P, *et al*. Heart-rate turbulence after ventricular premature beats as a predictor of mortality after acute myocardial infarction. *Lancet* 1999; **353**: 1390–1396.

27. Guzik P, Schmidt G. A phenomenon of heart-rate turbulence, its evaluation, and prognostic value. *Card Electrophysiol Rev* 2002; **6**: 256–261.

28. Armour JA. Intrinsic cardiac neurons. *J Cardiovasc Electrophysiol* 1991; **2**: 331–341.

29. Randall WC, Ardell JL. Selective parasympathectomy of automatic and conductile tissues of the canine heart. *Am J Physiol* 1985; **248**: H61–H68.

30. Chiou CW, Eble JN, Zipes DP. Efferent vagal innervation of the canine atria and sinus and atrioventricular nodes. The third fat pad. *Circulation* 1997; **95**: 2573–2584.

31. Armour JA. Myocardial ischaemia and the cardiac nervous system. *Cardiovasc Res* 1999; **41**: 41–54.

32. Stevens MJ, Raffel DM, Allman KC, *et al*. Cardiac sympathetic dysinnervation in diabetes: implications for enhanced cardiovascular risk. *Circulation* 1998; **98**: 961–968.

33. Elvan A, Zipes DP. Right ventricular infarction causes heterogeneous autonomic denervation of the viable peri-infarct area. *Circulation* 1998; **97**: 484–492.

34. Cao JM, Fishbein MC, Han JB, *et al*. Relationship between regional cardiac hyperinnervation and ventricular arrhythmia. *Circulation* 2000; **101**: 1960–1969.

35. Cao JM, Chen LS, KenKnight BH, *et al*. Nerve sprouting and sudden cardiac death. *Circ Res* 2000; **86**: 816–821.

36. Tsai J, Cao JM, Zhou S, *et al*. T wave alternans as a predictor of spontaneous ventricular tachycardia in a canine model of sudden cardiac death. *J Cardiovasc Electrophysiol* 2002; **13**: 51–55.

37. Liu YB, Wu CC, Lu LS, *et al*. Sympathetic nerve sprouting, electrical remodeling, and increased vulnerability to ventricular fibrillation in hypercholesterolemic rabbits. *Circ Res* 2003; **92**: 1145–1152.

38. Zhou S, Chen LS, Miyauchi Y, *et al*. Mechanisms of cardiac nerve sprouting after myocardial infarction. *Circ Res* 2004; **94**: 76–83.

39. Schwartz PJ. The rationale and the role of left stellectomy for the prevention of malignant arrhythmias. *Ann NY Acad Sci* 1984; **427**: 199–221.

40. Schwartz PJ. QT prolongation, sudden death, and sympathetic imbalance: the pendulum swings. *J Cardiovasc Electrophysiol* 2001; **12**: 1074–1077.

41. Verrier RL, Nearing BD, La Rovere MT, *et al*. Ambulatory electrocardiogram-based tracking of T wave alternans in postmyocardial infarction patients to assess risk of cardiac arrest or arrhythmic death. *J Cardiovasc Electrophysiol* 2003; **14**: 705–711.

42. Lampert R, Joska T, Burg MM, *et al*. Emotional and physical precipitants of ventricular arrhythmia. *Circulation* 2002; **106**: 1800–1805.
43. Kovach JA, Nearing BD, Verrier RL. Angerlike behavioral state potentiates myocardial ischemia-induced T-wave alternans in canines. *J Am Coll Cardiol* 2001; **37**: 1719–1725.
44. Kop WJ, Krantz DS, Nearing BD, *et al*. Effects of acute mental and exercise stress on T-wave alternans in patients with implantable cardioverter defibrillators and controls. *Circulation* 2004; **109**: 1864–1869.
45. Rashba EJ, Cooklin M, MacMurdy L, *et al*. Effects of selective autonomic blockade on T-wave alternans in humans. *Circulation* 2002; **105**: 837–842.
46. Lanfranchi PA, Somers VK, Braghiroli A, Corra U, Eleuteri E, Giannuzzi P. Central sleep apnea in left ventricular dysfunction: prevalence and implications for arrhythmic risk. *Circulation* 2003; **107**: 727–732.
47. Teo KK, Yusuf S, Furberg CD. Effects of prophylactic antiarrhythmic drug therapy in acute myocardial infarction. An overview of results from randomized controlled trials. *JAMA* 1993; **270**: 1589–1595.
48. Schwartz PJ, Verrier RL, Lown B. Effect of stellectomy and vagotomy on ventricular refractoriness. *Circ Res* 1977; **40**: 536–540.
49. Schwartz PJ, Motolese M, Pollavini G, *et al*. Prevention of sudden cardiac death after a first myocardial infarction by pharmacologic or surgical antiadrenergic interventions. *J Cardiovasc Electrophysiol* 1992; **3**: 2–16.
50. Schwartz PJ, Priori SG, Cerrone M, *et al*. Left cardiac sympathetic denervation in the management of high-risk patients affected by the long QT syndrome. *Circulation* 2004; **109**: 1826–1833.
51. Billman GE, Schwartz PJ, Stone HL. The effects of daily exercise on susceptibility to sudden cardiac death. *Circulation* 1984; **69**: 1182–1189.
52. Hull SS Jr, Vanoli E, Adamson PB, Verrier RL, Foreman RD, Schwartz PJ. Exercise training confers anticipatory protection from sudden death during acute myocardial ischemia. *Circulation* 1994; **89**: 548–552.
53. La Rovere MT, Bersano C, Gnemmi M, Specchia G, Schwartz PJ. Exercise-induced increase in baroreflex sensitivity predicts improved prognosis after myocardial infarction. *Circulation* 2002; **106**: 945–949.
54. Verrier RL, Lown B. Sympathetic–parasympathetic interactions and ventricular electrical stability. In: Schwartz PJ, Brown AM, Malliani A, & Zanchetti A, eds. *Neural Mechanisms in Cardiac Arrhythmias*. Raven Press, New York, 1978: 75–85.
55. Schwartz PJ, Billman GE, Stone HL. Autonomic mechanisms in ventricular fibrillation induced by myocardial ischemia during exercise in dogs with healed myocardial infarction. An experimental preparation for sudden cardiac death. *Circulation* 1984; **69**: 790–800.
56. Vanoli E, De Ferrari GM, Stramba-Badiale M, Hull SS Jr, Foreman RD, Schwartz PJ. Vagal stimulation and prevention of sudden death in conscious dogs with a healed myocardial infarction. *Circ Res* 1991; **68**: 1471–1481.

CHAPTER 6

Clinical characteristics of sudden cardiac death victims and precipitating events

Christine M. Albert and Stuart M. Cobbe

Clinical characteristics

Incidence and demographic features

The acute and chronic complications of coronary artery disease are the predominant cause of sudden cardiac death (SCD), hence the age and gender distribution of SCD parallels that of coronary artery disease (Figure 6.1). Population incidence rates of SCD ranging between 0.36 and 1.28/1000/annum have been reported [1]. The estimated SCD rates in blacks and whites are similar up to an age of 40 years. However, with increasing age, the rate in blacks increases compared with whites, and was 1.5 times greater by the seventh decade [2]. The greater prevalence of hypertension in black compared with white men may explain their greater incidence of SCD despite a lower prevalence of coronary artery disease [1].

Risk factors

The risk factors for SCD are predominantly those of atherosclerotic coronary disease, namely increasing age, male gender, family history of coronary artery disease, increased LDL cholesterol, hypertension, smoking, and diabetes mellitus [1,3]. Although the absolute risk of SCD is lower than in men, coronary heart disease (CHD) risk factors also predict SCD risk in women [4]. In subjects without recognized heart disease, increased heart rate and heavy alcohol consumption are additional predictors of SCD [1]. As well as being a risk factor for CHD, hypertension plays a disproportionate role in increasing the risk of SCD [5]. The principal mechanism by which hypertension predisposes to SCD is via left ventricular hypertrophy (LVH). The risk of sudden death in the presence of electrocardiographic LVH was comparable to that of coronary artery disease or heart failure [1].

Among newer risk factors, elevated levels of C-reactive protein (CRP) predict increased risk of SCD over a 17-year follow-up period. Men in the highest quartile of CRP had a 2.65-fold increase in risk compared with those in the lowest quartile, after adjustment for other risk factors [6]. In patients dying

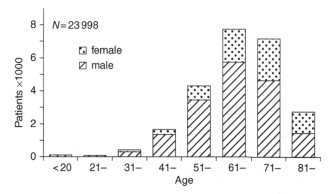

Figure 6.1 Age and gender distribution in 23 998 attempted resuscitations for sudden cardiac arrest in Scotland 1991–2001.

suddenly with severe coronary artery disease, serum CRP levels were significantly elevated both in the presence and absence of coronary thrombosis, and correlated with staining intensity for CRP in macrophages and plaque lipid core, and with the numbers of thin-cap atheromatous plaques [7].

Although a genetic predisposition to sudden death is usually considered among monogenic disorders such as hypertrophic cardiomyopathy or long-QT syndrome, there is evidence of a genetic "susceptibility factor" predisposing to SCD in unselected population studies. Family history was a predictor of SCD after correction for conventional CHD risk factors in two reports, with odds ratios of 1.57 and 1.8, respectively [1,3]. In families with a parental history of SCD on both sides, the relative risk for SCD increases to 9.4.

Prevalence of clinically diagnosed cardiac disease in SCD victims

Community or autopsy series have reported that 50–80% of SCD victims have no clinical history of heart disease [1,4,8]. However, epidemiological studies have reported a high prevalence of unrecognized myocardial infarction (MI) and left ventricular dysfunction in the community [1], hence the proportion of SCD that is genuinely the first manifestation of cardiac disease is impossible to define. Among SCD victims with prior cardiac disease, a history of previous MI or heart failure is common. In the Maastricht community study, overt heart failure was present in 26% of the group with a cardiac history [8]. Other reports have confirmed the prognostic value of ST-segment depression or T-wave inversion or the presence of bifascicular or trifascicular bundle branch block as risk markers for SCD, emphasizing the role of subclinical left ventricular hypertrophy/dysfunction and coronary artery disease as risk factors for SCD [1].

Documented rhythm at time of arrest

The first recorded rhythm in patients presenting with a sudden cardiovascular collapse is ventricular fibrillation (VF) in 75–80% of both men and women, with bradyarrhythmias (asystole or electromechanical dissociation) in the remainder [1,4]. Among patients with advanced cardiac disease, the proportion of nonarrhythmic deaths, commonly due to electromechanical dissociation, is greater [1].

Predisposing cardiac disorders

The diseases responsible for SCD vary according to the age, gender, and racial characteristics of the study population. In unselected series, coronary artery disease and its complications predominate [1,9], whereas in younger subjects or special groups such as athletes, a wider range of inherited and acquired cardiac disease is reported [10,11].

Coronary artery disease

The mechanisms responsible for SCD have been investigated by autopsy studies, as well as clinical, angiographic, and electrophysiological data from SCD survivors. The proportion of SCD victims with active coronary lesions (plaque rupture or erosion and/or coronary thrombosis) has varied from <20% to >80% in different autopsy series, with widely varying prevalence of acute or old MI according to case selection [1] (see Chapter 2). These data suggest that acute myocardial ischemia, with or without evidence of acute or old MI, is the major cause of SCD in patients with coronary artery disease.

Survivors of SCD due to coronary artery disease are classified into those with acute (ST elevation or Q wave) MI, those with ischemic events (ischemia/non-ST elevation MI), and those with primary ventricular tachyarrhythmias. Examples of the respective proportions in different series are: acute MI 44–51%, ischemia 20–34% and primary arrhythmic event 22% [12–14]. In one series, 27% of the acute MI, 55% of the ischemic event, and 71% of the primary arrhythmic event, patients had a prior history of infarction. SCD was the first cardiac event in 35%, 16%, and 6% of the groups respectively [12].

Survivors of cardiac arrest due to acute MI have a lower risk of recurrent SCD than those with acute ischemic events or primary arrhythmias [13,15]. Two explanations are advanced for this observation. First, following recovery from acute MI, the coronary arteries and myocardium are more stable than that following ischemic events or primary arrhythmias. Second, as mentioned above, acute MI patients have a lower burden of prior MI and left ventricular dysfunction than the other groups. In support of the latter point, a prior history of cardiac disease in resuscitated SCD victims is negatively associated with long-term survival [14]. SCD survivors commonly have extensive coronary atherosclerosis and left ventricular dysfunction [16]. Patients who developed recurrent SCD had more triple vessel coronary artery disease and poorer left ventricular function than long-term survivors. In a series of 680 SCD survivors, the independent predictors of subsequent mortality were cardiac arrest not due to definite MI, treatment for heart failure, and increased age [13].

There is often difficulty in distinguishing acute ischemia from primary arrhythmia, as the mechanism of SCD, in those without ST elevation/Q-wave MI. Patients in both categories commonly have multivessel coronary disease and left ventricular dysfunction. Prodromal symptoms may be lacking, or not recollected owing to amnesia caused by cerebral hypoxia. Minor T-wave changes and elevation in cardiac markers or enzymes may occur either as a cause or as a consequence of the cardiac arrest. The induction of sustained ventricular tachycardia or fibrillation by programmed ventricular stimulation denotes the presence of an arrhythmic substrate, and favors a primary arrhythmic mechanism. In contrast, non-MI SCD survivors who do *not* have inducible ventricular tachyarrhythmias have a high prevalence of complex lesions at angiography, suggesting plaque rupture as the mechanism of acute ischemia [17]. In view of the difficulty in establishing the exact mechanism of SCD in non-MI patients, they have been grouped together in clinical trials of the implantable cardioverter-defibrillator (ICD), as discussed in Chapter 15. Although not supported by randomized controlled trials, it is normal practice to attempt revascularization in SCD survivors, particularly if evidence of reversible ischemia is present. Adequate revascularization plus a negative postoperative electrophysiology study predicts a very low risk of recurrent SCD [18].

Other structural heart disease

Although coronary artery disease and its complications are the commonest causes of SCD, any structural heart disease that results in ventricular hypertrophy or dysfunction may also result in sudden death. Thus, patients with symptomatic chronic heart failure due to idiopathic dilated cardiomyopathy are at a similar risk of SCD like those with ischemic cardiomyopathy, and obtain similar benefit from an implantable defibrillator. Symptomatic chronic heart failure patients are already likely to be under medical care. A more problematic group is young subjects with asymptomatic structural heart disease, in whom sudden death may be the first presentation. A list of the commonest causes of sudden death in young adults is given in Table 6.1.

The death of a young, previously asymptomatic person is rightly regarded as a tragedy for the individual and family, and raises issues as to how such events can be prevented, and how the risk of future events in family members is assessed and managed. In the absence of a family history of SCD, the difficulty of identifying those at risk among healthy, asymptomatic young adults is enormous. For example, the calculated risk for sudden death in competitive high school athletes was 0.46/100 000 per academic year [19], and that in US Air Force recruits was 1.18/100 000 during a 42-day basic training period [20]. It is clearly impractical to screen every young person, or even every athlete for a risk of sudden death. Attention should be directed to those with cardiac symptoms, a family history of premature sudden death, or a family history of inherited cardiac disease.

Table 6.1 Principal causes of SCD in young adults.

Structural	Electrical	Toxic
Premature coronary artery disease	Long-QT syndrome	Cocaine, amphetamines, alcohol QT-prolonging drugs
Hypertrophic cardiomyopathy	Brugada syndrome	
Arrhythmogenic right ventricular cardiomyopathy	Catecholamine-induced polymorphic ventricular, tachycardias	
Anomalous coronary artery origin	Short-QT syndrome	
Acute myocarditis	Wolff–Parkinson–White syndrome	
Congenital aortic valve stenosis	Conducting system disorders	
Other congenital heart disease		

Hypertrophic cardiomyopathy

Estimates of the risk of sudden death in hypertrophic cardiomyopathy vary according to the characteristics of the patient cohort. In a tertiary referral registry, the 6-year SCD risk was 9% (95% CI = 5–13%). The variables predictive of risk were syncope, family history of SCD, nonsustained ventricular tachycardia, exercise blood pressure response, and left ventricular wall thickness. The estimated 6-year SCD risks for patients with zero, one, two, and three risk factors were 5% (95% CI = 1–9%), 7% (1–13%), 18% (4–33%), and 64% (25–100%) respectively [21]. In contrast, the annual SCD mortality in a community-based study was only 0.6% (5.4% at 6 years), suggesting that hypertrophic cardiomyopathy is a relatively benign disease in an unselected population [22].

Sudden death in the absence of structural heart disease

The estimated incidence of SCD in white Caucasians aged 16–64 years was 11/100 000/annum in England. Of these, 4.1% (0.45/100 000/annum) had no cause, found at autopsy [9]. The cause of SCD is not identified in as much as 31% of cases aged <35 years [10]. Among SCD victims aged 35 to 44 years, a higher proportion of women (50%) than of men (24%) had no cause of death determined [23]. These deaths are presumed to be due to primary arrhythmogenic disorders [24]. Although inherited ion channel defects, such as long- or short-QT syndromes, Brugada syndrome, and catecholamine-induced polymorphic ventricular tachycardias (see Chapter 9), account for a proportion of these cases, it is likely that other unrecognized disorders also occur. Early attempts at screening for ion channel mutations in SCD victims with no identifiable cause of death have shown only small proportions with known arrhythmia-inducing mutations [25].

Precipitating events

Diurnal/seasonal variation

Muller *et al.* [26] first demonstrated a circadian pattern of out-of-hospital SCD, with a peak incidence from 7 to 11 AM. A similar pattern was subsequently demonstrated in several other studies. A metaanalysis involving over 19 000 subjects reported a morning increase of SCD in all 19 studies surveyed, thus firmly establishing that SCD is more frequent in the morning hours between 6 AM and noon [27]. In an analysis that adjusted for individual wake-times of the decedents, Willich *et al.* [28] demonstrated that the relative risk of SCD was highest during the initial 3 h after awakening compared with other times of the day (Figure 6.2). A remarkably similar relationship with wake-time has also been demonstrated for nonfatal MI, suggesting that plaque rupture and/or thrombosis secondary to sympathetic nervous system activation in associated with assuming an upright posture and starting the day's activities contributes to SCD onset. It is well established that catecholamine blood levels, coronary resistance, and platelet aggregability all exhibit circadian rhythms, which alone or in aggregate could precipitate ischemia, plaque rupture, and/or thrombosis resulting in SCD.

Additionally, there appears to be periodicity in myocardial vulnerability to ventricular arrhythmias independent of ischemia. Several studies have documented similar morning peaks in the incidence of rapid ventricular tachyarrhythmias and/or appropriate shocks among patients with ICDs, even among those without CHD [29]. This morning peak in ventricular tachyarrhythmias and SCD appears to be blunted by beta-blockers [30], supporting the concept that excessive activation of the sympathetic nervous system in the morning hours may be responsible for SCD. Possible contributing factors include documented diurnal variations in PVC frequency, heart rate variability, and dispersion of repolarization, which may all be explained by an increase in sympathetic activity. In addition to the morning peak, there also appears to be a second smaller peak in the late afternoon, both in the incidence of out-of-hospital VF arrests [31] and in ventricular tachyarrhythmic events among ICD patients [32]. This excess may be due to an increase in activities that may trigger ventricular tachyarrhythmias during this time period (see section below).

In addition to the above diurnal variations, there are also weekly and seasonal patterns to SCD onset. The risk of out-of-hospital cardiac arrest [33] and SCD [34] appears to be highest on Monday with a nadir over the weekend [33]. Strikingly similar patterns have been reported for rapid ventricular tachyarrhythmias among ICD patients [35] and for nonfatal MI in the working population. These patterns of onset suggest that activity and

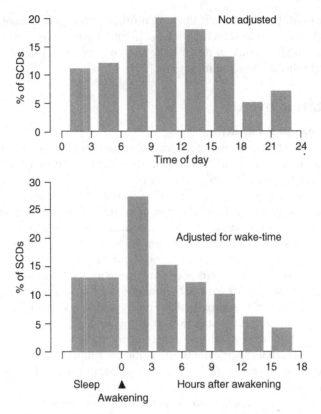

Figure 6.2 Wake-time adjusted analysis of community-based SCDs in Massachusetts. Time of SCD demonstrated a circadian variation with an increased incidence during the late morning compared with other times of the day (upper panel). Time of SCD adjusted for individual wake-times demonstrated an increased relative risk of 2.6 (95% CI = 1.6–4.2) during the initial 3 h after awakening compared with other times of the day (lower panel). (Reproduced from Reference 28 with permission from Elsevier.)

psychological exposures play roles in triggering SCD. There have also been reports of seasonal variation in SCD rates with lower rates in the summer months (July–September) and higher rates in winter (December–January) [34]. Again, parallel patterns have been documented for ventricular tachycardia episodes requiring ICD shocks [35]. These findings suggest that the onset of sudden death may be associated with endogenous rhythms and external factors including climatic conditions.

Activities preceding SCD
Individual exposure to potential triggers may also result in SCD at any time of the day. A number of studies have reported "triggering" of SCD by either physical or mental stress.

Vigorous exertion

Although there are many well-established cardiovascular benefits of exercise, it is also well known that SCD appears to occur with a higher than average frequency during or shortly after vigorous exertion. In various case series, from 6% to as high as 30% of SCDs occur in association with acute exertion. In Rhode Island, an examination of mortality records revealed 12-recorded cases of SCD during jogging during a 6-year period. The authors assessed the community exposure to jogging, and estimated that the age-adjusted relative risk of SCD during jogging was 7 (95% CI = 4–26) compared with the risk during sedentary activities [36]. These findings were extended using a prospective nested case-crossover design within the Physicians' Health Study [37]. Men who exercised less than weekly had a 74-fold increased risk of SCD in the period during and 30 min after exertion compared to the risk observed during other activities. In comparison, men who exercised at least five times per week had an 11-fold increased risk. However, this risk was still significantly elevated compared to the risk during periods of lesser exertion. A retrospective case–control study involving cardiac arrest victims in Seattle and King County came to similar conclusions [38].

The effect of vigorous exertion on the sympathetic nervous system and/or plaque vulnerability could account for both the transiently increased risk of SCD during a bout of exertion and the ability of habitual vigorous exercise to modify this excess risk. In an autopsy study of men with CHD who died suddenly, the findings showed that men who died during exertion were more likely to have plaque rupture than those who died at rest [39]. Alternatively, chronic exercise has known beneficial effects on lipids that may improve plaque stability and also has direct electrophysiologic effects through the sympathetic nervous system. Acute bouts of exercise, decrease vagal activity leading to an acute increase in susceptibility to VF, whereas habitual exertion increases basal vagal tone resulting in increased cardiac electrical stability.

Reassuringly, the absolute risk of SCD during any particular episode of vigorous exertion is extremely low in all studies (e.g. 1 SCD per 1.51 million episodes in the Physicians' Health Study [38]). So, despite large magnitude increases in the relative risk, SCD during vigorous exertion is a rare event. Little is currently known about whether more moderate levels of exertion might trigger SCD. Preliminary data from the Triggers of Ventricular Arrhythmia Study suggest that both moderate and vigorous exertion may trigger shocks for ventricular tachyarrhythmias among ICD patients.

Mental stress

Both acute and chronic mental stresses have been proposed as triggers of ventricular arrhythmias and SCD. However, there are inherent difficulties in assessing exposure to mental stress prior to a SCD event. In most cases, the exposure information is based on retrospective second-hand accounts, which may be unreliable for many reasons. Nevertheless, several retrospective

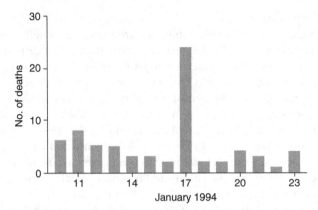

Figure 6.3 Daily numbers of sudden deaths related to CHD from January 10 through 23, 1994. On January 17, the day of the earthquake, there were 24 cases of sudden death related to atherosclerotic cardiovascular disease ($p < .001$). (Reproduced from Reference 41 with permission from Massachusetts Medical Society.)

studies have found increases in informant-reported objective life stresses, such as death of a spouse and loss of job, either acutely or during the weeks before the SCD [40]. On a population level, acute increases in the incidence of SCD have been documented after disasters such as earthquakes or wars. One such example is, the Northridge earthquake; there was a sharp increase in the number of sudden deaths due to CHD on the day of the earthquake followed by an unusually low incidence of such deaths in the week after [41] (Figure 6.3). This "natural experiment" exemplifies how emotional stress may precipitate cardiac events in those who may be predisposed to such events. Of the types of mental stress, anger may be a particularly potent trigger of ventricular arrhythmias. One small study of 49 ICD patients found that anger was the only emotion associated with ICD shocks for ventricular arrhythmias [42]. Recently, mental stress induced by anger recall and mental arithmetic has been demonstrated to induce cardiac electrical instability by increasing T-wave alternans among ICD patients with CHD. Interestingly, these same stressors did not increase T-wave alternans among controls [43]. Therefore, as suggested by the earthquake example, an underlying arrhythmic vulnerability is also required for these potentially "triggering" events/emotions to result in life-threatening arrhythmias.

With respect to chronic mental stresses, depression, anxiety, and social isolation have all been linked to increases in CHD mortality in diverse populations; and anxiety has been directly linked to SCD risk in three separate populations [44]. In the US Health Professionals Follow-up Study, high levels of phobic anxiety as measured by the Crown-Crisp Index were associated with a three-fold increase in risk of CHD death, which was entirely due to a six-fold increase in SCD [45]. We have found similar results among women enrolled in the Nurses' Health Study, but the magnitude of the risk elevation was less

(RR = 1.6; p = .03). Individuals with high levels of anxiety have reduced heart rate variability compared to normal subjects, and the mechanism underlying the increased risk of SCD is again thought to involve alterations in autonomic tone [44] similar to those described above for other triggers.

Sleep

Along with the morning peak in SCD incidence, most studies have reported a nadir during the nighttime sleeping hours [31,34]. In one review, only 12% of SCDs occurred during sleep [40]. This would be less than half of the number of cases expected to occur if the events were uniformly distributed throughout the 24-h period. However, since deaths that occur during the usual hours of sleep are less likely to be witnessed, these deaths are also less likely to be classified as sudden. Temporal patterns of ventricular tachyarrythmias in ICD patients should be free from this potential bias, and most studies have documented a similar decrease in ventricular tachyarrhythmias during sleep [29,32]. Since vagal tone and ventricular refractory periods are the highest during sleep, the mechanism underlying the majority of the 12% of SCDs that occur during sleep is unclear. Some of the rare forms of SCD not associated with structural heart disease described above occur preferentially during sleep. These include long QT3, where ventricular arrhythmias appear to be triggered by bradycardia, and Brugada syndrome. Mutations in the cardiac sodium channel gene, *SCN5A*, have been described in both of these disorders and have also been linked to cases of sudden infant death syndrome, which also occur during sleep [46].

Pharmacologic agents and SCD

In addition to other activities, pharmacologic agents can also trigger ventricular arrhythmias and SCD. The classic example of a drug-induced arrhythmia is *torsades de pointes* (TdP), a potentially lethal polymorphic ventricular tachycardia seen in the setting of QT-prolongation. Antiarrhythmic drugs (class IA and class III agents) and nonantiarrhythmic drugs that prolong the QT interval can induce this arrhythmia. Examples of nonantiarrhythmic drugs that can prolong the QT interval include macrolide antibiotics, antipsychotics, histamine receptor antagonists (Terfenadine), and cholinergic antagonists (Cisapride) [47]. A full listing is available at www.qtdrugs.org. Although TdP secondary to nonantiarrhythmic drugs is exceedingly rare (<1 case per 10 000 or 100 000 exposures) [48], rates of TdP in association with antiarrhythmic drugs range from 2% to as high as 8% in association with Quinidine [47]. Again, as for psychological triggers, the underlying vulnerability to ventricular arrhythmias influences risk. Patients with structural heart disease, particularly left ventricular systolic dysfunction and/or hypertrophy, are at an elevated risk of drug-induced TdP. In addition, there may be genetic factors that influence risk. Poorly penetrant mutations and/or polymorphisms in the genes that result in congenital long-QT syndrome have been found in 10–15% of patients with drug-associated long QT [49]. Therefore, there may be individuals carrying silent mutations and/or predisposing polymorphisms on *LQTS* genes who may manifest ventricular arrhythmias only when the arrhythmogenic substrate is destabilized further by QT-prolonging drugs.

Type IC antiarrhythmic agents can result in proarrhythmia through other mechanisms not dependent on QT-prolongation. Although these agents are safely utilized in younger patients without structural heart disease for a variety of supraventricular arrhythmias, the same agents can result in devastating consequences when used in patients with known ischemic heart disease. In this setting, otherwise nonfatal ischemic events can result in fatal ventricular arrhythmias and SCD [50]. Other classes of pharmacologic agents that can induce ventricular arrhythmias and SCD through a variety of mechanisms include sympathomimetic agents (cocaine, amphetamines, etc.), digoxin, diuretics, and heavy alcohol consumption (>5 drinks/day).

References

1. Priori SG, Aliot E, Blomstrom-Lundqvist C *et al.* Task force on sudden cardiac death of the European Society of Cardiology. *Eur Heart J* 2001; **22**: 1374–1450.
2. Burke AP, Farb A, Pestaner J *et al.* Traditional risk factors and the incidence of sudden coronary death with and without coronary thrombosis in blacks. *Circulation* 2002; **105**: 419–424.
3. Jouven X, Desnos M, Guerot C, Ducimetiere P. Predicting sudden death in the population: the Paris Prospective Study I. *Circulation* 1999; **99**: 1978–1983.
4. Albert CM, Chae CU, Grodstein F *et al.* Prospective study of sudden cardiac death among women in the United States. *Circulation* 2003; **107**: 2096–2101.
5. Weijenberg MP, Feskens EJ, Kromhout D. Blood pressure and isolated systolic hypertension and the risk of coronary heart disease and mortality in elderly men (the Zutphen Elderly Study). *J Hypertens* 1996; **14**: 1159–1166.
6. Albert CM, Ma J, Rifai N, Stampfer MJ, Ridker PM. Prospective study of C-reactive protein, homocysteine, and plasma lipid levels as predictors of sudden cardiac death. *Circulation* 2002; **105**: 2595–2599.
7. Burke AP, Tracy RP, Kolodgie F *et al.* Elevated C-reactive protein values and atherosclerosis in sudden coronary death: association with different pathologies. *Circulation* 2002; **105**: 2019–2123.
8. Gorgels AP, Gijsbers C, de Vreede-Swagemakers J, Lousberg A, Wellens HJ. Out-of-hospital cardiac arrest – the relevance of heart failure. The Maastricht Circulatory Arrest Registry. *Eur Heart J* 2003; **24**: 1204–1209.
9. Bowker TJ, Wood DA, Davies MJ *et al.* Sudden, unexpected cardiac or unexplained death in England: a national survey. *Quart J Med* 2003; **96**: 269–279.
10. Doolan A, Langlois N, Semsarian C. Causes of sudden cardiac death in young Australians. *Med J Aust* 2004; **180**: 110–112.
11. Maron BJ, Carney KP, Lever HM *et al.* Relationship of race to sudden cardiac death in competitive athletes with hypertrophic cardiomyopathy. *J Am Coll Cardiol* 2003; **41**: 974–980.
12. Goldstein S, Landis JR, Leighton R *et al.* Characteristics of the resuscitated out-of-hospital cardiac arrest victim with coronary heart disease. *Circulation* 1981; **64**: 977–984.

13. Cobbe SM, Dalziel K, Ford I, Marsden AK. Survival of 1476 patients initially resuscitated from out of hospital cardiac arrest. *Brit Med J* 1996; **312**: 1633–1637.
14. de Vreede-Swagemakers JJ, Gorgels AP, Dubois-Arbouw WI *et al.* Circumstances and causes of out-of-hospital cardiac arrest in sudden death survivors. *Heart* 1998; **79**: 356–361.
15. Schaffer WA, Cobb LA. Recurrent ventricular fibrillation and modes of death in survivors of out-of-hospital ventricular fibrillation. *N Engl J Med* 1975; **293**: 259–262.
16. Weaver WD, Lorch GS, Alvarez HA, Cobb LA. Angiographic findings and prognostic indicators in patients resuscitated from sudden cardiac death. *Circulation* 1976; **54**: 895–900.
17. Lo YS, Cutler JE, Blake K, Wright AM, Kron J, Swerdlow CD. Angiographic coronary morphology in survivors of cardiac arrest. *Am Heart J* 1988; **115**: 781–785.
18. Mangi AA, Boeve TJ, Vlahakes GJ *et al.* Surgical coronary revascularization and antiarrhythmic therapy in survivors of out-of-hospital cardiac arrest. *Ann Thorac Surg* 2002; **74**: 1510–1516.
19. Maron BJ, Gohman TE, Aeppli D. Prevalence of sudden cardiac death during competitive sports activities in Minnesota high school athletes. *J Am Coll Cardiol* 1998; **32**: 1881–1884.
20. Phillips M, Robinowitz M, Higgins JR, Boran KJ, Reed T, Virmani R. Sudden cardiac death in Air Force recruits. A 20-year review. *JAMA* 1986; **256**: 2696–2699.
21. Elliott PM, Poloniecki J, Dickie S *et al.* Sudden death in hypertrophic cardiomyopathy: identification of high risk patients. *J Am Coll Cardiol* 2000; **36**: 2212–2218.
22. Kofflard MJ, Ten Cate FJ, van der Lee C, van Domburg RT. Hypertrophic cardiomyopathy in a large community-based population: clinical outcome and identification of risk factors for sudden cardiac death and clinical deterioration. *J Am Coll Cardiol* 2003; **41**: 987–993.
23. Chugh SS, Chung K, Zheng ZJ, John B, Titus JL. Cardiac pathologic findings reveal a high rate of sudden cardiac death of undetermined etiology in younger women. *Am Heart J* 2003; **146**: 635–639.
24. Wever EF, Robles de Medina EO. Sudden death in patients without structural heart disease. *J Am Coll Cardiol* 2004; **43**: 1137–1144.
25. Chugh SS, Senashova O, Watts A *et al.* Postmortem molecular screening in unexplained sudden death. *J Am Coll Cardiol* 2004; **43**: 1625–1629.
26. Muller JE, Ludmer PL, Willich SN *et al.* Circadian variation in the frequency of sudden cardiac death. *Circulation* 1987; **75**: 131–138.
27. Cohen MC, Rohtla KM, Lavery CE, Muller JE, Mittleman MA. Meta-analysis of the morning excess of acute myocardial infarction and sudden cardiac death. *Am J Cardiol* 1997; **79**: 1512–1516.
28. Willich SN, Goldberg RJ, Maclure M, Perriello L, Muller JE. Increased onset of sudden cardiac death in the first three hours after awakening. *Am J Cardiol* 1992; **70**: 65–68.
29. Englund A, Behrens S, Wegscheider K, Rowland E (for the European 7219 Jewel Investigators). Circadian variation of malignant ventricular arrhythmias in patients with ischemic and nonischemic heart disease after cardioverter defibrillator implantation. *J Am Coll Cardiol* 1999; **34**: 1560–1568.

30. Peters RW, Muller JE, Goldstein S, Byington R, Friedman LM (for the BHAT Study Group). Propranolol and the morning increase in the frequency of sudden cardiac death (BHAT Study). *Am J Cardiol* 1989; **63**: 1518–1520.
31. Peckova M, Fahrenbruch CE, Cobb LA, Hallstrom AP. Circadian variations in the occurrence of cardiac arrest: initial and repeat episodes. *Circulation* 1998; **98**: 31–39.
32. Kozak M, Krivan L, Semrad B. Circadian variations in the occurrence of ventricular tachyarrhythmias in patients with implantable cardioverter defibrillators. *Pacing Clin Electrophysiol* 2003; **26**: 731–735.
33. Peckova M, Fahrenbruch CE, Cobb LA, Hallstrom AP. Weekly and seasonal variation in the incidence of cardiac arrests. *Am Heart J* 1999; **137**: 512–515.
34. Arntz HR, Willich SN, Schreiber C, Bruggemann T, Stern R, Schultheiss HP. Diurnal, weekly and seasonal variation of sudden death. Population-based analysis of 24,061 consecutive cases. *Eur Heart J* 2000; **21**: 315–320.
35. Muller D, Lampe F, Wegscheider K, Schultheiss HP, Behrens S. Annual distribution of ventricular tachycardias and ventricular fibrillation. *Am Heart J.* 2003; **146**: 1061–1065.
36. Thompson PD, Funk EJ, Carleton RA, Sturner WQ. Incidence of death during jogging in Rhode Island from 1975 through 1980. *JAMA* 1982; **247**: 2535–2538.
37. Albert CM, Mittleman MA, Chae CU, Lee I-M, Hennekens CH, Manson JE. Triggering of sudden cardiac death by vigorous exertion. *N Engl J Med* 2000: **343**: 1351–1361.
38. Siscovick DS, Weiss NS, Fletcher RH, Lasky T. The incidence of primary cardiac arrest during vigorous exercise. *N Engl J Med* 1984; **311**: 874–847.
39. Burke AP, Farb A, Malcom GT, Llang Y-H, Smialek J, Virmani R. Plaque rupture and sudden death related to exertion in men with coronary artery disease. *JAMA* 1999; **281**: 921–926.
40. Willich SN, Maclure M, Mittleman M, Arntz H-R, Muller JE. Sudden cardiac death: support for a role of triggering in causation. *Circulation* 1993; **87**: 1442–1450.
41. Leor J, Poole WK, Kloner RA. Sudden cardiac death triggered by an earthquake. *N Engl J Med* 1996; **334**: 413–419.
42. Lampert R, Joska T, Burg MM, Batsdord WP, McPherson CA, Jain D. Emotional and physical precipitants of ventricular arrhythmia. *Circulation* 2002; **106**: 1800–1805.
43. Kop WJ, Krantz DS, Nearing BD *et al.* Effects of acute mental stress and exercise on T-wave alternans in patients with implantable cardioverter defibrillators and controls. *Circulation* 2004; **109**: 1864–1869.
44. Kubzansky LD, Kawachi I. Going to the heart of the matter: negative emotions and coronary heart disease. *J Psychosom Res* 2000; **48**: 323–337.
45. Kawachi I, Colditz GA, Ascherio A *et al.* Coronary heart disease/myocardial infarction: prospective study of phobic anxiety and risk of coronary heart disease in men. *Circulation* 1994; **89**: 1992–1997.
46. Moric E, Herbert E, Trusz-Gluza M, Filipecki A, Mazurek U, Wilczok T. The implications of genetic mutations in the sodium channel gene (*SCN5A*). *Europace* 2003; **5**: 325–334.
47. Viskin S. Long QT syndromes and *torsade de pointes*. *Lancet* 1999; **354**: 1625–1633.
48. Haverkamp W, Breithardt G, Camm AJ *et al.* The potential for QT prolongation and proarrhythmia by non-antiarrhythmic drugs: clinical and regulatory implications.

Report on a policy conference of the European Society of Cardiology. *Eur Heart J* 2000; **21**: 1216–1231.

49. Yang P, Kanki H, Drolet B *et al.* Allelic variants in long-QT disease genes in patients with drug-associated *torsades de pointes. Circulation* 2002; **105**: 1943–1948.

50. Greenberg HM, Dwyer EM, Hochman JS, Steinberg JS, Echt DS, Peters RW. Interaction of ischemia and encainide/flecainide treatment: a proposed mechanism for the increased mortality in CAST1. *Br Heart J* 1995; **74**: 631–635.

Section two:
Disease states and special populations

CHAPTER 7

Ischemic heart disease

William Wijns and Elliott M. Antman

Epidemiology/scope of problem

Although considerable advances have occurred in the management of patients with cardiovascular diseases over the last 50 years, it still remains the single most common cause of natural death in industrialized countries. It is difficult to obtain precise estimates of the worldwide incidence of sudden cardiac death (SCD), but it is generally accepted that about 50% of cardiovascular deaths in industrialized countries are due to SCD [1]. Therefore, extension of the pandemic of ischemic heart disease to developing countries may lead to an increase in the incidence of SCD in developing nations of the world as well.

Epidemiologic studies have established ventricular tachycardia/ventricular fibrillation (VT/VF) as the typical sequence of electrical events leading to SCD. The pathophysiologic construct that has been proposed to explain SCD holds that patients experiencing SCD have an underlying high-risk substrate upon which certain triggers are superimposed (transient ischemia, hemodynamic fluctuations, neurocardiovascular influences, environmental factors) followed by precipitation of the fatal sequence of electrical events. Ischemic heart disease is estimated to be the cause of the high-risk underlying substrate in 80% of patients suffering from SCD [1,2] (Figure 7.1). Two broad patterns of initiation of the fatal arrhythmia have been reported in patients with ischemic heart disease: (1) acute myocardial ischemia triggers a ventricular tachyarrhythmia in patients who may or may not have a preexisting myocardial scar, and (2) a ventricular tachyarrhythmia occurs in the setting of a myocardial scar from a previous infarction but without evidence of acute myocardial ischemia occurring at the time of the ventricular tachyarrhythmia.

The important factors for identification of patients at risk when considering strategies for prevention of SCD in patients with ischemic heart disease include: (1) the size of the population subgroup at risk and (2) the time dependence of risk of SCD. Figure 7.2 illustrates the challenge of predicting and managing patients at risk of SCD [3]. While the overall incidence of SCD in the adult population is low, the large denominator of patients in that subgroup results in a large contribution to the total number of SCD events per year. Similarly, patients at high risk, such as those with a previous out-of-hospital cardiac arrest or those with a previous myocardial infarction (MI), reduced ejection fraction, and history of VT/VF, have a higher incidence of SCD

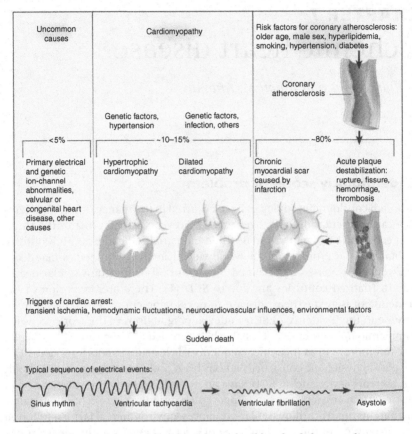

Figure 7.1 Pathophysiology and epidemiology of sudden death from cardiac causes. Reproduced from Reference 1 (p. 1475), with permission from the Massachusetts Medical Society.

when considered as a specific subgroup, but the smaller absolute number of patients relative to the overall adult population results in a relatively smaller contribution to the total number of sudden cardiac events per year.

The risk of SCD following a major cardiovascular (CV) event varies in a nonlinear fashion after the acute event. The idealized survival curves shown in Figure 7.3 emphasize that the highest risk of mortality is in the first 6–18 months after which the slope of the survival curve in high-risk patients appears to be roughly parallel to the slope of the survival curve for low-risk patients. Of note, the data on which these curves are based may not reflect the impact of contemporary interventions in patients with ischemic heart disease. For example, aggressive interventions at limitation of infarct size in patients with ST elevation myocardial infarction (STEMI) theoretically would decrease the proportion of patients with a large myocardial scar, putting them at risk for a VT. On the other hand, the increasing age of the

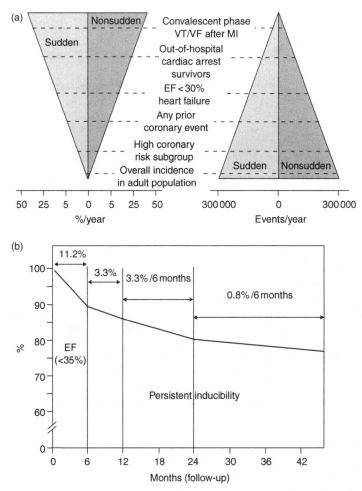

Figure 7.2 Incidence of sudden and nonsudden cardiac deaths in population subgroups, and the relation of total number of events per year to incidence figures. Approximations of subgroup incidence figures, and the related population pool from which they are derived, are presented. Approximately 50% of all cardiac deaths are sudden and unexpected. The incidence triangle on the left ("percent/year") indicates the approximate percentage of sudden and nonsudden deaths in each of the population subgroups indicated, ranging from the lowest percentage in unselected adult populations (0.1–2% per year) to the highest percentage in patients with VT or VF during convalescence after an MI (approximately 50% per year). The triangle on the right indicates the total number of events per year in each of these groups, to reflect incidence in context with the size of the population subgroups. The highest risk categories identify the smallest number of total annual events, and the lowest incidence category accounts for the largest number of events per year (EF = ejection fraction; VT = ventricular tachycardia; VF = ventricular fibrillation; MI = myocardial infarction). Reproduced from Reference 3 (p. 1620), with permission from the McGraw-Hill Company.

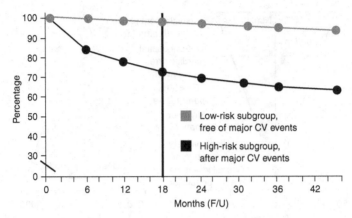

Figure 7.3 Idealized curves of survival from sudden death are shown for a population of patients with known cardiovascular disease but at low risk because of freedom from major cardiovascular (CV) events (top curve) and for populations of patients who have survived a major cardiovascular event (bottom curve). Attrition over time is accelerated in both absolute and relative terms for the initial 6–18 months after the major cardiovascular event. After the initial attrition, the slopes of the curves for the high-risk and low-risk populations parallel each other, highlighting both the early attrition and the attenuation of risk after 18–24 months. These relations have been observed in diverse high-risk subgroups (cardiac arrest survivors, post-myocardial infarction patients with high-risk markers, recent onset of heart failure), and highlight the changing risk pattern as a function of time and the importance of the time dimension for recognition and intervention in strategies designed to alter outcome. Reproduced from Reference 4 with permission from Elsevier.

population results in an expanding epidemiologic cohort at increased risk for SCD events. Finally, the impact of primary prevention strategies with an implantable cardioverter-defibrillator (ICD) is not reflected in the curves shown in Figure 7.3.

Diagnostic modalities

Table 7.1 shows a summary of clinical markers that have been identified as placing patients at increased risk of SCD [1]. With the exception of specific ECG abnormalities indicative of the Brugada or Wolff–Parkinson–White syndromes, all of the markers listed are applicable to evaluation of patients with ischemic heart disease. However, a fundamental problem in using the indicators listed in the table is the unsatisfactory predictive power in an individual patient. While the indicators shown in Table 7.1 are valid when discussing risk from a broad population perspective, the sensitivity and specificity of the indicators in an individual patient are far from ideal. This has inspired clinicians to continue in their search for additional indicators of risk of SCD and also to seek alternative treatment strategies, especially those that focus on

Table 7.1 Indicators of an increased risk of sudden death from arrhythmia.

Variable	Measure	Predictive power
Conventional coronary risk factors High cholesterol High blood pressure Smoking Diabetes	Risk of underlying disease	Low power to discriminate the individual person at risk for sudden death from arrhythmia
Clinical markers NYHA functional class Ejection fraction	Extent of structural disease	High power to predict death from cardiac causes; relatively low specificity at predictors of death from arrhythmia
Ambient ventricular arrhythmia Frequency of premature ventricular depolarizations Nonsustained ventricular tachycardia Sustained ventricular tachycardia	Presence of transient triggers	Low overall power if not combined with other variables Higher predictive power, with low ejection fraction
Electrocardiographic variables Standard ECG Left ventricular hypertrophy Width of QRS complex QT dispersion Specific abnormalities (e.g. prolonged QT interval, right bundle-branch block plus ST-segment elevation in lead V1 (Brugada syndrome), ST-segment and T-wave abnormalities in leads V1 and V2 (right ventricular dysplasia), delta waves (Wolff–Parkinson–White syndrome))	Presence of electrical abnormalities	Low power to predict death from arrhythmia High degree of accuracy in identifying specific electrical abnormalities
High resolution ECG Late potentials on signal-averaged electrocardiography T-wave alternans		High negative predictive value but low positive predictive value Primary predictive value unknown

(Continued)

Table 7.1 (Continued).

Variable	Measure	Predictive Power
Markers of autonomic nervous function 　Heart-rate variability 　Baroreflex sensitivity	Presence of conditioning factors	Exact predictive value unknown
Electrophysiological testing 　Inducibility of sustained tachyarrhythmia by programmed electrical stimulation	Presence of permanent substrate for ventricular arrhythmias	High degree of accuracy in specific high-risk subgroups

Notes: ECG, electrocardiogram; NYHA, New York Heart Association.
Source: Reproduced from Reference 1, with permission from the Massachusetts Medical Society.

primary prevention of SCD. The ICD, although expensive, has emerged as an important and effective treatment strategy not only for primary prevention but also for secondary prevention of SCD.

In addition, even in the absence of anginal symptoms, 55–60% of patients with ischemic cardiomyopathy present with areas of myocardium that suffer from chronic ischemic damage, the so-called hibernating myocardium [5].

The assessment of myocardial hibernation in view of defining the need for subsequent revascularization requires the use of specific imaging techniques, to be integrated with the roadmapping information that is provided by coronary angiography [6]. Nuclear techniques (positron tomography with fluorodeoxyglucose, thallium SPECT using a reinjection or a rest-redistribution protocol, or technetium SPECT) are more sensitive (higher negative predictive value) while stress echocardiography is more specific (higher positive predictive value) in predicting functional improvement following revascularization [7]. The choice of technique most often depends on local availability and expertise.

Treatment strategies

General medical treatment and role of nonantiarrhythmic drugs

Given the major contribution of ischemic heart disease to the global burden of SCD, it is critically important that clinicians rigorously screen for and treat established risk factors for the development of coronary atherosclerosis. The INTERHEART study of 15 152 cases of acute MI and 14 820 controls across 52 countries found that the following nine risk factors were strongly associated with the development of acute MI worldwide: current smoking, diabetes, hypertension, abdominal obesity, psychosocial index, non-consumption of fruits and vegetables daily, exercise, alcohol intake, and the ratio of ApoB/ApoA1 [8]. Although no data are available specifically documenting that treatment strategies favorably impacting on the constellation of risk factors listed above will have a significant impact on the incidence of SCD, a plausible argument can be made that treatments retarding the development and progression of coronary atherosclerosis will reduce the burden of infarct-related scars and ischemia and thereby favorably impact the risk of SCD [9].

The foundation of general medical treatment for ischemic heart disease is antiplatelet therapy. Although certain antiplatelet agents such as sulfin-pyrazone have been reported to reduce SCD, the data on which that observation is based is over 20 years old, and its accuracy and relevance to contemporary management of ischemic heart disease is uncertain [10]. In a large systematic overview of antiplatelet therapies in patients at high risk of vascular disease, the Antiplatelet Trialists' Collaboration reported a 22% reduction in MI, stroke, or vascular death with the use of antiplatelet therapy [11]. The majority of the data in that overview involved aspirin treatment, which underscores the rationale for the class I recommendation on both sides of the Atlantic for prescription of aspirin to patients with known ischemic heart disease or who are at risk for it [12–14]. Alternative antiplatelet agents such as clopidogrel have only marginal benefit when compared directly to aspirin but do contribute significantly to mortality reduction in patients with Non ST segment Elevation Acute Coronary Syndrome (NSTE-ACS) when combined with aspirin [14]. The precise quantitative impact of aspirin alone or combined with other antiplatelet agents on SCD cannot be estimated from the available literature but we believe it is likely to be substantial.

More specific evidence of a reduction in SCD has been reported in some prior primary prevention trials with beta-blockers. Although reductions in arrhythmic deaths were initially reported for the subgroup of patients with prior MI and reduced LV ejection fraction, the benefits of beta-blockade in reducing SCD have been reported to extend to a wider range of patients with varying levels of risk including those with coexistent heart failure and diabetes [9,15–17]. Angiotensin converting enzyme (ACE) inhibitors are an established class of drugs for lowering mortality in patients with ischemic heart disease and have been shown in a metaanalysis to be associated with a significant reduction in SCD after MI (OR 0.80; 95% CI = 0.70–0.92) [18]. The aldosterone inhibitors spironolactone and eplerenone have both been reported to reduce SCD by about 20% when added to ACE inhibitors in patients with heart failure that in the majority of cases was associated with ischemic heart disease [19,20]. Dietary supplementation with n-3 polyunsaturated fatty acids has been reported to reduce the risk of SCD [21]. Finally, although the data has not been established conclusively, use of statins has been reported to be associated with lower rates of VT/VF in patients with ischemic heart disease [22,23]. An observational study in high-risk patients treated with an ICD showed a reduced incidence of recurrent ventricular arrhythmias from 57% to 22% in patients off-versus on-lipid lowering drugs [24].

Myocardial revascularization: necessary but not sufficient

Animal models have shown that myocardial ischemia contributes to the development of VT/VF. Revascularization of ischemic myocardial zones in patients has been shown to reduce the incidence of future episodes of ischemia and may also reduce the risk of arrhythmias [25].

In patients shortly after MI, it has been argued that one of the late benefits of an open infarct artery of MI even in the absence of ischemia is greater electrical stability of the myocardium. However, the DECOPI trial (DEsobstruction COronaire en Post-Infarctus) could not establish that opening an occluded infarct artery in asymptomatic patients in the subacute phase after an MI is associated with reductions of either total mortality or SCD [26]. The larger ongoing Occluded Artery Trial (OAT) will provide information to address this important question [12].

The coronary artery bypass graft (CABG-PATCH) trial evaluated the importance of revascularization in patients scheduled for CABG with an ejection fraction less than 36% and an abnormal signal-averaged ECG (SAECG). After cardiopulmonary bypass, patients were randomized to a control group or implantation of an epicardial ICD [27]. There was no difference in total mortality. The reasons for the lack of mortality reduction are unclear, but possibilities include the failure of the SAECG to identify a high-risk cohort, the benefits of revascularization, and lack of power in the trial to detect any effect or SCD – the only mode of death that could potentially be reduced by an ICD.

Thus, the benefits of revascularization alone in preventing SCD have not been demonstrated conclusively, especially in patients with a history of SCD. Natale [28] has reported cases of ICD shocks in patients who survived SCD and underwent successful CABG surgery for significant coronary stenoses. Similar observations were made in patients with sustained ventricular tachyarrhythmias receiving both CABG and ICD [29]. New insights were recently provided by a 3-year follow-up study of 153 patients after aborted sudden death in whom ischemia, hibernating myocardium, and scar tissue were evaluated by stress-rest perfusion imaging using Technetium-99m tetrofosmin gated SPECT [30]. Patients with death or recurrence exhibited depressed ejection fraction below 30%, more extensive scar tissue, less ischemic/viable myocardium, and less frequently underwent revascularization.

In a pooled analysis of 18 studies involving 1749 patients and using either nuclear or echocardiographic preoperative evaluation, revascularization alone was associated with improved outcome and reduced mortality only in patients with hibernation (annual mortality rate of 7%). The annual mortality rate was 20% in patients with hibernation not undergoing revascularization and 17% in patients without hibernation, irrespective of medical or revascularization treatment (Figure 7.4). Taken together, these observations suggest that both the presence of scar and hibernating myocardium portend increased risk of SCD. Revascularization alone can only be recommended in the absence

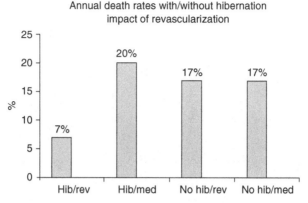

Figure 7.4 Pooled analysis from retrospective studies evaluating annual mortality rates in patient groups based on the selected therapy (medical versus revascularization) and the presence/absence of hibernating myocardium at preoperative testing (Hib = hibernation; rev = revascularization; med = medical therapy only). Reproduced from Reference 6.

of significant residual scar tissue. However, it is important to consider that after revascularization of hibernating myocardium, the ejection fraction is reported to increase by 6–10% in absolute units. Under these circumstances, depending on the preoperative value, the 40% threshold value for considering ICD implantation may no longer be reached [6]. These working hypotheses are currently being tested in two ongoing large, prospective, randomized trials [31,32].

Antiarrhythmics drugs

The role of antiarrhythmic drugs is discussed in detail in Chapter 14. As it pertains to post-MI patients, the premise that suppressing ectopic beats might confer survival benefit was invalidated by the results of several trials (Table 7.2). Results with amiodarone are either neutral or suggest reduction in arrhythmic deaths. However, in patients with heart failure and reduced ejection fraction, there is no indication for reduced total mortality.

Implantable cardioverter-defibrillator

A major advance in the management of SCD was the development of the ICD. Evidence for prevention of SCD using the ICD is quite robust and undoubtedly has contributed to the sharp increase in the use of ICDs. For example, in the EUROHEART survey, the implantation of ICDs occurred at a rate between 5 and 20 per 1 million inhabitants per year in 1995, but in just over 5 years rose to between 20 and 110 per 1 million inhabitants per year across a range of European countries [42].

Table 7.2 Clinical trials of antiarrhythmic drugs.

	Study Name	Year	Patients (n)	Inclusion	Test Drug	Primary Endpoint	p-Value	Placebo/drug
1	D-sotalol after MI	1982	1456	Post-MI	Placebo/D-sotalol	Mortality at 1 year	NS	8.9%/7.3%
2	IMPACT group	1984	630	Post-MI	Placebo/mexiletine	Mortality at 1 year	NS	4.8 %/7.6%
3	CAST I[a]	1991	1498	Post-MI	Placebo/encainide/flecainide	Mortality at 1 year	.0004	2.1%/5.7%
4	CAST II[a]	1992	2699	Post-MI	Placebo/moricizine	Mortality and SCD	NS	Early: 0.5%/2.6% Late: 3.2%/3.6%
5	STATCHF	1995	674	CHF EF < 40%	Placebo/amiodarone	Mortality at 2 year	NS	29.2%/30.6%
6	SWORD[a]	1996	3121	Post-MI/HF EF ≤ 40%	Placebo/D-sotalol	Mortality	.006	3.1%/5.0%
7	EMIAT	1997	1486	Post-MI EF ≤ 40%	Placebo/amiodarone	Mortality at 1 year	NS	13.7%/13.9%
8	CAMIAT	1997	1202	Post-MI	Placebo/amiodarone	Arrhythmic death and aborted VF	.029	6.9%/4.5%
9	SCD-HeFT	2005	2521	CHF EF ≤ 35%	Placebo/amiodarone/ICD	Mortality at 60 m	NS	7.2%/year CI: 1.06 (0.86–1.30)[b]

Notes: ICD = implantable cardioverter defibrillator; MI = myocardial infarction; EF = ejection fraction; CI = confidence interval; VPB = ventricular premature beat; VPS = ventricular premature stimulus.
[a] These studies were stopped prematurely.
[b] This hazard ratio compares patients who received amiodarone on top of conventional treatment, but no ICD ("placebo").

Trials of ICD therapy initially focused on secondary prevention of SCD in patients who had already sustained an episode of VT/VF. Three major randomized trials for secondary prevention among survivors of out-of-hospital cardiac arrest or high risk VT/VF have been completed: Antiarrhythmics Versus Implantable Defibrillators (AVID) [43], Canadian Implantable Defibrillator Study (CIDS) [44], and Cardiac Arrest Study Hamburg (CASH) [45]. Although the focus of these studies was not specifically on patients with ischemic heart disease, as expected from the epidemiologic discussions earlier in this chapter, the cohorts of patients enrolled in these three trials had a high prevalence of coronary disease and prior MI (Table 7.3). A metaanalysis combining AVID, CIDS, and CASH demonstrated directionally consistent observations and strong evidence favoring ICD therapy. The summary hazard ratio for total mortality was 0.72 (95% CI $= 0.60$–0.87, $p = .0006$) and for arrhythmic death was 0.50 (95% CI $= 0.37$–0.67, $p < .0001$) [47]. Based upon the secondary prevention trials noted above, we believe that patients with ischemic heart disease should have an ICD implanted, if they experience VF or hemodynamically compromising sustained VT more than 2 days after an MI, provided the arrhythmia is not judged to be due to transient or reversible ischemia or reinfarction.

Patients surviving the acute phase of MI enter the phase of chronic ischemic heart disease where they remain at risk for SCD. The risk of SCD is highest in the first few months after recovering from MI (annualized rate of 5–30 events per 100 patient-years depending upon ejection fraction) and then falls sharply over the ensuing months to years but remains in a range of 2–3 events per 100 patient-years [48]. Given the large cohort of patients who are at risk for SCD by virtue of recovering from an acute MI, primary prevention strategies are of utmost importance. Four randomized trials studied the use of an ICD in a primary prevention strategy following MI: Multicenter Automatic Defibrillator Implantation Trial (MADIT) [49], Multicenter Unsustained Tachycardia Trial (MUSTT) [50], MADIT II [51], Sudden Cardiac Death in Heart Failure Trial (SCD-HeFT) [41], and Defibrillators in Acute Myocardial Infarction Trial (DINAMIT) [53]. A consistent pattern of significant improvement in overall mortality was observed in the first three trials (Table 7.4).

In an effort to focus on first months after MI, the DINAMIT [53] investigators enrolled patients with an acute MI within the preceding 6–40 days if they had a left ventricular ejection fraction less than 35% and evidence of abnormal heart-rate variability (standard deviation of normal beat to beat intervals less than 70 ms (SDNN)). Patients with sustained VT more than 48 h after MI and those with class IV heart failure were excluded, as were those with CABG surgery or three-vessel Percutaneous Coronary Intervention (PCI) after MI. Most patients had large anterior MIs, and attempts at reperfusion were undertaken in more than 60% of patients. Of the 674 patients randomised, 332 were allocated to ICD therapy and 342 to no ICD therapy. The ICD was implanted a median of 7 days after the index MI. The primary endpoint of all-cause mortality did not differ between treatment arms (7.5% per year in the ICD arm

Table 7.3 Clinical trials of secondary prevention of SCD with ICDs.

Study	N	Patient Inclusion Criteria	% Patients with Prior-MI	EF % (Mean)	Endpoint(s)	Treatment Arms	Key Results
AVID	1016	Survivor of cardiac arrest VT with syncope Symptomatic sustained VT with LVEF ≤ 0.40	61	32	Total mortality Mode of death Quality of life Cost benefit	Amiodarone or sotalol	Significant improvement in overall survival with ICD (RRR = 29%)
CASH	191	Survivor of cardiac arrest	51	45	Total mortality Recurrences of arrhythmias requiring CPR Recurrence of unstable VT	ICD; amiodarone, propafenone, or metoprolol	Trend toward 23% improvement in survival with ICD
CIDS	659	Survivor of cardiac arrest Syncope with symptomatic sustained VT with LVEF ≤ 0.35 or syncope with inducible VT	77	34	Total mortality	Amiodarone	Trend toward 20% improvement in survival with ICD

Notes: AVID = Antiarrhythmics Versus Implantable Defibrillators; CASH = Cardiac Arrest Study Hamburg; CIDS = Canadian Implantable Defibrillator Study; RRR = relative risk reduction.

Source: Modified from Reference 46 with permission from Elsevier.

Table 7.4 Clinical trials of primary prevention of sudden death with ICDs: applicability to the post-MI population.

Study Name	Year	Patients (n)	Days After MI	Qualifying Arrhythmia	EF Upper Limit (Mean)	EPS	Mortality Hazard ICD Versus No ICD (95% CI)
MADIT [49]	1996	196	More than 20	3–30 VPBs; rate greater than 120 bpm	35%, 26%	Yes[a]	0.46 (0.26–0.82)
MUSTT [50]	1999	704	More than 3[b]	Greater than 2 VPS; rate greater than 100 bpm	40%, 30%	Yes[c]	0.42 (0.28–0.62)[d]
MADIT II [51]	2002	1232	More than 29	None necessary	30%, 23%	No	0.69 (0.51–0.93)
SCD-HeFT[e] [41]	2005	2531	—	None necessary	35%, 25%	No	0.77 (0.62–0.96)
DINAMIT [53]	2004	674	6–40	None necessary	35%	No	1.08 (0.76–1.55)

Notes: ICD = implantable cardioverter-defibrillator; MI = myocardial infarction; EP = electrophysiological; EF = ejection fraction; EPS = EP study; CI = confidence interval; VPB = ventricular premature beat; VPS = ventricular premature stimulus.

Source: Modified from table 27 in Reference 12, with permission from the ACC/AMA.

[a] Randomized MADIT patients had inducible VT not suppressed by a procainamide infusion during EP study.

[b] Only 16% of the overall MUSTT population was randomized within 1 month of MI.

[c] Randomized MUSTT patients had inducible VT and were randomized to antiarrhythmic drug therapy. On the basis of clinical indications, some patients received ICDs during the course of follow-up.

[d] This hazard ratio compares MUSTT patients in the antiarrhythmic arm who received ICDs with those who received only EP-guided antiarrhythmic therapy.

[e] SCD-HeFT included a population of heart failure patients with ischemic (52%) and non ischemic cardiomyopathies.

versus 6.9% per year in the control arm). Death due to arrhythmia was lower in the ICD arm (1.5% per year versus 3.5% per year; hazard ratio 0.42, 95% CI = 0.22–0.83, p = .009). However, nonarrhythmic deaths were higher in the ICD arm (6.1% per year versus 3.5% per year; hazard ratio 1.75, 95% CI = 1.11–2.76, p = .016).

The reason that ICD therapy was associated with an increased risk of nonarrhythmic death in DINAMIT is speculative. Potential causes include worsened hemodynamics induced by back-up right ventricular apical pacing, change in the mode of death shifting it from arrhythmic death to pump failure related mortality because of recurrent ischemia and infarction, and potential recovery of ventricular function after the first 3 months placing patients in a lower-risk group with no established benefit from an ICD. Also, implantation of an ICD may involve interruption of anticoagulation, induction of VF for testing, and delayed patient mobilization that could increase early mortality in ICD recipients.

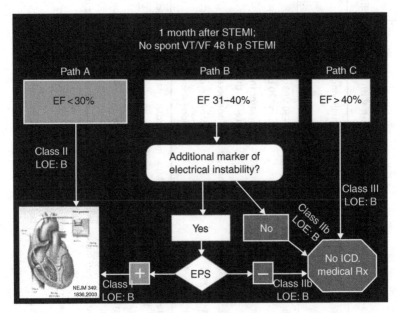

Figure 7.5 An evidence-based algorithm for primary prevention of SCD in post-STEMI patients without spontaneous VF or sustained VT at least 1 month post-STEMI to aid in selection of ICD in patients with STEMI and diminished ejection fraction. The appropriate management path is selected based upon left ventricular ejection fraction (LVEF) measured at least 1 month after STEMI. All patients, whether an ICD is implanted or not, should receive medical therapy (EF = ejection fraction; VF = ventricular fibrillation; VT = ventricular tachycardia; STEMI = ST-elevation myocardial infarction; NSVT = nonsustained VT; LOE = level of evidence; EPS = electrophysiological study). Reproduced from Reference 12, with permission from Oxford University Press.

An evidence-based algorithm for primary prevention of SCD in patients following STEMI without spontaneous VF or sustained VT at least 1 month post-STEMI is shown in Figure 7.5. The ejection fraction should be measured at least 1 month post-STEMI and then patients are managed according to three pathways. Path A includes those patients with ejection fraction less than or equal to 30% – they should be referred for ICD implantation without other testing. Path C involves those patients with ejection fraction greater than 40%; no ICD is recommended in such patients but evidence-based medical therapy following STEMI should be provided. Patients whose ejection fraction falls between 31% and 40% are managed according to pathway B. These patients with an intermediate level ejection fraction should be screened for additional evidence of electrical instability. This might include nonsustained VT on ECG monitoring, abnormal SAECG, abnormalities on autonomic baroreflex testing, or microvolt T-wave alternans. When there is additional evidence of electrical instability, patients should be referred for an electrophysiology study. If the VT/VF is inducible, an ICD should be implanted. If the electrophysiology study shows no inducible VT/VF, the usefulness of an ICD is not well established.

References

1. Huikuri HV, Castellanos A, Myerburg RJ. Sudden death due to cardiac arrhythmias. *N Engl J Med* 2001; **345**: 1473–1482.
2. Chugh SS, Jui J, Gunson K, *et al.* Current burden of sudden cardiac death: multiple source surveillance versus retrospective death certificate-based review in a large U.S. community. *J Am Coll Cardiol* 2004; **44**: 1268–1275.
3. Myerburg RJ, Castellanos A. Cardiovascular collapse, cardiac arrest, and sudden cardiac death. In: Kasper DL, Braunwald E, Fauci AS, Hauser SL, Longo DL, & Jameson JL, eds. *Harrison's Principles of Internal Medicine*, 16th edn. McGraw-Hill, New York, 2005: 1618–1624.
4. Myerburg RJ, Castellanos A. Cardiac arrest and sudden cardiac death. In: Braunwald E, Zipes DP, & Libby P, eds. *Heart Disease: A Textbook of Cardiovascular Medicine*, 6th edn. WB Saunders, Philadelphia, PA, 2001: 892.
5. Wijns W, Vatner SF, Camici PG. Hibernating myocardium. *N Engl J Med* 1998; **339**: 173–1781.
6. Underwood SR, Bax JJ, vom Dahl J, *et al.* Imaging techniques for the assessment of myocardial hibernation. Report of a study group of the European Society of Cardiology. *Eur Heart J* 2004; **25**: 815–836.
7. Bax JJ, Poldermans D, Elhendy A, *et al.* Sensitivity, specificity and predictive accuracies of various non-invasive techniques for detecting hibernating myocardium. *Curr Probl Cardiol* 2001; **26**: 141–188.
8. Yusuf S, Hawken S, Ounpuu S, *et al.* Effect of potentially modifiable risk factors associated with myocardial infarction in 52 countries (the INTERHEART study): case–control study. *Lancet* 2004; **364**: 937–952.
9. Priori SG, Aliot E, Blomstrom-Lundqvist C, *et al.* Task force on sudden cardiac death of the European Society of Cardiology. *Eur Heart J* 2001; **22**: 1374–1450.
10. Sherry S. The Anturane reinfarction trial. *Circulation* 1980; **62**: V73–V78.

11. Antithrombotic Trialists' Collaboration. Collaborative meta-analysis of randomised trials of antiplatelet therapy for prevention of death, myocardial infarction, and stroke in high risk patients. *BMJ* 2002; **324**: 71–86.
12. Antman EM, Anbe DT, Armstrong PW, *et al.* ACC/AHA guidelines for the management of patients with ST-elevation myocardial infarction: a report of the American College of Cardiology/American Heart Association Task Force on Practice Guidelines (Committee to Revise the 1999 Guidelines for the Management of Patients With Acute Myocardial Infarction). Available at www.acc.org/clinical/guidelines/stemi/index.pdf. In: 2004.
13. Braunwald E, Antman EM, Beasley JW, *et al.* ACC/AHA 2002 guideline update for the management of patients with unstable angina and non-ST-segment elevation myocardial infarction – summary article: a report of the American College of Cardiology/American Heart Association task force on practice guidelines (Committee on the Management of Patients With Unstable Angina). *J Am Coll Cardiol* 2002; **40**: 1366–1374.
14. Patrono C, Bachmann F, Baigent C, *et al.* Expert consensus document on the use of antiplatelet agents. The task force on the use of antiplatelet agents in patients with atherosclerotic cardiovascular disease of the European society of cardiology. *Eur Heart J* 2004; **25**: 166–181.
15. Friedman LM, Byington RP, Capone RJ, *et al.* Effect of propranolol in patients with myocardial infarction and ventricular arrhythmia. *J Am Coll Cardiol* 1986; **7**: 1–8.
16. Gottlieb SS, McCarter RJ, Vogel RA. Effect of beta-blockade on mortality among high-risk and low-risk patients after myocardial infarction. *N Engl J Med* 1998; **339**: 489–497.
17. Myerburg RJ, Spooner PM. Opportunities for sudden death prevention: directions for new clinical and basic research. *Cardiovasc Res* 2001; **50**: 177–185.
18. Domanski MJ, Exner DV, Borkowf CB, *et al.* Effect of angiotensin converting enzyme inhibition on sudden cardiac death in patients following acute myocardial infarction. A meta-analysis of randomized clinical trials. *J Am Coll Cardiol* 1999; **33**: 598–604.
19. Pitt B, Zannad F, Remme WJ, *et al.* The effect of spironolactone on morbidity and mortality in patients with severe heart failure. Randomized Aldactone Evaluation Study Investigators. *N Engl J Med* 1999; **341**: 709–717.
20. Pitt B, Remme W, Zannad F, *et al.* Eplerenone, a selective aldosterone blocker, in patients with left ventricular dysfunction after myocardial infarction. *N Engl J Med* 2003; **348**: 1309–1321.
21. Dietary supplementation with n-3 polyunsaturated fatty acids and vitamin E after myocardial infarction: results of the GISSI-Prevenzione trial. Gruppo Italiano per lo Studio della Sopravvivenza nell'Infarto miocardico. *Lancet* 1999; **354**: 447–455.
22. Downs JR, Clearfield M, Weis S, *et al.* Primary prevention of acute coronary events with lovastatin in men and women with average cholesterol levels: results of AFCAPS/TexCAPS. Air Force/Texas Coronary Atherosclerosis Prevention Study. *JAMA* 1998; **279**: 1615–1622.
23. Mitchell LB, Powell JL, Gillis AM, *et al.* Are lipid-lowering drugs also antiarrhythmic drugs? An analysis of the Antiarrhythmics Versus Implantable Defibrillators (AVID) trial. *J Am Coll Cardiol* 2003; **42**: 81–87.
24. De Sutter J, Tavernier R, De Buyzere M, *et al.* Lipid lowering drugs and recurrences of life-threatening ventricular arrhythmias in high-risk patients. *J Am Coll Cardiol* 2000; **36**: 766–772.

25. Ganz LI. Primary prevention of sudden cardiac death. *Curr Cardiol Rep* 2004; **6**: 339–347.
26. Smiseth OA, Steg PG, Sipido K, *et al.* News from the European Society of Cardiology Congress in Vienna, August 30 to September 3, 2003. *J Am Coll Cardiol* 2004; **43**: 691–697.
27. Bigger JT Jr. Prophylactic use of implanted cardiac defibrillators in patients at high risk for ventricular arrhythmias after coronary-artery bypass graft surgery. Coronary Artery Bypass Graft (CABG) Patch Trial Investigators. *N Engl J Med* 1997; **337**: 1569–1575.
28. Natale A, Sra J, Axtell K, *et al.* Ventricular fibrillation and polymorphic ventricular tachycardia with critical coronary artery stenosis: does bypass surgery suffice? *J Cardiovasc Electrophysiol* 1994; **5**: 988–994.
29. Geelen P, Primo J, Wellens F, *et al.* Coronary artery bypass grafting and defibrillator implantation in patients with ventricular tachyarrhythmias and ischemic heart disease. *Pacing Clin Electrophysiol* 1999; **22**: 1132–1139.
30. van der Burg AE, Bax JJ, Boersma E, *et al.* Impact of viability, ischemia, scar tissue, and revascularization on outcome after aborted sudden death. *Circulation* 2003; **108**: 1954–1959.
31. Cleland JG, Freemantle N, Ball SG, *et al.* The heart failure revascularisation trial (HEART): rationale, design and methodology. *Eur J Heart Fail* 2003; **5**: 295–303.
32. Jones RH. Surgical treatment for ischemic heart failure (STICH). Available from: http://www.clinicaltrials.gov/ct/gut/show/NCT00023595. In: 2004.
33. Julian DG, Jackson FS, Prescott RJ, *et al.* Controlled trial of sotalol for one year after MI. *Lancet* 1982; **1**: 1142–1147.
34. Impact Research Group. International mexiletine and placebo antiarrhythmic Coronary trial: I. report on arrhythmia and other findings. *J Am Coll Cardiol* 1984; **4**: 1148–1163.
35. Echt DS, Liebson PR, Mitchell LB, *et al.* CAST I. *N Engl J Med* 1991; **324**: 781–788.
36. The Cardiac Arrhythmia Suppression Trail II Investigators. Effect of antiarrhythmic agen moricizine of survival after myocardial infarction. *N Engl J Med* 1992; **327**: 227–233.
37. Singh SN, *et al. STAT CHF. N Engl J Med* 1995; **333**: 77–82.
38. Waldo AL, Camm AJ, deRuyter H, *et al.* SWORD. *Lancet* 1996; **348**: 7–12.
39. Julian DG, Camm AJ, Frangin G, *et al.* EMIAT. *Lancet* 1997; **349**: 667–674.
40. Cairns JA, Connolly SJ, Roberts R, *et al.* CAMIAT. *Lancet* 1997; **349**: 675–682.
41. Bardy GH, Lee KL, Mark DB, *et al.* Amiodarone or an implantable cardioverter-defibrillator for congestive heart failure. *N Engl J Med* 2005; **352**: 225–237.
42. Euro Heart Survey. Cardiovascular Diseases in Europe 2004. Available at http://www.escardio.org/knowledge/ehs/slides. Slides. Accessed on September 21, 2004.
43. The Antiarrhythmics Versus Implantable Defibrillators (AVID) Investigators. A comparison of antiarrhythmic-drug therapy with implantable defibrillators in patients resuscitated from near-fatal ventricular arrhythmias. *N Engl J Med* 1997; **337**: 1576–1583.
44. Connolly SJ, Gent M, Roberts RS, *et al.* Canadian implantable defibrillator study (CIDS): a randomized trial of the implantable cardioverter defibrillator against amiodarone. *Circulation* 2000; **101**: 1297–1302.
45. Kuck KH, Cappato R, Siebels J, *et al.* Randomized comparison of antiarrhythmic drug therapy with implantable defibrillators in patients resuscitated from cardiac arrest: the Cardiac Arrest Study Hamburg (CASH). *Circulation* 2000; **102**: 748–754.

46. Hayes DL, Zipes DP. Cardiac pacemakers and cardioverter-defibrillators. In: Zipes DW, Libby P, Bonow RO, & Braunwald E, eds. *Braunwald's Heart Disease: A Textbook of Cardiovascular Medicine*, 7th edn. Elsevier Inc., Philadelphia, PA, 2005: 788.
47. Connolly SJ, Hallstrom AP, Cappato R, *et al.* Meta-analysis of the implantable cardioverter defibrillator secondary prevention trials. AVID, CASH and CIDS studies. Antiarrhythmics Versus Implantable Defibrillator study. Cardiac Arrest Study Hamburg. Canadian Implantable Defibrillator Study. *Eur Heart J* 2000; **21**: 2071–2078.
48. Solomon SD, Zelenkofske S, McMurray JJ, *et al.* Valsartan in Acute Myocardial Infarction Trial (VALIANT) Investigators. Sudden death in patients with myocardial infarction and left ventricular dysfunction, heart failure, or both. *N Engl J Med* 2005; **352**: 2581–8.
49. Moss AJ, Hall WJ, Cannom DS, *et al.* Improved survival with an implanted defibrillator in patients with coronary disease at high risk for ventricular arrhythmia. Multicenter Automatic Defibrillator Implantation Trial Investigators. *N Engl J Med* 1996; **335**: 1933–1940.
50. Buxton AE, Lee KL, Fisher JD, *et al.* A randomized study of the prevention of sudden death in patients with coronary artery disease. Multicenter Unsustained Tachycardia Trial Investigators. *N Engl J Med* 1999; **341**: 1882–1890.
51. Moss AJ, Zareba W, Hall WJ, *et al.* Prophylactic implantation of a defibrillator in patients with myocardial infarction and reduced ejection fraction. *N Engl J Med* 2002; **346**: 877–883.
52. Bardy GH, Lee KL, Mark DB, *et al.* Amiodarone or an implantable cardioverter-defibrillator for congestive heart failure. *N Engl J Med* 2005; **352**: 225–237.
53. Hohnloser SH, Kuck KH, Dorian P, *et al.* DINAMIT Investigators. Prophylactic use of an implantable cardioverter-defibrillator after acute myocardial infarction. *N Engl J Med* 2004; **351**: 2481–8.

CHAPTER 8

The cardiomyopathies

William J. McKenna, Srijita Sen-Chowdhry, and Barry J. Maron

The cardiomyopathies are genetically determined heart muscle disorders that represent the leading cause of sudden cardiac death (SCD) after coronary artery disease (CAD). Hypertrophic cardiomyopathy (HCM), dilated cardiomyopathy (DCM), and arrhythmogenic right ventricular cardiomyopathy (ARVC) are the three main diseases in this group [1]. HCM and ARVC are particularly noteworthy as SCD is often the first clinical manifestation, particularly in young people engaged in strenuous activity. A fourth cardiomyopathy, isolated left ventricular non-compaction, is newly recognized and relatively few cases have been reported. It is thought to be caused by the arrest of normal myocardial compaction during embryogenesis, resulting in persistence of prominent ventricular trabeculation and deep intertrabecular recesses. Isolated non-compaction may be associated with congestive heart failure, thromboembolism, arrhythmia, and SCD [2]; however, risk stratification remains poorly defined and is not covered in further detail here.

Patients with cardiomyopathy are often young and otherwise in good health. In HCM and ARVC, the arrhythmic risk may be significant without concurrent systolic dysfunction or debilitating symptoms. Thus, prevention of SCD in this group yields an exceptional number of quality-adjusted life years. The implantable cardioverter-defibrillator (ICD) can theoretically nullify this risk; however, the need for lifelong device maintenance and lead replacements increases the likelihood of complications, underscoring the importance of accurate risk stratification. The role of antiarrhythmic agents in the ICD era should not be discounted. Beta-blockers and amiodarone can be safely administered to patients with structural heart disease and may be of particular value in controlling arrhythmic symptoms. Drug therapy is also indicated for suppressing electrical storm in patients with devices. This chapter aims to provide an overview of the underlying mechanisms, predictors, and prevention of SCD in HCM, DCM, and ARVC.

Hypertrophic cardiomyopathy

Hypertrophic cardiomyopathy is caused by mutations in sarcomeric proteins, which may result in myocardial hypertrophy, myocyte disarray, fibrosis, and small vessel disease. Autosomal dominant transmission is typical. Penetrance in a genotyped population was 55% between the ages of 10 and 29 and 75% by the age of 50 [3]. The clinical features often develop during puberty, although late-onset forms are also recognized, particularly in association with mutations in myosin-binding protein C. When a genetic diagnosis is not available, relatives are encouraged to undergo annual cardiac evaluation throughout adolescence and 5-yearly thereafter. This should comprise a full history, with particular focus on symptoms such as chest pain, dyspnoea, palpitation, and syncope; 12-lead electrocardiogram (ECG); and two-dimensional (2D) echocardiogram. First-degree relatives of probands with HCM have a 50% chance of carrying the disease-causing mutation; minor cardiac abnormalities are thus more likely to represent disease expression than in the general population. Modified diagnostic criteria have therefore been proposed for the diagnosis of familial HCM [4].

Phenocopies of HCM have been observed in Noonan's syndrome, mitochondrial myopathies, Friedreich's ataxia, Anderson–Fabry disease, and glycogen storage disorders. The clinical profile of these disease states is frequently distinct from that of sarcomeric HCM; mutations in AMP kinase, for example, may be associated with preexcitation, conduction system disease, and propensity towards cavity dilation and heart failure [5]. The advent of specific therapies, such as enzyme replacement in Fabry's disease, further underlines the need for early recognition. Energy depletion has been proposed as the central unifying mechanism [5].

Natural history of HCM

The estimated prevalence of HCM in the general adult population is around 1:500. Much of our initial understanding of natural history and prognosis was derived from tertiary center studies, which inevitably included a high proportion of patients with severe disease expression. The annual mortality rate was reported as 2–3% in adults and up to 6% in children. Conversely, in community-based populations without referral bias, the annual cardiac mortality may be less than 1% [6]. Thus, HCM is a common disease that follows a prolonged stable clinical course in the majority of patients. Complications include left ventricular outflow tract obstruction (LVOTO), diastolic dysfunction, ischemia, embolic stroke, and left ventricular failure (LVF). The latter, also known as the "burnt-out" phase, occurs in less than 5% of patients, and is characterized by left ventricular (LV) wall thinning and systolic dysfunction. SCD remains nonetheless the most frequent cause of premature mortality in HCM, with high-risk patients constituting an important minority of the overall population.

Mechanisms of SCD in HCM

Sudden cardiac death in HCM is frequently not preceded by premonitory symptoms. A bimodal pattern of circadian variability has been observed, with a notable peak in the morning hours after awakening, similar to that described in patients with CAD; a second, less prominent peak is observed in the early evening. Adolescents and young adults below the age of 35 show the highest incidence of SCD, although this does not translate into low risk through mid-life and beyond. The majority of deaths occur during mild exertion, sedentary activities, or even sleep; however, strenuous activity is not uncommonly a precipitant. HCM is consistently reported as the most common aetiology of SCD among athletes [7]. A noteworthy exception is the Veneto region of northern Italy, where ARVC is the leading cause of sports-related fatalities and deaths from HCM appear to be less frequent. This difference may be a direct consequence of preparticipation screening with electrocardiography, underscoring the effectiveness of such programmes in reducing deaths from HCM in trained athletes [8]. It is also apparent that timely diagnosis of ARVC may be more problematic.

Analysis of appropriate ICD interventions and fortuitously recorded arrhythmic events suggests that ventricular tachyarrhythmia is the most common mechanism of SCD in HCM [9]. The role of bradyarrhythmia is less clear from ICD interrogation as backup pacing may obscure its presence. Ventricular fibrillation (VF) may be spontaneous, or triggered by monomorphic or polymorphic ventricular tachycardia (VT), paroxysmal atrial fibrillation (AF), or rapid atrioventricular conduction via an accessory pathway. Myocyte disarray and fibrosis provide the arrhythmogenic substrate; precipitating factors include ischemia, LVOTO, and vascular instability. The contribution and interaction of these determinants will be complex, variable, and highly dependent on clinical status and circumstances.

Predictors of SCD in HCM

Noninvasive predictors of adverse outcome in HCM are summarized in Table 8.1 [1]. All patients with HCM should be offered comprehensive cardiac evaluation on an annual basis, comprising personal and family history, 12-lead ECG, 2D echocardiography, 24- or 48-h ambulatory ECG monitoring, and maximal upright exercise testing. The current algorithm identifies the majority of high-risk patients; however, up to 3% of sudden deaths occur in the absence of conventional prognostic indicators [10]. Definitive risk stratification for all HCM patients therefore remains elusive, although considerable progress has been made over the past two decades. The clinical markers of increased risk are discussed individually below.

Previous cardiac arrest or spontaneous sustained VT

An ICD is mandatory for secondary prevention in all cardiac arrest survivors with any form of cardiomyopathy, be it HCM, DCM, or ARVC. Spontaneous, sustained VT is rare in HCM and DCM, but an important predictor of adverse outcome in both, with a prognostic impact paralleling that of previous VF. In patients with HCM, sustained monomorphic VT should additionally raise suspicion of a left ventricular apical aneurysm.

Table 8.1 Risk factors for sudden cardiac death in hypertrophic cardiomyopathy.

Major Risk Factors	Possible in Individual Patients
Previous VF arrest	Atrial fibrillation
Spontaneous sustained VT	Myocardial ischemia
Family history of premature sudden death	LV outflow obstruction
(particularly, in a first-degree relative	High-risk mutation
and/or multiple in occurrence)	Intense competitive
Syncope one or more episode (particularly if	physical exertion
recurrent, exertional, or in the young)	"Burnt out" stage
LV thickness ≥30 mm	
Abnormal blood pressure response to exercise (a fall or	
failure to rise ≥25 mm Hg during maximum upright	
exercise testing in patients <50 years of age)	
Nonsustained ventricular tachycardia	
(3 or more consecutive beats at ≥120 bpm)	

Source: Reproduced from Reference 1.

Family history of HCM-related death

The prognostic impact of a malignant family history is greatest when deaths have occurred among close relatives, or multiple instances are documented. In smaller families, a single death may have greater bearing on management decisions. Although fatalities under the age of 40 are of particular significance, sudden and unexpected deaths in older relatives may also be relevant, particularly in families with late-onset disease.

Syncope

Ventricular tachyarrhythmia with hemodynamic compromise is a harbinger of SCD in many patients with cardiomyopathy, be it HCM, DCM, or ARVC. Thus, episodes of impaired consciousness in the context of cardiac disease may warrant investigation to establish the underlying cause. Conversely, it should be noted that the sensitivity and specificity of unexplained syncope as a prognostic indicator in HCM are low, probably because the majority of these events are not secondary to ventricular tachyarrhythmia. Supraventricular arrhythmia and LVOTO will account for a proportion of syncopal episodes in HCM patients. Exercise stress echocardiography may be indicated if exertional obstruction is suspected in a patient without evidence of a resting gradient. As in the general population, however, syncope in patients with HCM is likely to be neurally mediated frequently and unrelated to the disease state. Extended monitoring with a loop recorder is the most unambiguous means of determining whether unexplained syncope has an arrhythmic aetiology. Nevertheless, when syncope is recurrent, exertional, or associated with other risk factors, an ICD may be preferred as a safeguard intervention against lethal arrhythmic events.

Extreme left ventricular hypertrophy

About 10% of patients with HCM have massive left ventricular hypertrophy (LVH), with a maximum wall thickness ≥30 mm. Long-term unfavorable prognosis with SCD has been reported in this subgroup, many of whom are young (mean age <30) and minimally symptomatic [10,11]. A subsequent study, however, suggested that marked LVH was a significant predictor of SCD but only in association with other risk factors [12]. The impact of marked LVH on management will therefore depend on the overall clinical profile of the patient.

It should be noted that lesser degrees of hypertrophy do not necessarily imply low risk; in fact, the majority of sudden deaths occur among patients with a maximum wall thickness of <30 mm. Furthermore, mutations in Troponin T and Troponin I have been linked to sudden deaths in some patients with minimal or no hypertrophy [13–14]. The distribution of hypertrophy appears to have no clear prognostic significance, although hypertrophy confined to the LV apex has been associated with a favorable outcome.

Abnormal blood pressure response to exercise

Failure of the systolic blood pressure to rise by at least 25 mm Hg, or a fall in blood pressure during exercise, is observed in about one third of patients with HCM. The underlying mechanism appears to be inappropriate vasodilation in nonexercising muscles, which causes an exaggerated fall in systemic vascular resistance. Increased baroreceptor activity, secondary to wall stress or ischemia, has been invoked as the initial trigger [15]. Vascular instability is associated with an increased risk of SCD, although its prognostic impact is confined largely to patients under the age of 50.

Nonsustained VT

Ventricular arrhythmia has been documented in 90% of adults with HCM on a 24-h ambulatory ECG monitoring. Of these one-fifth have in excess of 200 ventricular extrasystoles and ventricular couplets are detected in at least 40%. Nonsustained ventricular tachycardia (NSVT), defined as three or more beats at a rate of ≥120 bpm, is found in about 20% of patients on Holter monitoring. The incidence of NSVT increases with age, although the associated risk is most prominent in young patients [16].

Other risk factors

Patients with LVOTO (gradient ≥30 mm Hg) at rest are at increased risk of death and progression to severe, disabling symptoms [17]. However, the positive predictive value of obstruction for SCD is not sufficient to justify prophylactic ICD insertion solely on this basis. Treatment should be directed towards gradient reduction; options include beta-blockers, disopyramide, alcohol septal ablation, and surgical myectomy.

In patients with symptoms of angina, coronary angiography may be indicated to identify coexisting CAD, which is associated with an increased risk of SCD. Risk factors for ischemic heart disease should also be optimized [18].

AF, either paroxysmal or chronic, has been documented in 20–25% of HCM patients. While AF is not a strong independent predictor of SCD, it may provoke ventricular tachyarrhythmia in susceptible patients and is associated with significant thromboembolic risk, warranting anticoagulation. Amiodarone is often effective in maintaining sinus rhythm.

The role of genotyping in risk stratification remains to be fully defined. Limited studies suggest that the clinical phenotype of troponin T mutations in some families is characterized by mild or subclinical hypertrophy [13], but a high incidence of SCD. In contrast, outcomes in families with β-myosin heavy chain mutations are heterogeneous and allele dependent [19]. It should be emphasized, however, that these inferences were drawn from relatively small numbers of genotyped families subject to referral bias. Increased availability of molecular genetic analysis in the future should facilitate elucidation of genotype–phenotype correlations, and the recent development of a rapid laboratory DNA test for HCM will undoubtedly contribute significantly. The Laboratory for Molecular Medicine (a clinical diagnostic testing facility within the Harvard Partners Center for Genetics and Genomics [http://www.hpcgg.org/LMM/tests.html]) currently analyses the five most common HCM genes (i.e. β-myosin heavy chain, myosin-binding protein C, cardiac troponin T, cardiac troponin I, and α-tropomyosin) for disease-causing mutations.

Electrophysiological study (EPS)

Programmed ventricular stimulation offers no advantage over noninvasive risk stratification in HCM. In contrast to CAD, monomorphic VT is rarely inducible in patients with HCM. Stimulation with three premature depolarizations in right and left ventricular sites commonly induces polymorphic VT or VF, a nonspecific response frequently observed in patients with CAD or nonischemic cardiomyopathy. Paradoxically, a substantial proportion of VF-arrest survivors with HCM are not inducible. Programmed ventricular stimulation is therefore of limited value in predicting arrhythmic risk in HCM. Conversely, EPS has an important role in the investigation and ablation of accessory pathways in patients with HCM and preexcitation.

Prevention

Patients with any form of cardiomyopathy, be it HCM, DCM, or ARVC, are generally discouraged from participating in competitive sports. Intense physical activity involving burst exertion (e.g. sprinting), strenuous isometric exercise (e.g. heavy lifting), or endurance training (e.g. marathon running) is best avoided, as are the dehydration and electrolyte imbalances to which athletes may be prone. Recreational activity and moderate levels of exercise may continue.

ICD therapy is strongly warranted for secondary prevention of SCD in HCM patients with a previous cardiac arrest or sustained, spontaneously occurring VT. A retrospective multicenter study reported an appropriate discharge rate of 11% per year in this high-risk subgroup [9]. Among patients who underwent device implantation for primary prevention, the annual intervention rate was about 5%. There may, however, be a substantial time lag between ICD insertion and discharge. Extended follow-up is therefore critical for assessing the survival benefit of ICDs in patients with HCM. An ongoing multicenter international study of HCM patients with ICDs is currently in progress to address this.

The presence of multiple clinical risk factors conveys greater likelihood for future sudden death events of sufficient magnitude to justify aggressive prophylactic treatment with the ICD for primary prevention of sudden death. Nevertheless, strong consideration should be afforded for a prophylactic ICD in any individual patient on the strength of at least one risk factor regarded to be major with respect to the clinical profile (e.g. a family history of sudden death in close relatives).

However, because the positive predictive value of any single risk factor for sudden death in HCM is low, such management decisions must often be based on individual judgment for the particular patient, by taking into account and integrating an overall clinical profile that includes age, the strength of the risk factor identified, the level of risk acceptable to the patient and family, and the potential complications largely related to the lead systems and to inappropriate device discharges. It is also worth noting that physician and patient attitudes toward ICDs (and the access to such devices within the respective health care system) can vary considerably among countries and cultures, and thereby impact importantly on clinical decision-making and the threshold for implant in HCM. The ACC/AHA/NASPE 2002 guidelines have designated the ICD for primary prevention of sudden death as a class IIb indication and for secondary prevention (after cardiac arrest) as a class I indication. The risk stratification pyramid in Figure 8.1 summarizes the contributing factors.

High-risk children with HCM pose a particularly difficult management problem. Device implantation at an early age will necessitate multiple upgrades, replacements, and lead revisions; growth can lead to displacement of transvenous leads. Paradoxically, the propensity towards SCD appears particularly high in childhood, often creating a clinical dilemma in management.

Dilated cardiomyopathy

Dilated carodiomyopathy is a chronic heart muscle disease characterized by enlargement and impaired systolic function of the LV or both ventricles. The degree of myocardial dysfunction is not explained by secondary causes such as systemic hypertension, valve disease, previous infarction, or ongoing ischemia. Patients with DCM typically present with symptoms of left ventricular failure such as dyspnoea, fatigue, and diminished exercise tolerance. Occasionally, however, stroke and SCD are the first clinical manifestations. Onset may be at any age, although the clinical impact of DCM is most

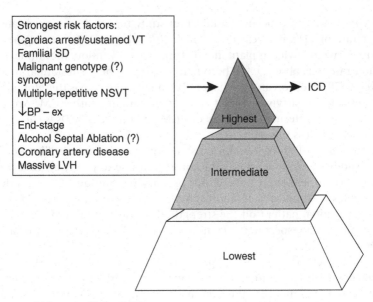

Strongest risk factors:
Cardiac arrest/sustained VT
Familial SD
Malignant genotype (?)
syncope
Multiple-repetitive NSVT
↓BP – ex
End-stage
Alcohol Septal Ablation (?)
Coronary artery disease
Massive LVH

Highest

Intermediate

Lowest

ICD

Figure 8.1 Risk pyramid for HCM.

prominent in young people, in whom it represents the leading indication for cardiac transplantation. Advances in pharmacological and device therapy over the past two decades have effected significant reductions in morbidity and mortality from the disease. Optimal identification of patients at risk of SCD continues to pose a major clinical challenge.

Aetiology of DCM

While the majority of cases of DCM were previously considered sporadic and idiopathic, the familial form is now recognized to account for at least 40–60% [20]. Pedigree analysis reveals autosomal dominant transmission in most families with DCM. Autosomal recessive, mitochondrial, and X-linked inheritance are also described. Since DCM is a genetically heterogeneous disease, multiple underlying molecular mechanisms have been invoked (Table 8.2) [21].

Other factors implicated in the pathogenesis of DCM include persistent viral infection, autoimmunity, infiltrative processes such as hemochromatosis, and toxins (notably alcohol and anthracycline derivatives such as doxorubicin). The final common pathway involves triggering neuroendocrine activation and local production of cytokines, causing maladaptive myocyte hypertrophy, apoptosis, and fibrosis, with consequent ventricular remodeling.

Familial evaluation

Variable penetrance and incomplete disease expression in relatives contribute to underestimation of the true prevalence of familial DCM. Isolated LV enlargement (LV end diastolic diameter ≥112% predicted) and mild contractile impairment are common among asymptomatic relatives [22],

Table 8.2 Molecular pathways underlying disease expression in DCM.

Mechanism	Mutations	Comments
Impaired transmission of force from sarcomere to extracellular matrix	*Cytoskeletal proteins* such as actin, desmin, metavinculin, dystrophin, and the sarcoglycans	May be associated with skeletal myopathy
Deficit in force generation	*Sarcomeric proteins* such as cardiac β-myosin and troponin T (autosomal dominant); troponin I (autosomal recessive)	More frequently associated with hypertrophic cardiomyopathy
Compromised cellular energy production	Recessive mutations in *carnitine*, required for transport of long-chain fatty acids into the mitochondria, and related proteins	
Nuclear envelope disruption, leading to myocyte damage and death	*Emerin* (X-linked) and *Lamin A/C* (autosomal dominant)	DCM with atrioventricular block +/− muscular dystrophy

many of whom have immunohistologic findings similar to those with established disease [23].

History and physical examination alone are therefore insufficient to detect the disease. Evaluation of family members with 12-lead ECG and 2D echocardiography is encouraged. Cardiopulmonary exercise testing is useful as an adjunct; peak oxygen consumption may be reduced in relatives with LV enlargement [24]. Abnormalities remain mild and static in most relatives, but a significant proportion develops overt DCM. Since predictors of disease progression are currently lacking, continued follow-up for all affected relatives is recommended. Whether adults with a normal evaluation should undergo periodic rescreening is unresolved. Although age-related penetrance is documented, the onset of overt disease expression is often unpredictable, even within the same family. However, a small proportion of adults will benefit from surveillance, leading some investigators to advocate serial assessment on a 3–5 yearly basis [25].

Pharmacological therapy for heart failure

Large-scale clinical trials have demonstrated the efficacy of angiotensin converting enzyme (ACE) inhibitors, angiotensin receptor antagonists, and beta-blockers in reducing morbidity and mortality in DCM. Spironolactone, an aldosterone receptor antagonist, is associated with a survival benefit in patients with advanced heart failure (New York Heart Association [NYHA] class IV) [26]. Anticoagulation is recommended in patients with moderate to severe LV dilation to reduce the risk of thromboembolism. Brain natriuretic peptide appears to correlate with LV dimensions and ejection fraction; monitoring of plasma levels may be of value in assessing the therapeutic response [27].

Interventional therapy for heart failure

Inter- and intraventricular conduction disturbances often occur in chronic heart failure, with prolongation of the QRS duration to >120 ms, most commonly observed as left bundle branch block (LBBB). Conduction delay appears to an independent predictor of increased risk in DCM [28], and the resulting mechanical dyscoordination is the target of cardiac resynchronization therapy (CRT). Between 7% and 14% of patients with DCM are candidates for CRT, depending on the stringency of the selection criteria [29]. A number of recent studies have shown improvements in LV ejection fraction, exercise capacity, and quality of life with atrial-synchronized biventricular pacing. The hemodynamic benefit appears to be related to decreased septal dyskinesia and mitral regurgitation, and increased LV filling time. Reversal of chamber remodeling and reduction in myocardial energy demand are also observed [30]. Evidence of mechanical dyssynchrony on tissue Doppler echocardiography is proving more reliable than electrical markers in the prospective identification of responders to CRT [31].

Arrhythmia in DCM

Atrial fibrillation affects 15–30% of patients with heart failure due to DCM, becoming more prevalent with increasing disease severity. New onset of AF may precipitate acute decompensation, particularly in the presence of a rapid ventricular response rate. However, the prognosis of patients with advanced heart failure and AF is becoming more favorable, consequent perhaps to avoidance of class I antiarrhythmic agents and more widespread use of ACE inhibitors, amiodarone, and warfarin [32].

Patients with DCM show a high incidence of ventricular arrhythmia. Almost half have frequent ventricular extrasystoles ($\geq$10/h) on ambulatory ECG monitoring; NSVT is present in up to 35%. However, sustained monomorphic VT is rare, occurring in 1–2% [33].

Arrhythmogenesis in DCM is generally attributed to the interstitial and replacement fibrosis observed on histology. Fractionated electrocardiograms suggest slow and inhomogeneous conduction in these areas, predisposing to reentrant arrhythmia. Indeed, mapping of explanted DCM hearts during VF has demonstrated epicardial reentrant wavefronts with conduction block at sites of increased fibrosis [34].

In contrast, VT in DCM does not appear to be related to reentry. Three-dimensional intraoperative mapping has been performed on hearts from patients undergoing transplantation for DCM. Both, spontaneous and induced ventricular extrasystoles and NSVT originated primarily in the subendocardium by a focal mechanism, the exact nature of which remains to be defined. There was no clear correlation with the histology at these locations [35]. However, abnormal conduction at sites of extensive collagen infiltration may play a key role in promoting acceleration of VT and deterioration into VF, with its hallmark multiple reentrant circuits. Deranged electrolytes and stretch-induced arrhythmia secondary to mechanical overload may also contribute to arrhythmogenesis in DCM.

SCD in DCM

Sudden cardiac death accounts for at least 30% of overall mortality from DCM. Ventricular tachyarrhythmia is the most prominent aetiology in other-wise stable patients. However, pulmonary or systemic embolization, brady-arrhythmia, and electromechanical dissociation (EMD) are also important precipitants, particularly in advanced disease. Cardiac arrest secondary to bradyarrhythmia or EMD may be more frequent in patients with NYHA class IV heart failure requiring treatment with intravenous inotropic drugs and high-dose loop diuretics [36].

An ICD is mandatory for DCM patients with a previous cardiac arrest or spontaneous sustained VT. Annual discharge rates of at least 12% have been reported in patients who underwent device implantation for secondary pre-vention [37]. The incidence of appropriate shocks was almost as high in DCM patients with unexplained syncope, which is also a compelling indication for an ICD [38]. Programmed ventricular stimulation is not useful in the risk stratification of these patients, and may unnecessarily delay ICD insertion [39].

The utility of programmed ventricular stimulation has also been assessed in DCM patients with nonsustained VT. Inducibility of sustained mono-morphic VT varies from 0–14%, with low positive and negative predictive value. A further 0–29% has inducible polymorphic VT or VF, which is widely considered a nonspecific response to aggressive stimulation protocols [40]. The low induction rate in DCM is in contrast to the myocardial infarction population, probably reflecting the lack of stable reentrant circuits in the former.

The prospective observational Marburg Cardiomyopathy Study (MACAS) was designed to determine the clinical value of noninvasive prognostic indicators in a large cohort of patients with DCM. The exclusion criteria included a history of sustained VT or VF, unexplained syncope within the previous 12 months, and amiodarone therapy. Over 340 patients were enrolled and underwent evaluation with echocardiography, signal-averaged ECG (SAECG), ambulatory ECG monitoring, and microvolt T-wave altern-ans. Heart-rate variability, baroreflex sensitivity, and QTc dispersion were also analyzed.

During a mean follow-up period of 52 months, major arrhythmic events, defined as sustained VT, VF, or SCD, occurred in 13%. The only significant predictor of arrhythmic risk was reduced LV ejection fraction. In addition, there was a tendency towards increased arrhythmic risk in patients with NSVT on Holter monitoring and those who were not on beta-blocker therapy at enrolment. The combination of LV ejection fraction <30% and nonsustained VT was associated with an 8.2-fold risk of major arrhythmic events [41].

Conversely, SAECG, baroreflex sensitivity, heart-rate variability, and T-wave alternans were not helpful in risk stratification. This is in apparent contrast to the findings from several previous reports; smaller study populations, inclusion of patients with sustained VT, and shorter follow-up periods have been cited as possible explanations [38].

ICD or amiodarone?

The Sudden Cardiac Death in Heart Failure Trial (SCD-HeFT) [42] compared placebo, amiodarone, and ICD insertion in >2500 patients with NYHA class II or III heart failure, and LV ejection fraction <35% in spite of optimal medical therapy. Approximately equal number of patients with ischemic heart failure and DCM were recruited. There was a 23% reduction in all-cause mortality at 5 years in the ICD group compared with placebo, while no effect was observed for amiodarone versus placebo. The findings appear to argue against the effectiveness of amiodarone in preventing SCD, and strengthen the case for ICD placement in patients with significant impairment of LV systolic function.

In contrast, the earlier Amiodarone Versus Implantable Defibrillator (AMIOVIRT) study [43] had failed to demonstrate a statistically significant difference in 1- and 3-year survival rates among DCM patients on amiodarone therapy compared with those who received an ICD. Indeed, a trend towards improved arrhythmia-free survival rates and cost of medical care was observed in the patients treated with amiodarone. All patients had LV ejection fraction ≤0.35, documented NSVT, and NYHA functional class I–III. However, both population size and duration of follow-up were considerably smaller than in SCD-HeFT.

Low-dose amiodarone may nonetheless have an important role in suppressing AF in patients with DCM. Furthermore, similar improvements in cardiac symptoms, function, and sympathetic nerve activity over a 1-year treatment period have been reported in patients treated with either beta-blockers or amiodarone [44]. Thus, amiodarone may be a useful alternative in patients with heart failure who cannot tolerate beta-blocker therapy.

At present, a pragmatic approach to risk stratification entails prioritizing patients with a prior cardiac arrest, sustained VT, or syncope for ICD insertion. For the remainder, medical therapy with serial assessment of LV function and ambulatory ECG monitoring is recommended. The evidence appears to support offering prophylactic ICD insertion to patients with LV ejection fraction <30% on optimal medical therapy, particularly in the presence of NSVT. Low-dose amiodarone therapy may be a useful adjunct to treatment in asymptomatic patients with improved LV function (>35%) and NSVT on ambulatory ECG monitoring. The current recommendations are summarized in Figure 8.2.

Arrhythmogenic right ventricular cardiomyopathy

Arrhythmogenic right ventricular cardiomyopathy has long been defined by its pathological hallmark of myocardial atrophy and fibrofatty replacement

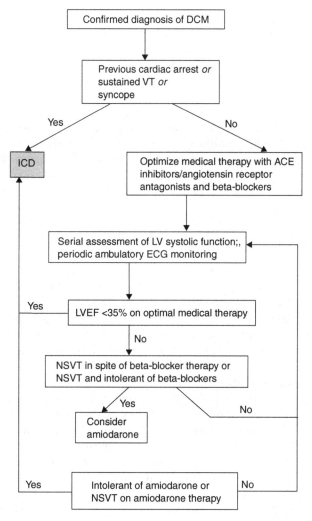

Figure 8.2 Flow chart of recommended approach to risk stratification in DCM.

within the right ventricle (RV). Initial clinical descriptions were of adults with monomorphic VT of LBBB morphology, indicating its right ventricular origin, and an enlarged RV in the presence of normal pulmonary vasculature. The condition was thought to arise from a developmental abnormality of the RV myocardium, leading to the original designation of right ventricular cardiomyopathy. This conception has evolved, over the last 25 years, into our current perspective of a genetically determined heart muscle disease with diverse phenotypic manifestations. Although heart failure is an important complication of advanced disease, ARVC exerts far greater clinical impact as a cause of ventricular arrhythmia and SCD, which represents a key distinction from DCM.

Natural history of ARVC

Four distinct phases have been described in the natural history of ARVC [45], although familial evaluation suggests that stepwise progression to advanced disease occurs in only a minority of patients:

1 The early "concealed" phase, which may be associated with minor ventricular arrhythmia. Patients are often asymptomatic, but may nonetheless be at risk of SCD, notably during extreme exertion. Structural changes, when present, are subtle and may be confined to one region of the so-called triangle of dysplasia: the inflow, outflow, and apical portions of the RV.

2 Overt electrical disorder, in which symptomatic ventricular arrhythmia is observed, accompanied by more obvious morphological and functional abnormalities of the RV. This is typically of LBBB morphology, indicating its RV origin, and ranges from isolated ventricular extrasystoles to nonsustained or sustained VT.

3 Progression of myocardial disease results in RV failure with relatively preserved LV function.

4 Significant LV involvement with biventricular failure occurs in the advanced stage, leading to a phenotype that resembles DCM. Fibrofatty substitution of the LV myocardium was present on histology in 76% of postmortem and explanted hearts in a multicenter study correlating clinical and pathologic features of ARVC [46]. Arrhythmic events, heart failure, and inflammatory infiltrates were more frequent in patients with disease involving the LV.

Genetic basis of ARVC

One of the landmarks in our understanding of the disease came with the identification of a mutation in plakoglobin as the cause of Naxos disease, an autosomal recessive variant of ARVC associated with palmoplantar keratoderma and woolly hair [47]. More recently, mutations in desmoplakin have been linked to autosomal dominant forms of ARVC [48]. Plakoglobin and desmoplakin are key components of desmosomes, the adhesive junctions between cells. Under conditions of mechanical stress, the inherent weakness of the mutant cell adhesion proteins results in myocyte detachment and death. An inflammatory response may accompany the injury; scattered foci of lymphocytes have been documented in up to 67% of hearts on post-mortem. Repair by fibrofatty replacement follows. The inverse relationship between wall stress and wall thickness may explain the increased susceptibility of the thin-walled RV, and the predilection of early ARVC for its thinnest portions: the triangle of dysplasia.

Clinical presentation of ARVC

Arrhythmogenic right ventricular cardiomyopathy typically presents with symptoms of arrhythmia, such as palpitation, presyncope, and syncope. Unfortunately, VF arrest is the first clinical manifestation of the disease in over 50% of index cases [49], often young people engaged in strenuous activity. This underscores the need to evaluate the family members of SCD victims for the disease. Since penetrance may be as low as 15–30% in some families, second-degree relatives should also be offered screening. Serial assessment of asymptomatic relatives is generally advised from early puberty; childhood cases of ARVC are documented but extremely rare. Contrary to traditional thinking, there is no age limit beyond which disease expression becomes unlikely. Presentation in later life is probably under-recognized; many older patients with ARVC undoubtedly have a presumptive diagnosis of heart failure secondary to CAD. From a practical standpoint, however, the frequency of evaluation may be reduced after middle age.

Affected relatives identified during familial assessment are increasingly represented among the ARVC population. Similarly, preparticipation screening of athletes consistently yields a small but significant proportion of cases. A minority of patients may present with RV failure in the absence of pulmonary hypertension, or biventricular failure mimicking DCM. There is growing appreciation of early biventricular involvement in ARVC. Disease variants that primarily affect the LV are also recognized, highlighting the potential overlap with DCM [50]. A family history of sudden premature death without previously established heart failure raises the suspicion of ARVC, as does prominent ventricular arrhythmia with minimal ventricular enlargement or dysfunction in a relative.

Clinical diagnosis of ARVC

Patients in whom ARVC is suspected should be evaluated with 12-lead ECG, SAECG, 2D echocardiography and/or cardiac magnetic resonance, and ambulatory ECG monitoring. Exercise testing may unmask ventricular arrhythmia and is also recommended. A similar noninvasive evaluation should be offered to all first and second-degree relatives of ARVC index cases.

The clinical features of ARVC tend to be nonspecific, and a single test is seldom diagnostic. To facilitate and standardize clinical diagnosis, an international task force proposed a criteria for ARVC in 1994 (Table 8.3)[42]. The guidelines were developed by expert consensus at a time when the prevailing perception of ARVC was dominated by experience with symptomatic index cases and SCD victims – that is, the severe end of the disease spectrum. Accordingly, the task force criteria are highly specific but lack sensitivity for the concealed phase of ARVC and the familial form, where disease expression is incomplete. As such, their main use is in establishing the diagnosis in index cases. Furthermore, the breadth of phenotypic variation in ARVC is only now being elucidated. Revision of existing guidelines will ultimately become a necessity, and has already been addressed to some extent in the setting of familial disease.

Prospective evaluation of the relatives of ARVC index cases has identified a subset with isolated, minor cardiac abnormalities that do not fulfill the task force criteria. Since these features are likely to represent disease expression within the context of autosomal dominant inheritance, modified criteria have been proposed for familial ARVC (Table 8.4)[51].

Table 8.3 Task force criteria for diagnosis of ARVC in *index cases*.

1. Family history
Major
Familial disease confirmed at necropsy or surgery.
Minor
Family history of premature sudden death (<35 years of age) due to suspected ARVC.
Family history – clinical diagnosis based on present criteria.

2. ECG depolarization/conduction abnormalities
Major
Epsilon waves or localized prolongation (>110 ms) of QRS complex in right precordial leads (V1–V3).
Minor
Late potentials on signal-averaged EKG.

3. ECG repolarization abnormalities
Minor
Inverted T waves in right precordial leads (V2 and V3) in people >12 years of age and in absence of right bundle branch block.

4. Arrhythmias
Minor
Sustained or nonsustained LBBB-type VT documented on EKG or Holter monitoring or during exercise testing.
Frequent ventricular extrasystoles (>1000/24 h on Holter monitoring).

5. Global or regional dysfunction and structural alterations
Major
Severe dilatation and reduction of right ventricular ejection fraction with no or mild left ventricular involvement.
Localized right ventricular aneurysms (akinetic or dyskinetic areas with diastolic bulgings).
Severe segmental dilatation of right ventricle.
Minor
Mild global right ventricular dilatation or ejection fraction reduction with normal left ventricle.
Mild segmental dilatation of right ventricle.
Regional right ventricular hypokinesia.

6. Tissue characteristics of walls
Major
Fibrofatty replacement of myocardium on endomyocardial biopsy.

ARVC or idiopathic right ventricular arrhythmia?

In evaluating a patient with arrhythmia of RV origin, the differential diagnosis is between ARVC and idiopathic right ventricular arrhythmia (IRVA), a focal arrhythmic disorder that is widely reported to have an excellent prognosis. The original description of "idiopathic right ventricular outflow tract tachycardia"

Table 8.4 Proposed modification of task force criteria for the diagnosis of *Familial* ARVC.

ARVC in first-degree relative plus one of the following:

ECG
T-wave inversion in right precordial leads (V2 and V3).

Signal-averaged electrocardiogram
Late potentials seen on signal-averaged electrocardiogram.

Arrhythmia
Left bundle branch block-type ventricular tachycardia on EKG, Holter monitoring or
  during exercise testing.
Extrasystoles >200 over a 24-h period.

Structural or functional abnormality of the right ventricle
Mild global right ventricular dilatation and/or reduction in ejection fraction with
normal left ventricle.
Mild segmental dilatation of the right ventricle.
Regional right ventricular hypokinesia.

Note: Applicability is confined to first-degree relatives who do not fulfil the original
task force guidelines.

reflected the significant proportion that arises from discrete sites in the free wall of the pulmonary infundibulum. An inferior-axis QRS configuration of the VT is typical but not requisite; 10% of cases of IRVA in a recent series did not map to the right ventricular outflow tract [52]. Conversely, VT associated with ARVC may be localized to the outflow tract, limiting the diagnostic value of this feature. Discrimination is critical, as management of the two diseases is quite distinct. IRVA frequently responds to verapamil and radio frequency ablation may be curative. Furthermore, a diagnosis of IRVA obviates the need for familial assessment since it has no hereditary basis.

In IRVA 12-lead ECG, SAECG, and imaging studies are unremarkable; however, this is also true of many patients with early ARVC. A history of premature SCD or unexplained heart failure in a relative, raises suspicion of ARVC. However, absence of a conspicuous family history does not exclude ARVC, owing to variable penetrance and the possibility of a *de novo* mutation.

Invasive EPS, while not a routine component of the diagnostic work-up for ARVC, may have a role in the differentiation of IRVA from ARVC. Consistent with a reentrant mechanism, VT in overt ARVC may be inducible by programmed ventricular stimulation, exhibits entrainment, and is associated with fragmented diastolic potentials. In contrast, VT in IRVA has electrophysiological characteristics compatible with the proposed focal mechanism, including the frequent requirement of an isoprenaline infusion and/or burst pacing for provocation. Nevertheless, a proportion of patients with spontaneous ventricular arrhythmia will not be inducible at EPS, regardless of the underlying diagnosis. Indeed, establishing a definitive diagnosis may not be possible at first presentation; patients have been assigned a diagnosis of IRVA until typical features of ARVC evolved some years later. Continued follow-up of patients with presumed IRVA is therefore recommended.

Risk stratification in ARVC

All patients with a confirmed diagnosis of ARVC are discouraged from participating in competitive sports and endurance training. The rationale for this is two-fold; sympathetic stimulation is known to precipitate arrhythmia, while excessive mechanical stress may aggravate the underlying disease process. As in HCM, however, the majority of deaths occur during sedentary activity [53]. Ventricular arrhythmia in ARVC may respond to beta-blockers, which are frequently prescribed first-line. Amiodarone may be used in conjunction or as lone therapy. Sotalol and mexiletine have also been advocated. Standard heart failure therapy is indicated for patients with ventricular dysfunction.

The annual mortality rate in ARVC patients on medical treatment has been reported as around 1%. Arrhythmic death accounts for the majority of fatalities; however, advanced heart failure and embolic stroke are causative in a small proportion. SCD may occur without premonitory symptoms and the disease course is often unpredictable. Consequently, recent years have seen a trend towards ICD insertion when the diagnosis of ARVC has been established. Follow-up studies have confirmed a high incidence of appropriate ICD shocks in certain high-risk groups, underscoring the significant survival benefit [54,55]. The annual discharge rate was 10% among ARVC patients with a previous cardiac arrest or hemodynamically unstable VT, and 8% in patients with unexplained syncope [54]. Conversely, intervention for VF occurred in only 3% of ARVC patients who underwent ICD placement for VT without hemodynamic compromise.

In patients without recognized predictors of SCD, the potential prognostic value of prophylactic ICD therapy may be somewhat tempered by a significant risk of complications. Only 56% of ARVC patients with ICDs remained free from severe adverse events 7 years after device implantation in one tertiary centre series [55]. Thus, indiscriminate ICD recommendations are unlikely to benefit the majority of patients. Even less is known about long-term outcomes in the growing cohort of patients with familial ARVC. The majority may have a favorable prognosis, analogous to the benign course of HCM in community-based populations without referral bias. Developing a risk stratification algorithm for ARVC will be one of the key challenges for the next decade.

Long-term follow-up of patients with Naxos disease has yielded the following predictors of SCD: arrhythmic syncope, LV involvement, early onset of symptoms, and early structural progression [41]. The 3% annual disease-related mortality was higher than that reported in other populations, suggesting that recessive ARVC may have a worse prognosis. Of note, QRS dispersion ≥40 ms, well-tolerated sustained VT, and a family history of SCD were not significantly related to adverse outcome.

Applicability of the Naxos data to autosomal dominant forms of the disease awaits validation. However, a multicenter study of 132 ARVC patients with ICDs confirmed that prior cardiac arrest, VT with hemodynamic compromise, and LV involvement (LV ejection fraction <55%) were independent predictors of ventricular flutter or fibrillation. Furthermore, younger patients with progressive disease appear more predisposed to VF [54], probably in association with so-called "hot phases"; recurrent bouts of myocyte loss and inflammation. Repair by fibrofatty replacement eventually leads to the formation of stable reentrant circuits; thus patients with later stages of the disease may have sustained monomorphic VT that is well tolerated and less likely to deteriorate into VF.

As in DCM and HCM, programmed ventricular stimulation was not helpful in risk assessment of patients with ARVC. Over 50% of patients with inducible VT did not experience ICD therapy in the 3-year follow-up period, whereas a similar proportion of patients who were not inducible had appropriate interventions.

At present, overwhelming indications for ICD insertion in ARVC include previous VF arrest, VT with impairment of consciousness, or sustained VT

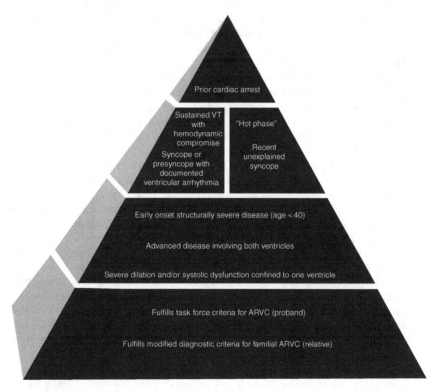

Figure 8.3 Risk stratification pyramid for ARVC.

that is refractory to drug treatment. The evidence also favors offering device implantation to patients with LV involvement or unexplained syncope. Young patients with prominent structural abnormalities, such as marked RV dilation or systolic dysfunction, may also be candidates, as are those with symptomatic exacerbation and/ or ECG changes suggestive of a "hot phase." A risk stratification pyramid illustrating these concepts is shown in Figure 8.3.

In contrast, the evidence supporting ICD therapy for sustained monomorphic VT without hemodynamic compromise is more limited. The exception is the patient who is intolerant to antiarrhythmic drugs and may benefit from antitachycardia pacing to terminate the events. Other proposed predictors of arrhythmic risk include inverted T waves beyond V3, which may correlate with LV involvement, and QRS dispersion $\geq$40 ms [56]. While prospective trials are lacking, clinical judgment on an individual basis should dictate the need for intervention in these instances.

References

1. Maron BJ, McKenna WJ, Danielson GK *et al.* Cardiology; Committee for Practice Guidelines. European Society of Cardiology. American College of Cardiology/European Society of Cardiology clinical expert consensus document on hypertrophic cardiomyopathy. A report of the American College of Cardiology Foundation Task Force on Clinical Expert Consensus Documents and the European Society of Cardiology Committee for Practice Guidelines. *J Am Coll Cardiol* 2003; **42**(9): 1687–1713.
2. Oechslin EN, Attenhofer Jost CH, Rojas JR, Kaufmann PA, Jenni R. Long-term follow-up of 34 adults with isolated left ventricular noncompaction: a distinct cardiomyopathy with poor prognosis. *J Am Coll Cardiol* 2000; **36**(2): 493–500.
3. Charron P, Carrier L, Dubourg O, *et al.* Penetrance of familial hypertrophic cardiomyopathy. *Genet Couns* 1997; **8**(2): 107–114.
4. McKenna WJ, Spirito P, Desnos M, Dubourg O, Komajda M. Experience from clinical genetics in hypertrophic cardiomyopathy: proposal for new diagnostic criteria in adult members of affected families. *Heart* 1997; **77**(2): 130–132.
5. Blair E, Redwood C, Ashrafian H, *et al.* Mutations in the gamma(2) subunit of AMP-activated protein kinase cause familial hypertrophic cardiomyopathy: evidence for the central role of energy compromise in disease pathogenesis. *Hum Mol Genet* 2001; **10**(11): 1215–1220.
6. Maron BJ, Casey SA, Poliac LC, *et al.* Clinical course of hypertrophic cardiomyopathy in a regional United States cohort. *JAMA* 1999; **281**(7): 650–655.
7. Maron BJ. Sudden death in young athletes. *N Engl J Med* 2003; **349**(11): 1064–1075.
8. Corrado D, Basso C, Schiavon M, Thiene G. Screening for hypertrophic cardiomyopathy in young athletes. *N Engl J Med* 1998; **339**(6): 364–369.
9. Maron BJ, Shen WK, Link MS, *et al.* Efficacy of implantable cardioverter-defibrillators for the prevention of sudden death in patients with hypertrophic cardiomyopathy. *N Engl J Med* 2000; **342**(6): 365–373.
10. Elliott PM, Poloniecki J, Dickie S, *et al.* Sudden death in hypertrophic cardiomyopathy: identification of high risk patients. *J Am Coll Cardiol* 2000; **36**(7): 2212–2218.

11. Spirito P, Bellone P, Harris KM, *et al*. Magnitude of left ventricular hypertrophy and risk of sudden death in hypertrophic cardiomyopathy. *N Engl J Med* 2000; **342**(24): 1778–1785.
12. Elliott PM, Gimeno Blanes JR, Mahon NG, Poloniecki JD, McKenna WJ. Relation between severity of left-ventricular hypertrophy and prognosis in patients with hypertrophic cardiomyopathy. *Lancet* 2001; **357**(9254): 420–424.
13. Varnava AM, Elliott PM, Baboonian C, *et al*. Hypertrophic cardiomyopathy: histopathological features of sudden death in cardiac troponin T disease. *Circulation* 2001; **104**(12): 1380–1384.
14. Mogensen J, Kubo T, Duque M, *et al*. Idiopathic restrictive cardiomyopathy is part of the clinical expression of cardiac troponin I mutations. *J Clin Invest* 2003; **111**(2): 209–216.
15. Lim PO, Morris-Thurgood JA, Frenneaux MP. Vascular mechanisms of sudden death in hypertrophic cardiomyopathy, including blood pressure responses to exercise. *Cardiol Rev* 2002; **10**(1): 15–23.
16. Monserrat L, Elliott PM, Gimeno JR, *et al*. Non-sustained ventricular tachycardia in hypertrophic cardiomyopathy: an independent marker of sudden death risk in young patients. *J Am Coll Cardiol* 2003; **42**(5): 873–879.
17. Maron MS, Olivotto I, Betocchi S, *et al*. Effect of left ventricular outflow tract obstruction on clinical outcome in hypertrophic cardiomyopathy. *N Engl J Med* 2003; **348**(4): 295–303.
18. Sorajja P, Ommen SR, Nishimura RA, Gersh BJ, Berger PB, Tajik AJ. Adverse prognosis of patients with hypertrophic cardiomyopathy who have epicardial coronary artery disease. *Circulation* 2003; **108**(19): 2342–2348.
19. Bonne G, Carrier L, Richard P, *et al*. Familial hypertrophic cardiomyopathy: from mutations to functional defects. *Circ Res* 1998; **83**(6): 580–593.
20. Mestroni L, Rocco C, Gregori D, *et al*. Familial dilated cardiomyopathy: evidence for genetic and phenotypic heterogeneity. Heart Muscle Disease Study Group. *J Am Coll Cardiol* 1999; **34**(1): 181–190.
21. Shaw T, Elliott P, McKenna WJ. Dilated cardiomyopathy: a genetically heterogeneous disease. *Lancet* 2002; **360**(9334): 654–655.
22. Baig MK, Goldman JH, Caforio AL, *et al*. Familial dilated cardiomyopathy: cardiac abnormalities are common in asymptomatic relatives and may represent early disease. *J Am Coll Cardiol* 1998; **31**(1): 195–201.
23. Mahon NG, Madden BP, Caforio AL, *et al*. Immunohistologic evidence of myocardial disease in apparently healthy relatives of patients with dilated cardiomyopathy. *J Am Coll Cardiol* 2002; **39**(3): 455–462.
24. Mahon NG, Sharma S, Elliott PM, *et al*. Abnormal cardiopulmonary exercise variables in asymptomatic relatives of patients with dilated cardiomyopathy who have left ventricular enlargement. *Heart* 2000; **83**(5): 511–517.
25. Crispell KA, Hanson EL, Coates K, Toy W, Hershberger RE. Periodic rescreening is indicated for family members at risk of developing familial dilated cardiomyopathy. *J Am Coll Cardiol* 2002; **39**(9): 1503–1507.
26. Pitt B, Zannad F, Remme WJ, *et al*. The effect of spironolactone on morbidity and mortality in patients with severe heart failure. Randomized Aldactone Evaluation Study Investigators. *N Engl J Med* 1999; **341**(10): 709–717.
27. Groenning BA, Nilsson JC, Sondergaard L, *et al*. Evaluation of impaired left ventricular ejection fraction and increased dimensions by multiple neurohumoral plasma concentrations. *Eur J Heart Fail* 2001; **3**(6): 699–708.

28. Iuliano S, Fisher SG, Karasik PE, Fletcher RD, Singh SN. Department of Veterans Affairs Survival Trial of Antiarrhythmic Therapy in Congestive Heart Failure. QRS duration and mortality in patients with congestive heart failure. *Am Heart J* 2002; **143**(6): 1085–1091.
29. Grimm W, Sharkova J, Funck R, *et al.* How many patients with dilated cardiomyopathy do potentially benefit from cardiac resynchronisation therapy using biventricular or left ventricular pacing? *PACE* 2003; **26**: 155–157.
30. St John Sutton MG, Plappert T, Abraham WT, *et al.* Effect of cardiac resynchronization therapy on left ventricular size and function in chronic heart failure. *Circulation* 2003; **107**(15): 1985–1990.
31. Penicka M, Bartunek J, De Bruyne B, *et al.* Improvement of left ventricular function after cardiac resynchronization therapy is predicted by tissue Doppler imaging echocardiography. *Circulation* 2004; **109**(8): 978–983.
32. Naccarelli GV, Hynes BJ, Wolbrette DL, *et al.* Atrial fibrillation in heart failure: prognostic significance and management. *J Cardiovasc Electrophysiol* 2003; **14**(Suppl. 12): S281–S286.
33. Priori SG, Aliot E, Blomstrom-Lundqvist C, *et al.* Update of the guidelines on sudden cardiac death of the European Society of Cardiology. *Eur Heart J* 2003; **24**(1): 13–15.
34. Wu TJ, Ong JJ, Hwang C, Lee JJ, *et al.* Characteristics of wave fronts during ventricular fibrillation in human hearts with dilated cardiomyopathy: role of increased fibrosis in the generation of reentry. *J Am Coll Cardiol* 1998; **32**(1): 187–196.
35. Pogwizd SM, McKenzie JP, Cain ME, *et al.* Mechanisms underlying spontaneous and induced ventricular arrhythmias in patients with idiopathic dilated cardiomyopathy. *Circulation* 1998; **98**(22): 2404–2414.
36. Faggiano P, d'Aloia A, Gualeni A, Gardini A, Giordano A. Mechanisms and immediate outcome of in-hospital cardiac arrest in patients with advanced heart failure secondary to ischemic or idiopathic dilated cardiomyopathy. *Am J Cardiol* 2001; **87**(5): 655–657, A10–A11.
37. Grimm W, Hoffmann J J, Muller HH, Maisch B. Implantable defibrillator event rates in patients with idiopathic dilated cardiomyopathy, nonsustained ventricular tachycardia on Holter and a left ventricular ejection fraction below 30%. *J Am Coll Cardiol* 2002; **39**: 780–787.
38. Fonarow GC, Feliciano Z, Boyle NG, *et al.* Improved survival in patients with nonischemic advanced heart failure and syncope treated with an implantable cardioverter-defibrillator. *Am J Cardiol* 2000; **85**(8): 981–985.
39. Brilakis ES, Shen WK, Hammill SC, *et al.* Role of programmed ventricular stimulation and implantable cardioverter-defibrillators in patients with idiopathic dilated cardiomyopathy and syncope. *Pacing Clin Electrophysiol* 2001; **24**(11): 1623–1630.
40. Grimm W, Hoffmann J, Menz V, Luck K, Maisch B. Programmed ventricular stimulation for arrhythmia risk prediction in patients with idiopathic dilated cardiomyopathy and nonsustained ventricular tachycardia. *J Am Coll Cardiol* 1998; **32**(3): 739–745.
41. Grimm W, Christ M, Bach J, Muller HH, Maisch B. Noninvasive arrhythmia risk stratification in idiopathic dilated cardiomyopathy: results of the Marburg cardiomyopathy study. *Circulation* 2003; **108**(23): 2883–2891.

42. Bardy GH, Lee KL, Mark DB, *et al.* Amiodarone or an implantable cardioverter-defibrillator for congestive heart failure. *N Engl J Med* 2005; **352**: 225–237.
43. Wijetunga M, Strickberger SA. Amiodarone Versus Implantable Defibrillator Randomized Trial (AMIOVIRT): background, rationale, design, methods, results and implications. *Card Electrophysiol Rev* 2003; **7**(4): 452–456.
44. Toyama T, Hoshizaki H, Seki R, *et al.* Efficacy of amiodarone treatment on cardiac symptom, function, and sympathetic nerve activity in patients with dilated cardiomyopathy: comparison with beta-blocker therapy. *J Nucl Cardiol* 2004; **11**(2): 134–141.
45. Corrado D, Fontaine G, Marcus FI, *et al.* Arrhythmogenic right ventricular dysplasia/cardiomyopathy: need for an international registry. *Circulation* 2000; **101**(11): E101–E106.
46. Corrado D, Basso C, Thiene G, *et al.* Spectrum of clinicopathologic manifestations of arrhythmogenic right ventricular cardiomyopathy/dysplasia: a multicenter study. *J Am Coll Cardiol* 1997; **30**(6): 1512–1520.
47. Protonotarios N, Tsatsopoulou A, Anastasakis A, *et al.* Genotype–phenotype assessment in autosomal recessive arrhythmogenic right ventricular cardiomyopathy (Naxos disease) caused by a deletion in plakoglobin. *J Am Coll Cardiol* 2001; **38**(5): 1477–1484.
48. Rampazzo A, Nava A, Malacrida S, *et al.* Mutation in human desmoplakin domain binding to plakoglobin causes a dominant form of arrhythmogenic right ventricular cardiomyopathy. *Am J Hum Genet* 2002; **71**(5): 1200–1206.
49. Nava A, Bauce B, Basso C, *et al.* Clinical profile and long-term follow-up of 37 families with arrhythmogenic right ventricular cardiomyopathy. *J Am Coll Cardiol* 2000; **36**: 2226–2233.
50. Michalodimitrakis M, Papadomanolakis A, Stiakakis J, Kanaki K. Left side right ventricular cardiomyopathy. *Med Sci Law* 2002; **42**: 313–317.
51. Hamid MS, Norman M, Quraishi A, *et al.* Prospective evaluation of relatives for familial arrhythmogenic right ventricular cardiomyopathy reveals a need to broaden diagnostic criteria. *J Am Coll Cardiol* 2002; **40**: 1445–1450.
52. Niroomand F, Carbucicchio C, Tondo C, *et al.* Electrophysiological characteristics and outcome in patients with idiopathic right ventricular arrhythmia compared with arrhythmogenic right ventricular dysplasia. *Heart* 2002; **87**(1): 41–47.
53. Tabib A, Loire R, Chalabreysse L, *et al.* Circumstances of death and gross and microscopic observations in a series of 200 cases of sudden death associated with arrhythmogenic right ventricular cardiomyopathy and/or dysplasia. *Circulation* 2003; **108**(24): 3000–3005.
54. Corrado D, Leoni L, Link MS, *et al.* Implantable cardioverter-defibrillator therapy for prevention of sudden death in patients with arrhythmogenic right ventricular cardiomyopathy/dysplasia. *Circulation* 2003; **108**(25): 3084–3091.
55. Wichter T, Paul M, Wollmann C, *et al.* Implantable cardioverter/defibrillator therapy in arrhythmogenic right ventricular cardiomyopathy: single-center experience of long-term follow-up and complications in 60 patients. *Circulation* 2004; **109**(12): 1503–1508.
56. Peters S, Peters H, Thierfelder L. Risk stratification of sudden cardiac death and malignant ventricular arrhythmias in right ventricular dysplasia-cardiomyopathy. *Int J Cardiol* 1999; **71**(3): 243–250.

CHAPTER 9
Inherited arrhythmogenic diseases

Silvia G. Priori and Charles Antzelevitch

Genetic disorders in the structurally normal heart

Cardiac arrhythmias developing in the absence of structural heart disease have often been referred to as "idiopathic" [1] or "primary" electrical disorders. Only recently it has become evident that most of these disorders are associated with defects in the genes that encode cardiac ion channels and other proteins involved in their regulation (Table 9.1). The presenting symptoms of these diseases include palpitations, syncope, and sudden cardiac death. All these syndromes are characterized by genetic heterogeneity that is, the same clinical phenotype is associated with multiple genetic "loci." To further increase the complexity of the genetic heterogeneity of the arrhythmogenic syndromes it has become clear that within each locus there are many different mutations that are distributed throughout the open reading frame of the gene. A continuously updated list of the mutations identified in these genes is provided on the website "Gene connection for the heart" (http://pc4.fsm.it:81/cardmoc). Since there are no "common" mutations that account for a substantial percentage of the disease-related genes, it is necessary to screen the entire coding sequence of each gene: this feature of the arrhythmogenic syndromes accounts for the long time required to complete molecular diagnosis in these diseases.

It is important to remember that not all the genes responsible for inherited arrhythmogenic diseases have been identified. Therefore not all patients with a clinical diagnosis of any of these diseases can be successfully genotyped. As a consequence, a "negative" result of DNA screening does not rule out the presence of the disease, it simply implies that the gene on which the mutation is located has not been discovered yet.

This chapter will examine the clinical, molecular, and cellular aspects of inherited arrhythmogenic diseases with specific focus on clinical management.

Long-QT syndrome

Clinical presentation
The long-QT syndrome (LQTS) is characterized by syncopal events caused by ventricular tachyarrhythmias (*torsades des pointes* (Tdp)) that begin manifesting

during childhood or adolescence. The estimated prevalence of this disorder is 1–2: 10 000. The ECG diagnosis is based on the presence of prolonged repolarization (QT interval) and abnormal T-wave morphology; cardiac events are often precipitated by physical or emotional stress but they may also occur at rest [2].

Patterns of inheritance and extracardiac manifestations

Two clinical variants of LQTS have been identified: one inherited as an autosomal dominant trait, the Romano Ward syndrome and the other inherited as an autosomal recessive trait, the Jervell and Lange-Nielsen syndrome that combines long-QT intervals, arrhythmia susceptibility, and neurosensorial deafness (Table 9.1). More recently two other forms of LQTS with extracardiac manifestations have been described: (1) Andersen syndrome or LQT7, that combines a skeletal muscle phenotype, prolonged QT interval, and arrhythmias [3,4]; and (2) Timothy syndrome or LQT8 [5,6] that is characterized by syndactyly, cardiac malformations, mental retardation, and other phenotypes in addition to long-QT intervals and arrhythmias.

As many as 35% of LQTS cases appear to occur in sporadic individuals, however molecular analysis has shown that in many of such cases the disease is inherited by parents who are carriers of the genetic defect without clinical manifestations of the disease [7]. More recently it has been reported that parental mosaicism may also account for apparently sporadic cases [6,8].

Genetic bases

In the early 1990s, four LQTS loci were identified on chromosomes 11, 3, 7, and 4 [9–11]. Subsequently positional cloning allowed the identification of *KCNQ1* as the gene of LQT1 on chromosome 11 [12]; shortly after the candidate gene approach led to the identification of *KCNH2* and *SCN5A* as the genes on chromosomes 7 (LQT2) and 3 (LQT3) [13,14]. More recently mutations in two additional genes on chromosome 21, *KCNE1* (LQT5) and *KCNE2* (LQT6) were identified. All the *LQT1–3* and *LQT5–6* genes encode for cardiac ion channels subunits and therefore it was suggested that LQTS is a cardiac ion channel disease. Recent data, however, showed that the gene associated with LQT4 is *ANK2* that encodes for an intracellular protein called Ankyrin that is responsible for "anchoring" ion channels to the cellular membrane [15]. At this point it is clear that the phenotype of LQTS may also be derived by mutations in protein that regulate assembly, trafficking, or function of cardiac ion channels.

The genetic bases of LQTS with extra-cardiac phenotypes has also been identified. One gene has been linked to Andersen's syndrome, *JCNJ2*, encoding for the ion channel Kir 2.1 conducting the inward rectifier current, mutations for these gene account for approximately 50% of cases of LQT7 [16]. The gene for Timothy syndrome is *CACNA1C*, that encodes for the cardiac L-type calcium-channel gene. All LQT8 patients carry the same mutation G406R: it is

Table 9.1 Genetic loci and genes of inherited disorders with normal heart.

Locus Name	Chromosomal Locus	Inheritance	Gene Symbol	Protein	Phenotype	OMIM ID
LQT1	11p15.5	AD	KCNQ1	I_{Ks} potassium channel alpha subunit (KvLQT1)	Long QT	192500
LQT2	7q35-q36	AD	KCNH2	I_{Kr} potassium channel alpha subunit (HERG)	Long QT	152427
LQT3	3p21	AD	SCN5A	Cardiac sodium channel alpha subunits (Nav 1.5)	Long QT	603830
LQT4	4q25-q27	AD	ANK2	Ankyrin B, anchoring protein	Long QT, atrial fibrillation	600919
LQT5	21q22.1-q22.2	AD	KCNE1	I_{Ks} potassium channel beta subunit (MinK)	Long QT	176261
LQT6	21q22.1-q22.2	AD	KCNE2	I_{Kr} potassium channel beta subunit (MiRP)	Long QT	603796
LQT7	17q23.1-q24.2	AD	KCNJ2	I_{K1} potassium channel (Kir2.1)	Long QT, Potassium sensitive periodic paralysis, dysmorphic features	170390
LQT8	12p13.3	AD	CACNA1C	ICa L-type	Long QT, syndactyly, hypoglicemia, hypothermia, mental retardation cardiac malformation	601005
JLNS1	11p15.5	AR	KCNQ1	I_{Ks} potassium channel alpha subunit (KvLQT1)	Long QT, Deafness	220400
JLNS2	21q22.1-q22.2	AR	KCNE1	I_{Ks} potassium channel beta subunit (MinK)	Long QT, Deafness	176261

	Locus	Inheritance	Gene	Protein	Phenotype	OMIM
BrS1	3p21	AD	SCN5A	Cardiac sodium channel (Nav 1.5)	ST segment elevation, RBBB	601144
BrS2	3p22-25	AD	Unknown	Unknown	ST segment elevation, RBBB	—
SQTS1	7q35-q36	AD	KCNH2	I_{Kr} potassium channel alpha subunit (HERG)	Short-QT interval	—
SQTS2	11p15.5	AD	KCNQ1	I_{Ks} potassium channel alpha subunit (KvLQT1)	Short-QT interval	—
SQTS3	17q23.1-q24.2	AD	KCNJ2	I_{K1} potassium channel (Kir2.1)	Short-QT interval	—
ATFB1	11p15.5	AR	KCNQ1	I_{Ks} potassium channel alpha subunit (KvLQT1)	Atrial fibrillation	607554
ATFB2	10q22-q24	AD	Unknown	Unknown	Atrial fibrillation	608583
ATFB3	6q14-16	AD	Unknown	Unknown	Atrial fibrillation	608988
ATFB4	21q22.1-q22.2	AD	KCNE2	I_{Kr} potassium channel beta subunit (MiRP)	Atrial fibrillation	607554
CPVT1	1q42.1-q43	AD	RyR2	Cardiac ryanondine receptor	Exercise-induced arrhythmias, normal resting ECG, bradycardia	604772
CPVT2	1p13.3-p11	AR	CASQ2	Cardiac calsequestrin	Exercise-induced arrhythmias, normal resting ECG, bradycardia	114251

Notes: AD = autosomal dominant; AR = autosomal recessive; RBBB = right bundle branch block.

too early to know if other genes or other mutations may also cause this form of LQTS [6].

Approximately 95% of patients with a known genetic defects are affected by LQT1, LQT2, or LQT3, accordingly a substantial body of genotype–phenotype correlations have been established in patients with these forms of the disease.

Genotype–phenotype correlation

LQT1 is the most prevalent variant of LQTS, accounting for approximately 50% of genotyped patients [17]. Loss of function of the ion channel that conducts the slowly activating delayed rectifier (I_{Ks}) underlies congenital LQT1. LQT1 patients have a typical ECG morphology with a broad-based T-wave with a smooth morphology [18], the prolongation of QT interval in LQT1 patients is often moderate and a high percentage of carriers of mutations have a normal QTc (incomplete penetrance). Patients with a QTc > 500 ms are at a higher risk of becoming symptomatic for cardiac events [19]. The majority of arrhythmic episodes are precipitated by physical exercise [20], for unknown reasons swimming is frequently implicated in arrhythmias development in LQT1 [21]. Interestingly LQT1 patients have a very good response to beta-blockers [22].

The typical features of LQT1 patients have been replicated in *in-vitro* models, in arterially-perfused wedge preparations, inhibition of I_{Ks} using chromanol 293B led to uniform prolongation of action potential duration (APD) in epicardial, M cells (M) and endocardial cells, causing little change in transmural dispersion of repolarization (TDR). Although the QT interval is prolonged, TdP never occurred under these conditions. Addition of isoproterenol resulted in abbreviation of epicardial and endocardial APD while in the M cells, APD either prolonged or remained the same, thus causing an increase in TDR and TdP [23]. The combination of I_{Ks} block and β-adrenergic stimulation created a broad based T wave in the perfused wedge, similar to that observed in patients. These findings help to provide us an understanding of the great sensitivity of LQT1 patients, to sympathetic influences [22,24].

LQT2

The distinguishing ECG feature of LQT2 patients is the presence of flattened T waves with typical second components of the T wave called "notches" [18]. As an average, the QT interval is more prolonged in LQT2 patients than in LQT1 and a smaller percentage of LQT2 patients than LQT1 patients have a normal QTc (incomplete penetrance). Patients with a QTc > 500 ms are at higher risk of becoming symptomatic for cardiac events [19]. The majority of arrhythmic episodes are precipitated by emotional stress [20]: interestingly, acoustic stimuli represent a specific trigger of cardiac events in LQT2 [25]. The response of LQT2 patients to beta-blockers is less remarkable than that of LQT1 patients and therefore in LQT2 patients with a longer QT interval or in those with the occurrence of syncopal events during childhood, the use of a prophylactic implantable cardioverter-defibrillator (ICD) may be considered in combination with beta-blockers [22].

KCNH2 (HERG; causing LQT2) gene encodes for the α subunit of the channel conducting the rapidly activating delayed rectifier potassium channel, I_{Kr}. I_{Kr} inhibition is also responsible for most cases of acquired or drug-induced LQTS thus suggesting that similar pathophysiological mechanisms link LQT2 and acquired LQTS. *In vitro* studies have provided very interesting insights on the electrophysiological mechanisms of LQT2. In the wedge, inhibition of I_{Kr} with D-sotalol produces a preferential prolongation of the M cell action potential, resulting in accentuation of TDR and spontaneous as well as stimulation-induced TdP. If I_{Kr} block is accompanied by hypokalemia, a deeply notched or bifurcated T wave is observed in the wedge preparation, similar to that seen in patients with LQT2. Isoproterenol further exaggerates TDR and increases the incidence of TdP in this model, but only transiently [26].

SCN5A (LQT3)

The prevalence of LQT3 is estimated to be 10–15% of all genotyped patients. For this reason, a much smaller number of LQT3 patients are available and data on genotype–phenotype correlation are therefore less solid than for the other two genotypes in which they are based on a large population of patients.

The ECG of LQT3 patients presents a typical pattern with a very prolonged ST segment and a small, peaked T wave [18]. Most of cardiac events in LQT3 occur at rest or during sleep. The response of LQT3 to therapy with beta-blockers is often incomplete and therefore the implant of an ICD should be considered in these patients for primary prevention of cardiac arrest.

In vitro studies have been able to explain several features of this form of LQTS. *SCN5A* mutations identified in LQT3 cause a gain of function by enhancing the late sodium current (late I_{Na}). *In vitro* augmentation of late I_{Na} using the sea anemone toxin ATX-II produced a preferential prolongation of the M cell action potential in the wedge, resulting in a marked increase in TDR and development of TdP. Because epicardial APD was also significantly prolonged, there was a delay in the onset of the T wave in the wedge, as observed in the clinical syndrome [27]. β-adrenergic stimulation abbreviates APD of all cell types under these conditions, reducing TDR and suppressing TdP [26]; thus providing an explanation for the prevalence of cardiac events at rest in LQT3 patients.

Management of LQTS

All patients with LQTS should be advised to restrict physical activity and exposure to stressful environments; they should avoid QT-prolonging drugs and should receive beta-blockers. In patients who have experienced a cardiac arrest, an ICD is indicated in addition to beta-blockers based on the evidence that these individuals remain at high risk of experiencing cardiac events while on therapy [28]. Patients genotyped as LQT3 and LQT2 may be candidates for an ICD as a primary prophylaxis of cardiac arrest [22].

Brugada syndrome

Clinical presentation

Brugada syndrome (BrS) is an inherited arrhythmogenic disease character-ized by ST segment elevation in the right precordial leads (more than 2 mm in leads V1,V2, and/or V3), with or without right bundle branch block and susceptibility to ventricular tachyarrhythmias. The age of onset of clinical manifestations (syncope or cardiac arrest) is the third to fourth decade of life, although malignant forms with onset during early childhood have been reported [29]. Cardiac events typically occur during sleep or at rest [30]. The disease is inherited as an autosomal dominant trait but there is a striking male to female ratio of 8 : 1 in the occurrence of clinical manifestations. The reason for the increased risk of males is not understood. Interestingly the diagnostic pattern of coved ST segment elevation is not spontaneously present in all affected patients and in some individuals a concealed form of BrS is present that can be unmasked by administration of sodium channel blocking drugs. These patients are at lower risk of cardiac arrhythmias than patients with an overt diagnostic ECG pattern.

Genetic basis and pathophysiology

In 1998, the gene responsible for at least some cases of BrS was identified as the cardiac sodium channel gene (*SCN5A*), thus defining BrS as an allelic disease to LQT3 [31]. Mutations in *SCN5A*, including missense mutations, in frame deletions or frameshifts leading to and early truncation of the protein, have been identified in approximately 20% of patients with BrS. Another BrS locus was reported [32] on the short arm of chromosome 3, but no gene has been identified.

SCN5A mutations identified in BrS cause a reduction of the sodium cur-rent that is believed to amplify the heterogeneities intrinsic to the early phases (phase 1-mediated notch) of the action potential of cells residing in different layers of the right ventricular wall of the heart. The presence of a transient outward current (I_{to})-mediated spike and dome morphology, or notch, in ventricular epicardium but not endocardium, creates a transmural voltage gradient that is responsible for the inscription of the electrocardio-graphic J wave [27,33]. Accentuation of the notch in RV epicardium underlies the accentuation of the J wave or ST segment elevation that characterizes BrS. The arrhythmogenic substrate develops when some RV epicardial site undergo an all-or-none repolarization at the end of phase 1, leading to loss of the action potential dome. Conduction of the action potential dome from sites at which it is maintained to sites at which it is lost causes local reexcitation via phase 2 reentry leading to the development of a closely coupled extrasystole capable of capturing the vulnerable window across the ventricular wall, thus triggering a circus movement reentry in the form of ventricular tachycardia/ventricular fibrillation (VT/VF) [33,34].

A rebalancing of currents active at the end of phase 1 also underlies the unmasking of the syndrome in response to drugs. Vagotonic agents, $I_{K\text{-ATP}}$ activators and hypokalemia achieve this by augmenting outward currents, whereas sodium channel blockers, beta-blockers, cocaine, antidepressants, and antihistamines like terfenadine are likely to accomplish this by reducing inward currents.

Management of BrS

There are no drugs with a proven efficacy in patients with BrS. As a consequence, the only treatment to prevent sudden death is represented by the ICD. To target the use of the ICD it is important to be able to identify patients at highest risk of cardiac events. There is consensus that patients who have experienced syncope and have a spontaneous ECG diagnostic for BrS are at high risk of cardiac events and should receive a defibrillator. The most difficult patients to manage are those who are diagnosed after provocative pharmacologic challenge (i.v. flecainide, propafenone, or ajmaline) or those who are asymptomatic. For these patients the use of programmed electrical stimulation has been proposed by some authors [35] but other groups failed to confirm that the test is of any value [36–38], therefore at present time the management of asymptomatic patients remains empirical.

Familial atrial fibrillation

Clinical presentation

Atrial fibrillation (AF) is the most common sustained arrhythmia encountered in clinical practice, most often it develops in the context of ischemic heart disease, hypertension, and congestive heart failure. However, in 3–30% of cases of AF no underlying cardiovascular disease can be detected and occasionally a familial segregation of the phenotype is observed [39]. Darbar *et al.* [40] recently reported that 5% of AF is familial and this percentage is even higher among patients with lone AF (15%).

Genetic bases and pathophysiology

Brugada *et al.* [41] in 1997, provided the first hint for a genetic predisposition to AF (also called familial atrial fibrillation, FAF). In this report an autosomal dominant inheritance was demonstrated and linkage analysis mapped the FAF locus to a 10cM region on the long arm of chromosome 10 (10q22-q24) in three families; the specific gene is yet to be identified. An additional locus was mapped [42] to chromosome 6q 14-16. More recently Chen *et al.* [43]. and Yang *et al.* [44] demonstrated two additional loci for FAF. In a four-generation Chinese family, AF mapped to chromosome 11p15.5 and a gain of function mutation in the *KCNQ1* gene was identified and shown to segregate with the clinical phenotype. Shortly after, the same authors identified mutations in the

KCNE2 in FAF patients [44]. It is therefore apparent that at least some forms of AF are allelic disorders to LQTS in which gain of function mutations cause an accelerated repolarization that predisposes to atrial arrhythmias.

Atrial fibrillation may also occur in families in the presence of cardiac channelopathies such as the long-QT [45], short-QT [46], and Brugada [47] syndromes; these congenital ion channelopathies may lead to enhanced spatial dispersion and phase 2 reentry in the atria, thus providing both the substrate and the trigger for the induction of AF. At present time, nothing is known on specific features that may distinguish patients with inherited AF from those with acquired forms of the disease.

Short-QT syndrome

Clinical presentation

The first anecdotal report of a disease characterized by abnormally abbreviated repolarization detected at the surface ECG was made by Gussak *et al.* in 2000 [48]. They described two siblings and their mother with persistently short-QT-interval ranging from 260 to 275 ms. Sudden death was also present in another unrelated patient showing a similar electrocardiographic pattern. More recently Gaita *et al.* [46], reported two additional families with a history of sudden cardiac death showing this phenotype in the absence of structural heart disease. VF was inducible with programmed electrical stimulation (PES) in all surviving affected individuals.

Another distinctive feature of the ECG identified in some patients with the short-QT syndrome (SQTS) is the appearance of tall peaked T waves, similar to those encountered with hyperkalemia. Patients are easily inducible into VF during programmed electrical stimulation. The ICD is a reasonable therapy even if more recently it has been suggested [49] that quinidine may provide a reasonable pharmacological treatment able to prolong repolarization and prevent arrhythmias inducibility. More data will be required to define the optimal risk stratification and treatment strategy for SQTS patients

Genetic bases and pathophysiology

The SQTS has been linked to mutations causing a gain of function in either I_{Kr} [50], I_{Ks} [51], or I_{K1} [52]. The augmented T_{peak}–T_{end} interval associated with the peaked T wave observed in SQTS suggests that a TDR underlies the arrhythmogenic substrate. Recent studies conducted using the wedge preparation have provided evidence in support of this hypothesis. The potassium channel opener pinacidil caused a heterogeneous abbreviation of action potential duration among the different cell types spanning the ventricular wall, thus creating the substrate for the genesis of VT under conditions associated with short-QT intervals. Polymorphic VT could be readily induced with PES. The increase in TDR was further accentuated by isoproterenol, leading to easier induction and more persistent VT/VF. The latter is likely due to the reduction in the wavelength of the reentrant circuit, which reduces the path length required for maintenance of reentry [53].

Catecholaminergic polymorphic ventricular tachycardia

Clinical presentation

The catecholaminergic polymorphic ventricular tachycardia (CPVT) is a disease described by Coumel *et al.* in 1978 [54], and characterized by exercize-induced polymorphic ventricular arrhythmias, syncope occurring during physical activity or acute emotion, a normal resting electrocardiogram, and the absence of structural cardiac abnormalities. Supraventricular tachyarrythmias are also part of the manifestations of CPVT. Family history of one or multiple sudden cardiac deaths is evident in 30% of cases [55]. Symptoms usually develop during childhood or adolescence, although cases in which the first symptoms appeared during adulthood have been reported. The resting ECG is unremarkable with the exception of sinus bradycardia and prominent "U" waves reported in some patients [54]. Therefore the diagnosis is not always straightforward. Given the fact that in approximately 15% of patients cardiac arrest is the first manifestation of the disease [56], in some patients it may be initially considered as "idiopathic ventricular fibrillation" (IFV) [55–57].

To establish the diagnosis of CPVT, it is critical to observe exercise or emotion induced polymorphic VT. These arrhythmias are reproducibly induced by exercise stress test, but not by PES. The most typical arrhythmias of CPVT is the so-called bidirectional VT in which the VT presents with an alternating 180° QRS axis on a beat-to-beat basis.

Genetic bases

CPVT1 – autosomal dominant

The first locus for CPVT was identified by Swan *et al.* who mapped the disease to chromosome 1q42-43 [58]. In 2001, Priori *et al.* demonstrated that the disease is caused by a mutation in the *RyR2* gene encoding for the cardiac Ryanodine receptor [55]. RyR2 is a large protein that tetramerizes across the membrane of the sarcoplasmic reticulum (SR) and forms the SR Ca^{2+} release channel in heart, essential for the regulation of the intracellular calcium and excitation–contraction coupling [59].

CPVT2 – autosomal recessive

Lahat *et al.* [60] in 2001, provided the first evidence for a variant of CPVT inherited as an autosomal dominant trait. They mapped the disease seven consanguineous Bedouin families in a 16 cM interval on chromosome 1p23-21 and subsequently identified *CASQ2* as the responsible gene [61]. *CASQ2* encodes calsequestrin, a protein that serves as a major Ca^{2+} binding protein and is localized in the terminal cisternae of the SR. Calsequestrin is bound to the Ryanodine receptor and participates in control of excitation–contraction coupling [62].

Pathophysiology

Several lines of evidence point to delayed afterdepolarization (DAD)-induced triggered activity (TA) as the mechanism underlying monomorphic or bidirectional VT in CPVT patients. These include the identification of genetic mutations involving Ca^{2+} regulatory proteins, a similarity of the ECG features to those associated with digitalis toxicity, and the precipitation by adrenergic stimulation. The cellular mechanisms underlying the various ECG phenotypes, and the transition of monomorphic VT to polymorphic VT or VF, were recently elucidated with the help of the wedge preparation [63].

The wedge was exposed to low-dose caffeine to mimic the defective calcium homeostasis encountered under conditions that predispose to CPVT. The combination of isoproterenol and caffeine led to the development of DAD-induced TA arising from epicardium, endocardium, or the M region. Migration of the source of ectopic activity was responsible for the transition from monomorphic to slow polymorphic VT. Alternation of epicardial and endocardial source of ectopic activity gave rise to a bidirectional VT. Epicardial VT was associated with an increased T_{peak}–T_{end} interval and TDR due to reversal of the normal transmural activation sequence, thus creating the substrate for reentry, which permitted the induction of a more rapid polymorphic VT with PES. Propranolol or verapamil suppressed arrhythmic activity [63].

Clinical management

Patients affected by CPVT should be treated with beta-blockers and they should be advised to limit physical activity and exposure to stressful situations. Beta-blockers often reduce the duration and the rate of VT elicited by exercise or emotion but rarely obtain complete suppression of ventricular arrhythmias. When sustained VT persists despite beta-blockers, the addition of an ICD may be considered [56]. Since several patients with CPVT also have supraventricular tachyarrhythmias, careful programming of the devise should be planned to avoid inappropriate ICD shocks; the use of dual chambers ICD may also be indicated.

References

1. Priori SG, Borggrefe M, Camm AJ, *et al.* Unexplained cardiac arrest. The need for a prospective registry. *Eur Heart J* 1992; **13**: 1445–1446.
2. Napolitano C, Priori SG. The long QT syndrome: molecular and genetic aspects. In: Gussak I & Antzelevitch C, eds. *Cardiac Repolarization*. Totowa, NJ: Humana Press, 2003: 169–185.
3. Andersen ED, Krasilnikoff PA, Overvad H. Intermittent muscular weakness, extrasystoles, and multiple developmental anomalies. A new syndrome? *Acta Paediatr Scand* 1971; **60**: 559–564.

4. Tawil R, Ptacek LJ, Pavlakis SG, *et al.* Andersen's syndrome: potassium-sensitive periodic paralysis, ventricular ectopy, and dysmorphic features. *Ann Neurol* 1994; **35**: 326–330.
5. Marks ML, Trippel DL, Keating MT. Long QT syndrome associated with syndactyly identified in females. *Am J Cardiol* 1995; **76**: 744–745.
6. Splawski I, Timothy KW, Sharpe LM, *et al.* Ca(V)1.2 calcium channel dysfunction causes a multisystem disorder including arrhythmia and autism. *Cell* 2004; **119**: 19–31.
7. Priori SG, Napolitano C, Schwartz PJ. Low penetrance in the long-QT syndrome: clinical impact. *Circulation* 1999; **99**: 529–533.
8. Miller TE, Estrella E, Myerburg RJ, *et al.* Recurrent third-trimester fetal loss and maternal mosaicism for long-QT syndrome. Circulation 2004; **109**: 3029–3034.
9. Keating MT, Atkinson D, Dunn C, Timothy K, Vincent GM, Leppert M. Linkage of a cardiac arrhythmia, the long QT syndrome, and the Harvey *ras-1* gene. *Science* 1991; **252**: 704–706.
10. Jiang C, Atkinson D, Towbin JA, *et al.* Two long QT syndrome loci map to chromosomes 3 and 7 with evidence for further heterogeneity. *Nat Genet* 1994; **8**: 141–147.
11. Schott JJ, Charpentier F, Peltier S, *et al.* Mapping of a gene for long QT syndrome to chromosome 4q25–27. *Am J Hum Genet* 1995; **57**: 1114–1122.
12. Wang Q, Curran ME, Splawski I, *et al.* Positional cloning of a novel potassium channel gene: *KVLQT1* mutations cause cardiac arrhythmias. *Nat Genet* 1996; **12**: 17–23.
13. Wang Q, Shen J, Splawski I *et al. SCN5A* mutations associated with an inherited cardiac arrhythmia, long QT syndrome. *Cell* 1995; **80**: 805–811.
14. Curran ME, Splawski I, Timothy KW, Vincent GM, Green ED, Keating MT. A molecular basis for cardiac arrhythmia: *HERG* mutations cause long QT syndrome. *Cell* 1995; **80**: 795–803.
15. Mohler PJ, Schott JJ, Gramolini AO, *et al.* Ankyrin-B mutation causes type 4 long-QT cardiac arrhythmia and sudden cardiac death. *Nature* 2003; **421**: 634–639.
16. Plaster NM, Tawil R, Tristani-Firouzi M, *et al.* Mutations in *Kir2.1* cause the developmental and episodic electrical phenotypes of Andersen's syndrome. *Cell* 2001; **105**: 511–519.
17. Splawski I, Shen J, Timothy KW, *et al.* Spectrum of mutations in long-QT syndrome genes: *KVLQT1, HERG, SCN5A, KCNE1,* and *KCNE2. Circulation* 2000; **102**: 1178–1185.
18. Moss AJ, Zareba W, Benhorin J, *et al.* ECG T-wave patterns in genetically distinct forms of the hereditary long QT syndrome. *Circulation* 1995; **92**: 2929–2934.
19. Priori SG, Schwartz PJ, Napolitano C, *et al.* Risk stratification in the long-QT syndrome. *N Engl J Med* 2003; **348**: 1866–1874.
20. Schwartz PJ, Priori SG, Spazzolini C, *et al.* Genotype–phenotype correlation in the long-QT syndrome: gene-specific triggers for life-threatening arrhythmias. *Circulation* 2001; **103**: 89–95.
21. Ackerman MJ, Tester DJ, Porter CJ. Swimming, a gene-specific arrhythmogenic trigger for inherited long QT syndrome. *Mayo Clin Proc* 1999; **74**: 1088–1094.
22. Priori SG, Napolitano C, Schwartz PJ, *et al.* Association of long QT syndrome loci and cardiac events among patients treated with beta-blockers. *JAMA* 2004; **292**: 1341–1344.

23. Shimizu W, Antzelevitch C. Cellular basis for the ECG features of the *LQT1* form of the long-QT syndrome: effects of beta-adrenergic agonists and antagonists and sodium channel blockers on transmural dispersion of repolarization and *torsade de pointes. Circulation* 1998; **98**: 2314–2322.
24. Ali RH, Zareba W, Moss AJ, *et al.* Clinical and genetic variables associated with acute arousal and nonarousal-related cardiac events among subjects with long QT syndrome. *Am J Cardiol* 2000; **85**: 457–461.
25. Moss AJ, Robinson JL, Gessman L, *et al.* Comparison of clinical and genetic variables of cardiac events associated with loud noise versus swimming among subjects with the long QT syndrome. *Am J Cardiol* 1999; **84**: 876–879.
26. Shimizu W, Antzelevitch C. Differential effects of beta-adrenergic agonists and antagonists in *LQT1, LQT2,* and *LQT3* models of the long QT syndrome. *J Am Coll Cardiol* 2000; **35**: 778–786.
27. Yan GX, Antzelevitch C. Cellular basis for the normal T wave and the electrocardiographic manifestations of the long-QT syndrome. *Circulation* 1998; **98**: 1928–1936.
28. Moss AJ, Zareba W, Hall WJ, *et al.* Effectiveness and limitations of beta-blocker therapy in congenital long-QT syndrome. *Circulation* 2000; **101**: 616–623.
29. Priori SG, Napolitano C, Giordano U, Collisani G, Memmi M. Brugada syndrome and sudden cardiac death in children. *Lancet* 2000; **355**: 808–809.
30. Brugada J, Brugada R, Brugada P. Right bundle-branch block and ST-segment elevation in leads V1 through V3: a marker for sudden death in patients without demonstrable structural heart disease. *Circulation* 1998; **97**: 457–460.
31. Chen Q, Kirsch GE, Zhang D, *et al.* Genetic basis and molecular mechanism for idiopathic ventricular fibrillation. *Nature* 1998; **392**: 293–296.
32. Weiss R, Barmada MM, Nguyen T, *et al.* Clinical and molecular heterogeneity in the Brugada syndrome: a novel gene locus on chromosome 3. *Circulation* 2002; **105**: 707–713.
33. Yan GX, Antzelevitch C. Cellular basis for the Brugada syndrome and other mechanisms of arrhythmogenesis associated with ST-segment elevation. *Circulation* 1999; **100**: 1660–1666.
34. Lukas A, Antzelevitch C. Phase 2 reentry as a mechanism of initiation of circus movement reentry in canine epicardium exposed to simulated ischemia. *Cardiovasc Res* 1996; **32**: 593–603.
35. Brugada J, Brugada R, Brugada P. Determinants of sudden cardiac death in individuals with the electrocardiographic pattern of Brugada syndrome and no previous cardiac arrest. *Circulation* 2003; **108**: 3092–3096.
36. Priori SG, Napolitano C, Gasparini M, *et al.* Clinical and genetic heterogeneity of right bundle branch block and ST-segment elevation syndrome: a prospective evaluation of 52 families. *Circulation* 2000; **102**: 2509–2515.
37. Priori SG, Napolitano C, Gasparini M, *et al.* Natural history of Brugada syndrome. Insights for risk stratification and management. *Circulation* 2002; **105**: 1342–1347.
38. Eckardt L, Probst V, Smits JP, *et al.* Long-term prognosis of individuals with right precordial ST-segment-elevation Brugada syndrome. *Circulation* 2005; **111**: 257–263.
39. Wolf L. Familial auricular fibrillation. *N Engl J Med* 1943; **229**: 396–397.
40. Darbar D, Herron KJ, Ballew JD, *et al.* Familial atrial fibrillation is a genetically heterogeneous disorder. *J Am Coll Cardiol* 2003; **41**: 2185–2192.

41. Brugada R, Tapscott T, Czernuszewicz GZ, *et al.* Identification of a genetic locus for familial atrial fibrillation. *N Engl J Med* 1997; **336**: 905–911.
42. Ellinor PT, Shin JT, Moore RK, Yoerger DM, MacRae CA. Locus for atrial fibrillation maps to chromosome 6q14–16. *Circulation* 2003; **107**: 2880–2883.
43. Chen YH, Xu SJ, Bendahhou S, Wang XL *et al. KCNQ1* gain-of-function mutation in familial atrial fibrillation. *Science* 2003; **299**: 251–254.
44. Yang Y, Xia M, Jin Q, *et al.* Identification of a *KCNE2* gain-of-function mutation in patients with familial atrial fibrillation. *Am J Hum Genet* 2004; **75**: 899–905.
45. Kirchhof P, Eckardt L, Franz MR, *et al.* Prolonged atrial action potential durations and polymorphic atrial tachyarrhythmias in patients with long QT syndrome. *J Cardiovasc Electrophysiol* 2003; **14**: 1027–1033.
46. Gaita F, Giustetto C, Bianchi F, *et al.* Short QT syndrome: a familial cause of sudden death. *Circulation* 2003; **108**: 965–970.
47. Morita H, Kusano-Fukushima K, Nagase S, *et al.* Atrial fibrillation and atrial vulnerability in patients with Brugada syndrome. *J Am Coll Cardiol* 2002; **40**: 1437–1444.
48. Gussak I, Brugada P, Brugada J, *et al.* Idiopathic short QT interval: a new clinical syndrome? *Cardiology* 2000; **94**: 99–102.
49. Wolpert C, Schimpf R, Giustetto C, *et al.* Further insights into the effect of quinidine in short QT syndrome caused by a mutation in *HERG*. *J Cardiovasc Electrophysiol* 2005; **16**: 54–58.
50. Brugada R, Hong K, Dumaine R, *et al.* Sudden death associated with short-QT syndrome linked to mutations in *HERG*. *Circulation* 2004; **109**: 30–35.
51. Bellocq C, van Ginneken AC, Bezzina CR, *et al.* Mutation in the *KCNQ1* gene leading to the short QT-interval syndrome. *Circulation* 2004; **109**: 2394–2397.
52. Priori SG, Pandit SV, Rivolta I, *et al.* A novel form of short QT syndrome (SQT3) is caused by a mutation in the *KCNJ2* gene. *Circulation Res* 2005; **96**(7): 800–807.
53. Extramiana F, Antzelevitch C. Amplified transmural dispersion of repolarization as the basis for arrhythmogenesis in a canine ventricular-wedge model of short-QT syndrome. *Circulation* 2004; **110**: 3661–3666.
54. Coumel P, Fidelle J, Lucet V, Attuel P, Bouvrain Y. Catecholaminergic-induced severe ventricular arrhythmias with Adams–Stokes syndrome in children: report of four cases. *Br Heart J* 1978; **40**: 28–37.
55. Priori SG, Napolitano C, Tiso N, *et al.* Mutations in the cardiac ryanodine receptor gene (*hRyR2*) underlie catecholaminergic polymorphic ventricular tachycardia. *Circulation* 2001; **103**: 196–200.
56. Priori SG, Napolitano C, Memmi M, *et al.* Clinical and molecular characterization of patients with catecholaminergic polymorphic ventricular tachycardia. *Circulation* 2002; **106**: 69–74.
57. Leenhardt A, Lucet V, Denjoy I, Grau F, Ngoc DD, Coumel P. Catecholaminergic polymorphic ventricular tachycardia in children. A 7-year follow-up of 21 patients. *Circulation* 1995; **91**: 1512–1519.
58. Swan H, Piippo K, Viitasalo M, *et al.* Arrhythmic disorder mapped to chromosome 1q42-q43 causes malignant polymorphic ventricular tachycardia in structurally normal hearts. *J Am Coll Cardiol* 1999; **34**: 2035–2042.
59. Marks AR, Priori S, Memmi M, Kontula K, Laitinen PJ. Involvement of the cardiac ryanodine receptor/calcium release channel in catecholaminergic polymorphic ventricular tachycardia. *J Cell Physiol* 2002; **190**: 1–6.

60. Lahat H, Eldar M, Levy-Nissenbaum E, *et al*. Autosomal recessive catecholamine-or exercise-induced polymorphic ventricular tachycardia. *Circulation* 2001; **103**: 2822–2827.
61. Lahat H, Pras E, Olender T, *et al*. A missense mutation in a highly conserved region of CASQ2 is associated with autosomal recessive catecholamine-induced polymorphic ventricular tachycardia in Bedouin families from Israel. *Am J Hum Genet* 2001; **69**: 1378–1384.
62. Zhang L, Kelley J, Schmeisser G, Kobayashi YM, Jones LR. Complex formation between junctin, triadin, calsequestrin, and the ryanodine receptor. Proteins of the cardiac junctional sarcoplasmic reticulum membrane. *J Biol Chem* 1997; **272**: 23389–23397.
63. Nam GB, Burashnikov A, Antzelevitch C. Cellular mechanisms underlying the development of catecholaminergic ventricular tachycardia. *Heart Rhythm* 2004; **1**: 188 (abs. suppl) (abs).

CHAPTER 10
Sudden cardiac death and valvular heart diseases

David Messika-Zeitoun, Bernard J. Gersh, Olivier Fondard, and Alec Vahanian

Sudden cardiac death is a major public health problem. In the United States, its incidence has been estimated as high as 400 000 each year. Despite progress made in resuscitation, treatment of sudden death is usually unsuccessful and apart from some notable exceptions, the vast majority of patients with cardiac arrest do not survive [1]. From a pathological registry of 1000 adults under 65 years of age with no previous history of cardiac disease, valvular heart disease was the fourth largest cause of sudden death after coronary artery disease, left and right cardiomyopathies, and tissue conduction abnormalities [2]. However, even if valvular diseases account for only a small proportion of sudden deaths overall, the relatively high frequency of valvular heart disease in the general population increases the importance of sudden cardiac death and valvular heart disease as a clinical entity. In this chapter, we present the currently available data regarding the incidence and determinants of sudden death for each major organic valvular disease, that is, aortic stenosis, aortic regurgitation, mitral regurgitation, and mitral stenosis.

Aortic stenosis

Aortic stenosis is the most common valvular disease in Western countries and its prevalence increases with aging population. Pioneering studies performed prior to the area of catheterization and cardiac surgery have shown that patients with aortic stenosis experienced sudden death.

Symptomatic patients with aortic stenosis

Development of symptoms is a turning point in a patient's history. In 1968, Ross and Braunwald, in their classic review of the natural history of aortic stenosis, underlined the critical importance of the functional status [3]. Fifty percent survival is 5 years in patients who present with angina, 3 years for those with syncope, and 2 years with dyspnoea or congestive heart failure. Approximately half of the deaths were sudden [4,5]. A specific cause of sudden death is often difficult to establish and sudden death in aortic stenosis is probably multifactorial. Several mechanisms have been suggested, such as malfunction of the baroreceptor mechanism [6], ventricular arrhythmias caused by ischemia or atrioventricular block due to aortic valve calcification extending into the conduction system. It is worthy to note that, myocardial ischemia may be observed in aortic stenosis even in the absence of coronary artery disease.

Thus, symptomatic patients with severe aortic stenosis must be operated on without delay. Patients with left ventricular dysfunction with or without low gradients [7,8], especially if there is a contractile reserve, should also be considered for surgery as well as patients with severe pulmonary hypertension [9].

Asymptomatic patients with aortic stenosis
In contrast, management of asymptomatic patients with severe aortic stenosis is more controversial.

Incidence of sudden death
Recent prospective studies provide important information regarding the incidence of sudden death. Results of major retrospective and prospective studies [4,5,10–17] are summarized in Table 10.1. All these studies show that sudden death is an uncommon complication of asymptomatic aortic stenosis – probably less than 1% [19,20]. In regard to the mortality and morbidity of surgery for aortic stenosis and the risk of serious prosthetic valve complication, surgery in all asymptomatic patients to prevent the risk of sudden death, should not be recommended.

However, several important facts need to be emphasized. First, the current definition of severe aortic stenosis (aortic valve gradient ≥ 50 mm Hg or aortic valve area ≤ 1 cm^2 or <0.6 cm^2/m^2 of body surface area) is not universally accepted [19,20]. Second, the correlation between the onset of symptoms and the severity of stenosis is highly variable [15]. Third, New York Heart Association (NYHA) classification is subjective and symptoms may be absent in sedentary patients or because patients progressively limit their physical activity. Finally, even if the occurrence of sudden death not preceded by symptoms in initially asymptomatic patients is rare, the interval between occurrence of symptoms and sudden death may be very short and the window for surgical correction may be missed [21]. Moreover, patients do not always report symptoms promptly, which highlights the critical importance of education and of periodic follow-up. Patients who understand the expected course of the disease and are aware of potential symptoms are more likely to report the onset of even mild symptoms promptly. Also, it has been shown that there is an important variability [15,18,22] in aortic stenosis progression and that even mild or moderate aortic stenosis incur an excess mortality [18]. Thus, because sudden death does not leave any opportunity for review of therapeutic options, it is essential to identify asymptomatic patients at high risk of sudden death

Table 10.1 Natural history of asymptomatic patients with aortic stenosis.

Study	Year	Number of Patients	Severity of Aortic Stenosis	Age, Years	Follow-up, Years	Deaths, Number of Patients			Event-free Survival[a]
						Total Death	Sudden Death	Sudden Death not Preceded by Symptoms	
Chizner et al. [4]	1980	8	AVA < 1.1 cm²	24	5.7	0	0	0	—
Turina et al. [11]	1987	17	AVA < 0.9 cm²	—	2.0	0	0	0	75% at 5 years
Horstkotte and Loogen [12]	1988	35	AVA = 0.8–1.5 cm²	—	"Years"	—	3	3	—
Kelly et al. [5]	1988	51	PV = 3.5–5.8 m/s	63	1.4	8	1	0	—
Pellikka et al. [13]	1990	113	PV ≥ 4.0 m/s	70	1.8	14	3	1 (aortic dissection)	74 ± 6% at 2 years
Kennedy et al. [10][b]	1991	28	AVA = 0.9 ± 0.1 cm²	69	2.0	NA	0	0	70% at 4 years
Faggiano et al. [14]	1992	37	AVA = 0.85 ± 0.15 cm²	72	1.7	3	1	0	—
Otto et al. [15]	1997	123	PV ≥ 2.5 m/s	63	2.5	8	0	0	76% at 2 years
Rosenhek et al. [16]	2000	128	PV > 4 m/s	60	1.8	8	1	1	56 ± 5% at 2 years
Amato et al. [17]	2001	66	AVA ≤ 1 cm²	50	0.7–2	NA	4	4	38 ± 6% at 2 years
Rosenhek et al. [18]	2004	176	PV = 2.5–4 m/s	58	4.6	34	NA	1	75 ± 3% at 5 years[c]

Notes: AVA = aortic valve area, NA = not available, PV = peak aortic velocity.

[a] Death or aortic valve replacement.

[b] No or minimal symptoms.

[c] Including perioperative and late deaths after aortic valve replacement.

(and/or of developing symptoms) who may benefit from a more aggressive strategy.

High-risk subgroups
Prospective studies have identified several criteria associated with high risk of developing symptoms and of requiring valve replacement.

Severity of the stenosis. Aortic jet velocity has been recognized in multiple studies as a reliable predictor of outcome [13,15,16]. For example, in 123 patients with aortic stenosis followed for 2.5 years, when the initial peak velocity was ≥4 m/s event-free survival (death or aortic valve replacement) was $21 \pm 18\%$ at 2 years compared to $84 \pm 16\%$ when the jet velocity was <3 m/s. Rapid increase of aortic jet velocity (≥0.3 m/s per year) is also an important predictor of poor outcome [15,16]. Amato *et al.* also identified an extremely reduced *aortic valve area* (<0.7 cm^2) as a predictor of poor outcome [17].

Exercise testing. Aortic stenosis, even moderate, has traditionally been regarded as a contraindication to exercise testing. Although exercise test should not be performed in symptomatic patients, recent studies show that, in asymptomatic patients, under strict medical supervision, it is safe and informative [15,17,23]. It can unmask symptoms in reputed asymptomatic patients and provide important prognostic information. Of note, in Amato's study [17], four patients (6%) experienced sudden death. None had preceding symptoms, but all had an aortic valve area <0.7 cm^2 and a positive exercise test.

Aortic valve calcification. Aortic valve calcification is the process that leads to aortic valve stenosis and its degree has been shown to provide important prognostic information[16,18,24]. In 128 asymptomatic patients with severe aortic stenosis, moderate or severe calcification, assessed by echocardiography, identifies patients with poor prognosis [16]. Similarly, in 100 patients with aortic stenosis, after adjustment for age, gender, symptoms, ejection fraction, and aortic valve area, degree of aortic valve calcification quantitatively assessed by Electron-Beam-Computed Tomography was independently predictive of event-free survival ($p < .001$) [24].

Associated coronary artery disease. There is an increasing body of both clinical and experimental data demonstrating a pathophysiological link between aortic stenosis and atherosclerosis, especially in the coronary bed. Thus, a 50% increase in cardiac mortality due to myocardial infarction has been reported in patients with aortic sclerosis – valve thickening without hemodynamic obstruction – suggesting an association between aortic valve disease and coronary artery disease [25]. More recently, in patients with mild or moderate aortic stenosis, associated coronary artery disease was an independent predictor of outcome [18].

It has not been fully proven that patients with these characteristics should be operated on but the risk of developing symptoms and of sudden death seem reasonable justifications for surgical intervention. These conditions have been included in the current recommendations of the European Society of Cardiology Working Group on valvular heart disease [20].

Recommendations for surgery in asymptomatic patients with aortic stenosis – European Society of Cardiology Working Group recommendations

Surgery should be considered in asymptomatic patients with severe aortic stenosis in the following circumstances:

1 Patients with an abnormal response to exercise: development of symptoms, drop in blood pressure, inadequate blood pressure rise, and markedly impaired exercise tolerance.

2 Patients with moderate to severe calcification, peak jet velocity >4 m/s, or accelerated rate of progression of peak velocity (≥0.3 m/s/year).

3 Patients with left ventricular dysfunction (left ventricular ejection fraction (LVEF) <50%). This situation is however rare in asymptomatic aortic stenosis.

Even if there is a lower level of evidence, surgery can probably also be considered in the following situations:

1 Severe left ventricular hypertrophy (>15 mm wall thickness) unless this is due to hypertension.

2 Severe ventricular arrhythmias for which no other cause than severe aortic stenosis can be identified.

Aortic regurgitation

Aortic regurgitation is a less common valvular disorder but still represents 10% of native valve disease in the recent Euro Heart Survey [26]. As with aortic stenosis, onset of symptoms marks an important shift in the course of the disease.

Symptomatic patients with aortic regurgitation

Symptoms in patients with severe aortic regurgitation are a major independent prognostic factor [27,28]. When not operated on, the prognosis of symptomatic patients is grim. Natural history studies of nonoperated patients who experienced symptoms of heart failure report very high mortality rates including sudden death [11,27–29]. Not operated on, mortality rate is as high as 72 ± 12% at 5 years (24.6% yearly) [27]. Even mild [27] or transient [11] symptoms are associated with an excess mortality and NYHA functional class II shows a significant association to subsequent sudden death [30]. Thus, symptomatic patients must be promptly referred for surgery [19,20]. When operated on early in the course of the disease, surgical correction of the regurgitation provides an excellent long-term outcome [28]. On the other hand, patients in NYHA class III/IV, even with markedly reduced ejection fraction, should also be considered for surgery. They incur excess operative and postoperative mortality rates but mid-term symptoms free is obtained in most patients [31].

Asymptomatic patients with aortic regurgitation
Incidence and determinants of sudden death

Asymptomatic patients with severe aortic regurgitation may also be at risk of sudden death. Table 10.2 summarizes the seven most important studies regarding the natural history of asymptomatic patients [30,32–37]. These studies show that the risk of sudden death in asymptomatic patients is low (<0.2% per year). However, the risk is not zero and subgroups at higher risk can be defined.

Extreme left ventricular dilatation and dysfunction are associated with sudden death. Turina reported five sudden deaths in patients awaiting for surgery [29], two of whom (not recorded in Table 10.2) were asymptomatic but with a severely enlarged left ventricle and low ejection fraction. Similarly, among 104 asymptomatic patients with severe aortic regurgitation, two sudden deaths were observed in patients with severely enlarged left ventricle (end-diastolic diameter ≥80 mm and end-systolic diameter ≥55 mm) and subnormal LVEF (40–45%) [34]. In another study of 104 asymptomatic or minimally symptomatic patients, four died suddenly [30]. These four deaths were not preceded by symptoms or the development of resting left ventricular dysfunction at their last evaluation 6–10 months before. In this study, the predictors of sudden cardiac death were the LVEF during exercise and particularly the ratio of Δ (exercise − rest) LVEF/Δ (exercise − rest) end-systolic wall stress that relates more closely to left ventricular contractility than ejection fraction. In the high-risk tercile, the 5-years rate of sudden death was 3.3%. Patients who demonstrate progression of left ventricular dilatation or progressive decline in ejection fraction on serial studies also represent a higher-risk group that requires careful monitoring [34].

Identification of such predictors is fully in agreement with a previous study showing that in patients with aortic valve diseases, the severity of ventricular arrhythmias (recorded by 24-h ambulatory ECG) is strongly associated with myocardial performance [38]. It is also important to note that left ventricular dimensions and function parameters can be dissociated from the functional status, and more than 40% of patients with severe aortic regurgitation and markedly reduced ejection fraction (<35%) [31] or severely enlarged left ventricle (≥80 mm) [39] had no or minimal symptoms.

Recommendations for surgery in asymptomatic patients with aortic regurgitation – European Society of Cardiology Working Group recommendations

Surgery is recommended in asymptomatic patients with severe aortic regurgitation and left ventricular dysfunction (≤50%) and/or severe dilatation (end-diastolic diameter >70 mm, end-systolic diameter >50 mm or even better >25 mm/m^2 of body surface area) [19,20]. A rapid increase in left ventricular diameters on serial testing is a further incentive to consider surgery.

Table 10.2 Natural history of asymptomatic patients with aortic regurgitation.

Study	Year	Number of Patients	Age, Years	Ejection Fraction, %	Functional Class	Follow-up, Years	Sudden Death, Number of Patients	Symptoms, Left Ventricular Dysfunction or Death, Annual Progression Rate
Henry et al. [32]	1980	37	35	—	I: 100%	2.8	0	38% "during follow-up"
Siemenczuk et al. [33]	1989	50	48 ± 16	67 ± 8	I or II	3.7	0	4%
Bonow et al. [34]	1991	104	36	55	I: 100%	8	2	<5%
Scognamiglio et al. [36]	1994	143[a] Digoxin: 69 Nifedipine: 74	35 ± 13	63	I: 100%	6	0	At 6 years 34 ± 6% 15 ± 3%
Tornos et al. [37]	1995	101	41 ± 14	58 ± 7	I: 100%	4.6	0	3%
Ishii et al. [35]	1996	27	42 ± 12	36 ± 5[b]	I: 100%	14.2	0	3.6%
Borer et al. [30]	1998	104	46 ± 15	55 ± 5	I: 80% "Early II": 20%	7.3	4	6.2%

[a] Patients enrolled in a prospective randomized pharmacological study (74 were assigned to digoxin and 69 to nifedipine).
[b] Fractional shortening.

In addition, aortic root dilatation is a common feature associated with aortic regurgitation (AR). Surgery should be undertaken, irrespective of the degree of AR or left ventricular function, in patients with aortic root dilatation >55 mm. In patients with bicuspid aortic valves or Marfan syndrome, a lower degree of root dilatation (50 mm) can be used as a threshold for surgery, in particular if a valve-sparing operation is possible or if there is a rapid increase of aortic diameter.

Mitral regurgitation

Organic mitral regurgitation is increasingly observed because of population aging and the high prevalence of degenerative lesions in the adult and elderly age strata.

Symptomatic patients with mitral regurgitation

As for aortic valve diseases, the development of symptoms is a critical turning point. Patients in NYHA class III–IV incur an excess mortality when conservatively managed [40] and postoperatively, they display an excess short- and long-term mortality [41]. This excess mortality encompasses sudden death. The prognosis of 216 patients with severe mitral regurgitation conservatively managed was poor ($33 \pm 9\%$ at 8 years), and 11 patients experienced sudden death (60% of cardiac deaths) [42]. More recently, Grigioni *et al.* [43] analyzed the occurrence of sudden death in 348 patients (age 67 ± 12 years) with mitral regurgitation due to flail leaflet, which represents the most common cause of mitral regurgitation requiring surgical correction. During a mean follow-up of 48 ± 11 months, 99 deaths occurred under conservative management. Among the 74 cardiac deaths, 25 were sudden (one quarter of all deaths). At 5 and 10 years, total mortality rates were $29 \pm 3\%$ and $53 \pm 5\%$, respectively; cardiac death rates $21 \pm 3\%$ and $43 \pm 5\%$; and sudden death rates $8.6 \pm 2\%$ and $18.8 \pm 4\%$ (yearly rate 1.8%). Yearly rate of sudden death was significantly higher ($p < .0001$) in patients in NYHA class III–IV (7.8%) than in those in class I (1.0%) or II (3.1%) (Figure 10.1(a)). Thus, patients who present with symptoms, even transient or regressive on diuretics, should be offered surgery whatever be their LVEF.

Asymptomatic patients with mitral regurgitation
Incidence and predictors of sudden death

However, sudden death can occur even in asymptomatic patients. In the Grigioni *et al.* study, in addition to symptoms, independent determinants of sudden death were LVEF and atrial fibrillation. Yearly rate of sudden death increased from 1.5% in patients with normal ejection fraction to 12.7% in patients with ejection fraction <50% ($p < .0001$) (Figure 10.1(b)) and from 1.3% in patients in sinus rhythm to 4.9% in patients in atrial fibrillation ($p = .0004$) (Figure 10.1(c)). A striking finding of this study was that even if independent predictors of sudden death could be identified, it remained

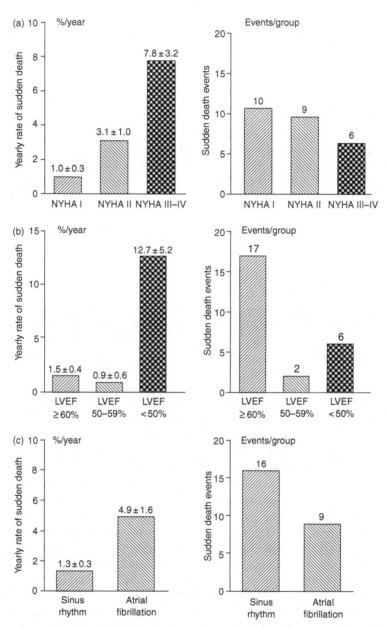

Figure 10.1 Relation between (a) NYHA functional class, (b) LVEF, (c) cardiac rhythm (sinus rhythm or atrial fibrillation) and sudden death. Left, yearly rates of sudden death (±SEE) according to functional classes I, II, and III or IV (a), LVEF classified as ≥60%, 50–59%, and <50% (b), and in sinus rhythm and atrial fibrillation (c). Right, Number of sudden death events according to NYHA class (a), LVEF (b), and rhythm (c). Reproduced from Reference 43, with permission from Elsevier.

a poorly predictable event and the majority of sudden deaths occurred among patients in NYHA functional class I or II, in sinus rhythm, and with ejection fraction ≥60%. Therefore, the risk of sudden death in this low-risk population (0.8% per year) should be balanced against the operative risk, especially in young patients when the valve is repairable [44].

To date, there are no randomized trials comparing the outcome after early surgery for organic mitral regurgitation to the outcome with medical management. However, survival of patients with severe mitral regurgitation when operated on in NYHA functional class I or II with normal LVEF is identical to expected [41] suggesting that early surgery, in this subgroup, may suppress the excess risk of sudden death. Also, mitral valve surgery (repair or replacement), was independently associated with a reduced risk of sudden death [43]. Finally, surgery prevents the occurrence of symptoms, left ventricular dysfunction [45,46], and atrial fibrillation [47] which, as mentioned above, are independent predictors of sudden death.

Mechanisms of sudden death

Mitral valve prolapse versus regurgitation

Mitral valve prolapse is a common feature in the general population (2.4% according to the Framingham Heart Study) [48] and is the most frequent cause of mitral regurgitation in Western countries [26]. The link between sudden death and mitral valve prolapse has been recognized for decades but, until recently, it remained highly debated. Previous reports have documented specific anatomic lesions associated with mitral valve prolapse – endocardial friction lesions and thrombotic lesions in the angle between the posterior leaflet and the left atrial wall – and leaflet lengths and valve thickness has been associated with an increased risk of sudden death.

Even if one cannot rule out a possible association between mitral valve prolapse and an increased incidence of sudden death, there are strong arguments suggesting that sudden death in mitral valve disease is related more to the regurgitation and its consequences on cardiac remodeling and function than to the valve prolapse itself. First, in 1000 autopsies performed on adults with no previous medical history, 14 patients with isolated mitral valve prolapse were observed and all presented with severe mitral regurgitation [2]. A second argument emanated from the recently published natural history of mitral valve prolapse [49]. In this community study, mortality and morbidity of 833 Olmsted County, MN, residents diagnosed with asymptomatic mitral valve prolapse by 2D-echocardiography were prospectively evaluated (4581 person-years of follow-up). At 10 years, cardiac mortality was 9±2% and was predicted by the severity of the regurgitation and, to a lesser degree, by LVEF. This analysis did not specifically state the rate of sudden death, but the survival of patients with neither a moderate to severe mitral regurgitation nor an LVEF <50% was similar to expected. Finally, major determinants of sudden death are the NYHA class, right or left ejection fraction, and atrial fibrillation, which are all direct consequences of the regurgitation [43].

Mitral regurgitation and ventricular arrhythmias
Even if the influence of bradyarrhythmia and electromechanical dissociation seems to have been underestimated, the majority of sudden deaths are caused by acute ventricular tachyarrhythmias. Thus, in the study by Grigioni *et al.* [43], in 10 patients in whom the cardiac rhythm could be ascertained during the episode of circulatory collapse, ventricular tachyarrhythmia was observed in all (ventricular fibrillation in seven and ventricular tachycardia in three). Of note, a high frequency of severe ventricular arrhythmia are observed in patients with mitral valve prolapse with and without mitral regurgitation (between 27% and 35%) and the predictive value of ambient ventricular arrhythmia and Holter monitoring remains controversial requiring future large prospective studies. Similarly, the role of heart-rate variability or programmed ventricular stimulation may also be of interest in the prediction of sudden death but needs to be further evaluated.

Recommendations for surgery in asymptomatic patients with mitral regurgitation – European Society of Cardiology Working Group recommendations

Surgery can be recommended in selected asymptomatic patients with severe mitral regurgitation:

1 Asymptomatic patients with signs of left ventricular dysfunction (ejection fraction <60% and/or left ventricular end-systolic dimension >45 mm), even in patients with a high likelihood of valve replacement, to prevent further deterioration of left ventricular function.
2 Patients with atrial fibrillation and "preserved" left ventricular function.
3 Patients with "preserved" left ventricular function and pulmonary hypertension (pulmonary systolic pressure >50 mm Hg at rest or 60 mm Hg on exercise) with a high likelihood of valve repair.

The other indications are controversial:

1 Asymptomatic patients with no signs of left ventricular dysfunction; surgical correction can be considered in patients younger than 75 years with high likelihood of valve repair and a low operative risk.
2 Patients with mitral valve prolapse and "preserved" left ventricular function with recurrent ventricular arrhythmias despite medical therapy.

Mitral stenosis

Rheumatic mitral stenosis is a frequent cause of valve disease in developing countries [26]. In Western countries, as a result of immigration trends from the developing world, it remains a significant problem despite the striking decrease in the prevalence of rheumatic fever. The natural history of untreated mitral stenosis had been carefully studied prior to the advent of cardiac surgical and percutaneous techniques. In those pioneering studies [50], the main causes of death were congestive heart failure or pulmonary edema, thrombo-embolic complications and infections. No sudden death relating to mitral stenosis has been reported. Absence of left ventricular remodeling in mitral stenosis probably explains this finding.

Conclusion

Sudden death is not an uncommon complication in patients with valvular heart disease but its occurrence in patients without significant symptoms is devastating. For the clinical management of those patients, the key is the timing of surgical intervention and the need to balance spontaneous risk under conservative management against the operative and long-term postoperative risk. Valvular diseases are conditions that can be "easily" and effectively treated by surgical interventions and therefore, it is essential to define subgroups at higher risk of sudden death in whom an aggressive strategy should be considered. Overall, development of symptoms and signs of left ventricular dysfunction are major predictors of sudden death and are by themselves strong indications for a surgical intervention. It should be emphasized that the database regarding sudden cardiac death in patients with valvular heart disease is quite limited and there exists a paucity of data with which to risk stratify in comparison to what is known in patients with ischemic heart disease and the cardiomyopathies. In the majority of trials of antiarrhythmic therapy and implantable cardioverter-defibrillator (ICD), patients with significant valvular heart disease were excluded. Currently, the only documented indication for an ICD in patients with valvular heart disease is a history of cardiac arrest or symptomatic ventricular arrhythmias. For the primary prevention of sudden cardiac death using an ICD, there is a dire lack of data and perhaps the best approach is to determine the optimal time for surgical intervention. This would be a fruitful and needed area of future investigation.

References

1. Bunch TJ, White RD, Gersh BJ, *et al.* Long-term outcomes of out-of-hospital cardiac arrest after successful early defibrillation. *N Engl J Med* 2003; **348**: 2626–2633.
2. Loire R, Tabib A. Unexpected sudden cardiac death: result of 1000 autopsies. *Arch Mal Coeur* 1996; **89**: 13–18.
3. Ross J Jr, Braunwald E. Aortic stenosis. *Circulation* 1968; **38**: 61–67.
4. Chizner MA, Pearle DL, deLeon AC Jr. The natural history of aortic stenosis in adults. *Am Heart J* 1980; **99**: 419–424.
5. Kelly TA, Rothbart RM, Cooper CM, Kaiser DL, Smucker ML, Gibson RS. Comparison of outcome of asymptomatic to symptomatic patients older than 20 years of age with valvular aortic stenosis. *Am J Cardiol* 1988; **61**: 123–130.
6. Grech ED, Ramsdale DR. Exertional syncope in aortic stenosis: evidence to support inappropriate left ventricular baroreceptor response. *Am Heart J* 1991; **121**: 603–606.
7. Monin JL, Monchi M, Gest V, Duval-Moulin AM, Dubois-Rande JL, Gueret P. Aortic stenosis with severe left ventricular dysfunction and low transvalvular

pressure gradients: risk stratification by low-dose dobutamine echocardiography. *J Am Coll Cardiol* 2001; **37**: 2101–2107.

8. Nishimura RA, Grantham JA, Connolly HM, Schaff HV, Higano ST, Holmes DR, Jr. Low-output, low-gradient aortic stenosis in patients with depressed left ventricular systolic function: the clinical utility of the dobutamine challenge in the catheterization laboratory. *Circulation* 2002; **106**: 809–813.

9. Malouf JF, Enriquez-Sarano M, Pellikka PA, *et al.* Severe pulmonary hypertension in patients with severe aortic valve stenosis: clinical profile and prognostic implications. *J Am Coll Cardiol* 2002; **40**: 789–795.

10. Kennedy KD, Nishimura RA, Holmes DR Jr, Bailey KR. Natural history of moderate aortic stenosis. *J Am Coll Cardiol* 1991; **17**: 313–319.

11. Turina J, Hess O, Sepulcri F, Krayenbuehl HP. Spontaneous course of aortic valve disease. *Eur Heart J* 1987; **8**: 471–483.

12. Horstkotte D, Loogen F. The natural history of aortic valve stenosis. *Eur Heart J* 1988; **9**(Suppl. E): 57–64.

13. Pellikka PA, Nishimura RA, Bailey KR, Tajik AJ. The natural history of adults with asymptomatic, hemodynamically significant aortic stenosis. *J Am Coll Cardiol* 1990; **15**: 1012–1017.

14. Faggiano P, Ghizzoni G, Sorgato A, *et al.* Rate of progression of valvular aortic stenosis in adults. *Am J Cardiol* 1992; **70**: 229–233.

15. Otto CM, Burwash IG, Legget ME, *et al.* Prospective study of asymptomatic valvular aortic stenosis. Clinical, echocardiographic, and exercise predictors of outcome. *Circulation* 1997; **95**: 2262–2270.

16. Rosenhek R, Binder T, Porenta G, *et al.* Predictors of outcome in severe, asymptomatic aortic stenosis. *N Engl J Med* 2000; **343**: 611–617.

17. Amato MC, Moffa PJ, Werner KE, Ramires JA. Treatment decision in asymptomatic aortic valve stenosis: role of exercise testing. *Heart* 2001; **86**: 381–386.

18. Rosenhek R, Klaar U, Schemper M, *et al.* Mild and moderate aortic stenosis. Natural history and risk stratification by echocardiography. *Eur Heart J* 2004; **25**: 199–205.

19. Bonow R, Carabello B, DeLeon A, *et al.* ACC/AHA guidelines for the management of patients with valvular heart disease. *Circulation* 1998; **98**: 1949–1984.

20. Iung B, Gohlke-Barwolf C, Tornos P, *et al.* Recommendations on the management of the asymptomatic patient with valvular heart disease. *Eur Heart J* 2002; **23**: 1252–1266.

21. Lund O, Larsen KE. Cardiac pathology after isolated valve replacement for aortic stenosis in relation to preoperative patient status. Early and late autopsy findings. *Scand J Thorac Cardiovasc Surg* 1989; **23**: 263–270.

22. Bellamy MF, Pellikka PA, Klarich KW, Tajik AJ, Enriquez-Sarano M. Association of cholesterol levels, hydroxymethylglutaryl coenzyme-A reductase inhibitor treatment, and progression of aortic stenosis in the community. *J Am Coll Cardiol* 2002; **40**: 1723–1730.

23. Das P, Rimington H, Smeeton N, Chambers J. Determinants of symptoms and exercise capacity in aortic stenosis: a comparison of resting haemodynamics and valve compliance during dobutamine stress. *Eur Heart J* 2003; **24**: 1254–1263.

24. Messika-Zeitoun D, Aubry MC, Detaint D, *et al.* Evaluation and clinical implications of aortic valve calcification by electron beam computed tomography. *Circulation* 2004; **110**: 356–362.

25. Otto CM, Lind BK, Kitzman DW, Gersh BJ, Siscovick DS. Association of aortic-valve sclerosis with cardiovascular mortality and morbidity in the elderly. *N Engl J Med* 1999; **341**: 142–147.
26. Iung B, Baron G, Butchart EG, *et al.* A prospective survey of patients with valvular heart disease in Europe: the Euro heart survey on valvular heart disease. *Eur Heart J* 2003; **24**: 1231–1243.
27. Dujardin KS, Enriquez-Sarano M, Schaff HV, Bailey KR, Seward JB, Tajik AJ. Mortality and morbidity of aortic regurgitation in clinical practice. A long-term follow-up study. *Circulation* 1999; **99**: 1851–1857.
28. Klodas E, Enriquez-Sarano M, Tajik AJ, Mullany CJ, Bailey KR, Seward JB. Optimizing timing of surgical correction in patients with severe aortic regurgitation: role of symptoms. *J Am Coll Cardiol* 1997; **30**: 746–752.
29. Turina J, Turina M, Rothlin M, Krayenbuehl HP. Improved late survival in patients with chronic aortic regurgitation by earlier operation. *Circulation* 1984; **70**: I147–I152.
30. Borer JS, Hochreiter C, Herrold EM, *et al.* Prediction of indications for valve replacement among asymptomatic or minimally symptomatic patients with chronic aortic regurgitation and normal left ventricular performance. *Circulation* 1998; **97**: 525–534.
31. Chaliki HP, Mohty D, Avierinos JF, *et al.* Outcomes after aortic valve replacement in patients with severe aortic regurgitation and markedly reduced left ventricular function. *Circulation* 2002; **106**: 2687–2693.
32. Henry WL, Bonow RO, Rosing DR, Epstein SE. Observations on the optimum time for operative intervention for aortic regurgitation. II. Serial echocardiographic evaluation of asymptomatic patients. *Circulation* 1980; **61**: 484–492.
33. Siemienczuk D, Greenberg B, Morris C, *et al.* Chronic aortic insufficiency: factors associated with progression to aortic valve replacement. *Ann Intern Med* 1989; **110**: 587–592.
34. Bonow RO, Lakatos E, Maron BJ, Epstein SE. Serial long-term assessment of the natural history of asymptomatic patients with chronic aortic regurgitation and normal left ventricular systolic function. *Circulation* 1991; **84**: 1625–1635.
35. Ishii K, Hirota Y, Suwa M, Kita Y, Onaka H, Kawamura K. Natural history and left ventricular response in chronic aortic regurgitation. *Am J Cardiol* 1996; **78**: 357–361.
36. Scognamiglio R, Rahimtoola SH, Fasoli G, Nistri S, Dalla Volta S. Nifedipine in asymptomatic patients with severe aortic regurgitation and normal left ventricular function. *N Engl J Med* 1994; **331**: 689–694.
37. Tornos MP, Olona M, Permanyer-Miralda G, *et al.* Clinical outcome of severe asymptomatic chronic aortic regurgitation: a long-term prospective follow-up study. *Am Heart J* 1995; **130**: 333–339.
38. von Olshausen K, Schwarz F, Apfelbach J, Rohrig N, Kramer B, Kubler W. Determinants of the incidence and severity of ventricular arrhythmias in aortic valve disease. *Am J Cardiol* 1983; **51**: 1103–1109.
39. Klodas E, Enriquez-Sarano M, Tajik AJ, Mullany CJ, Bailey KR, Seward JB. Aortic regurgitation complicated by extreme left ventricular dilation: long-term outcome after surgical correction. *J Am Coll Cardiol* 1996; **27**: 670–677.
40. Ling H, Enriquez-Sarano M, Seward J, *et al.* Clinical outcome of mitral regurgitation due to flail leaflets. *N Eng J Med* 1996; **335**: 1417–1423.

41. Tribouilloy C, Enriquez-Sarano M, Schaff H, *et al*. Impact of preoperative symptoms on survival after surgical correction of organic mitral regurgitation: rationale for optimizing surgical indications. *Circulation* 1999; **99**: 400–405.
42. Delahaye JP, Gare JP, Viguier E, Delahaye F, De Gevigney G, Milon H. Natural history of severe mitral regurgitation. *Eur Heart J* 1991; **12**(Suppl. B): 5–9.
43. Grigioni F, Enriquez-Sarano M, Ling LH, *et al*. Sudden death in mitral regurgitation due to flail leaflet. *J Am Coll Cardiol* 1999; **34**: 2078–2085.
44. Enriquez-Sarano M, Schaff H, Orszulak T, Tajik A, Bailey K, Frye R. Valve repair improves the outcome of surgery for mitral regurgitation. *Circulation* 1995; **91**: 1264–1265.
45. Enriquez-Sarano M, Tajik A, Schaff H, Orszulak T, Bailey K, Frye R. Echocardiographic prediction of survival after surgical correction of organic mitral regurgitation. *Circulation* 1994; **90**: 830–837.
46. Enriquez-Sarano M, Tajik A, Schaff H, *et al*. Echocardiographic prediction of left ventricular function after correction of mitral regurgitation: results and clinical implications. *J Am Coll Cardiol* 1994; **24**: 1536–1543.
47. Grigioni F, Avierinos JF, Ling LH, *et al*. Atrial fibrillation complicating the course of degenerative mitral regurgitation: determinants and long-term outcome. *J Am Coll Cardiol* 2002; **40**: 84–92.
48. Freed LA, Levy D, Levine RA, *et al*. Prevalence and clinical outcome of mitral-valve prolapse. *N Engl J Med* 1999; **341**: 1–7.
49. Avierinos JF, Gersh BJ, Melton LJ, 3rd, *et al*. Natural history of asymptomatic mitral valve prolapse in the community. *Circulation* 2002; **106**: 1355–1361.
50. Rowe JC, Bland EF, Sprague HB, White PD. The course of mitral stenosis without surgery: ten- and twenty-year perspectives. *Ann Intern Med* 1960; **52**: 741–749.

CHAPTER 11
Heart failure

William G. Stevenson and Helmut Drexler

Introduction

Sudden death is an important cause of mortality in patients with heart failure, with 20% to more than 50% of all deaths occurring suddenly. The term heart failure includes a wide variety of cardiac disorders characterized by symptoms related to elevated cardiac filling pressures and, in some cases diminished cardiac output that are associated with a number of other physiological derangements. The incidence and causes of sudden death varies with the type of heart disease and the severity of heart failure.

Heart failure with preserved systolic function

Heart failure with preserved systolic function encompasses a heterogeneous group of patients with valvular heart disease, restrictive cardiomyopathies, hypertrophic cardiomyopathy, and endomyocardial fibrosis. Sudden death in hypertrophic cardiomyopathy has been well studied (Chapter 8). In the other syndromes, knowledge is limited. Most patients with heart failure and preserved systolic function, however, do not have these causes, but rather are elderly patients, often with diabetes mellitus, long standing hypertension, and ventricular hypertrophy. Although mortality is only slightly less than that for patients with depressed systolic function, the risk of sudden death and markers for risk are not well defined. In the DIG trial, 2.8% of 395 patients with heart failure and left ventricular (LV) ejection fraction >0.55 died due to a presumed arrhythmic cause during a median follow-up of 37 months, accounting for 12% of all deaths in that subgroup [1].

Sudden death in heart failure with depressed systolic function

For chronic heart failure and depressed systolic function, the incidence of sudden death increases with the severity of heart failure as reflected in New York Heart Association (NYHA) functional classification and LV ejection fraction (Figure 11.1) [1,2]. Patients with minimal to modest symptoms (class I–II) have a sudden death risk that ranges from 2% to 6% per year. With more advanced symptoms (class III to IV), the risk increases from 5% to 12%

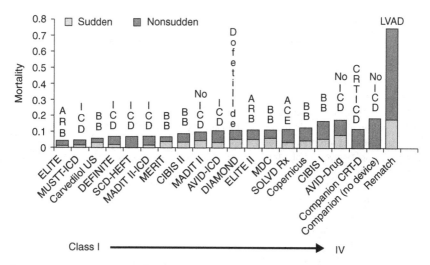

Figure 11.1 One-year mortality in recent trials enrolling heart failure patients or patients with arrhythmias and depressed ventricular function is shown. For each bar the lower portion is sudden death (if reported). The upper segment is nonsudden death. Trials are arranged according to predominant NYHA functional class of the patients enrolled as indicated by the arrow below the graph from left to right, unless specified results are shown for the treatment group with the therapy specified above the bar. ACE = angiotensin converting enzyme inhibitor, ARB = angiotensin receptor blocker, BB = beta-blocker, CRT-ICD = cardiac resynchonization therapy-ICD, ICD = implantable cardioverter-defibrillator.

per year. As heart failure severity increases, deaths from pump failure increase to a greater extent than sudden deaths and the proportion of deaths that are sudden decreases from 50% or more for mild to moderate heart failure, to 5% to 30% for severe heart failure. Of patients with advanced ventricular dysfunction but sufficient stability to be accepted onto out-patients waiting lists for cardiac transplantation, the risk of sudden death ranges from 10% to 20% per year [3,4].

Left ventricular ejection fraction, LV dilation, and natriuretic peptides that are markers of heart failure severity, ventricular dysfunction, and mortality also predict sudden death [1,5]. Elevated natriuretic peptide levels predict an increased risk of sudden death in survivors of myocardial infarction and in patients with chronic heart failure [6,7]. Left bundle branch block has been associated with greater mortality and sudden death in heart failure [8].

Causes of arrhythmias in heart failure

Ventricular tachycardia (VT) and ventricular fibrillation (VF) are probably the most frequent arrhythmias that cause sudden death in heart failure. However, different pathophysiologic mechanisms can lead to these arrhythmias (Table 11.1).

Table 11.1 Causes of sudden death in heart failure.

Primary arrhythmias
  Monomorphic VT
  Polymorphic VT
  VF
  AV block without sufficient escape rhythm
  Sinus arrest without sufficient escape rhythm
Causes of secondary cardiac arrests
  Acute myocardial infarction
  Stroke
  Pulmonary emboli
  Ruptured abdominal aortic aneurysm
  Hyperkalemia
  Hypokalemia
  Hypoglycemia
  Drug induced arrhythmias
    Torsade de pointes with QT prolongation
    Ventricular flutter – sodium channel blockade
    Bradyarrhythmias
    Beta-blockers, amiodarone, others
  Sleep apnea?

Scar-related reentry

Patients with prior myocardial infarction and heart failure typically have large areas of infarction (Chapter 3). Programmed stimulation studies suggest that more than a third of large infarcts can support reentry circuits [9]. The VTs that result are typically monomorphic, but can degenerate to VF. The arrhythmia substrate is relatively stable over time, such that victims that survive are subject to recurrences and VT is usually inducible at electrophysiologic testing, allowing this method to be potentially used to select high-risk patients for treatment.

In nonischemic cardiomyopathy, large areas of scar or infarction are usually absent. Sustained monomorphic VT is uncommon, but patients who do develop monomorphic VT are often found to have areas of low voltage consistent with scar, similar to those that are identified in areas of infarction [10]. The scar may be a consequence of replacement fibrosis due to the myopathic process itself or coronary embolism from left ventricular or atrial thrombus.

Bundle branch reentry VT

Approximately 8% of monomorphic VTs in patients with depressed ventricular function are due to reentry involving the his Purkinje system [10]. In the most common form, the reentrant excitation wavefront propagates up the left bundle branch, down the right bundle branch, and then through the interventricular septum to reenter the left bundle. These VTs are often rapid, causing syncope or cardiac arrest. They should be particularly suspected in patients who have sustained monomorphic VT associated with valvular heart disease, cardiomyopathy, or muscular dystrophy.

Hypertrophy

Chronic heart failure is usually accompanied by ventricular hypertrophy, with changes in myocardial structure and myocyte function that promote arrhythmias (Chapter 3). Action potential duration is prolonged due to reduced repolarizing potassium currents (reduced I_K, I_{K1}, and I_{to} have all been described) and abnormal intracellular calcium handling including increased Na–Ca exchanger expression and activity [11,12]. These changes are likely to increase susceptibility to the polymorphic VT *torsade de pointes*.

Hypertrophy is also accompanied by interstitial fibrosis, replacement fibrosis, and decreased gap junction surface area. Electrical coupling between myocytes is reduced, conduction slowing that results would be expected to promote reentry [13].

Myocardial ischemia and infarction

Acute myocardial ischemia and infarction are important causes of sudden death in patients with chronic heart failure [14]. Evidence of acute myocardial infarction or coronary artery lesions were identified in 42% of autopsies in sudden death victims from one heart failure trial [14].

Sympathetic nervous system activation, neurohumoral, and electrolyte abnormalities

Heart failure is associated with sympathetic activation and parasympathetic withdrawal, which increase susceptibility to VF during acute ischemia and promote automaticity [5,15]. Diuretic induced hypokalemia and magnesium depletion cause QT prolongation and promote arrhythmias [16–18]. Hyperkalemia is also a risk from treatment with medications that antagonize secretion and actions of aldosterone, administration of potassium supplements, and renal impairment [19,20]. One survey observed a 12% incidence of hyperkalemia >6.0 meq/L with the addition of spironolactone to heart failure regimens [20]. Hyperkalemia can present as either VT or bradyarrhythmias.

Sleep apnea with peripheral oxygen desaturation occurs in upto approximately 50% of patients with chronic heart failure and can contribute to sympathetic activation, exacerbation of heart failure, bradyarrhythmias, and ventricular ectopy and is a marker for increased mortality [21,22]. However, a relation of sleep apnea to sudden death has not been established.

Bradyarrhythmias

Atrio-ventricular (AV) block, and prolonged QRS duration are common in patients with heart failure [23,24]. In a series of 94 patients with nonischemic dilated cardiomyopathy, first or second degree AV block on ambulatory electrocardiogram monitoring was seen in 28% of patients and was associated with a greater than four-fold increase in sudden death [24]. Bradyarrhythmias at the time of cardiac arrest are more common in end-stage heart failure, in nonischemic cardiomyopathy, and in hospitalized patients [25].

Nonarrhythmia-dependent causes of sudden death

Although the majority of sudden deaths are probably due to VT/VF, causes that would not be addressed by a strategy that focuses on treatment of ventricular arrhythmias also occur, including thromboemboli from left atrium or ventricle causing stroke or myocardial infarction, pulmonary emboli, and ruptured aortic aneurysms. These events are consistent with implantable cardioverter-defibrillator (ICD) interrogations in patients who die suddenly, that often suggest pulseless electrical activity either after termination of VT or VF, or with no detected tachyarrhythmia [26,27].

Patients with chronic heart failure who survive a cardiac arrest that is due to a presumed "secondary" cause, such as pulmonary edema, myocardial ischemia, or hyperkalemia remain at high risk for sudden death even if the precipitating cause is recognized and treatment instituted. Whether ICDs reduce sudden death in this population is not yet known.

Identifying patients at high risk for arrhythmic sudden death

Identifying patients at greatest risk of arrhythmic sudden death is of great interest with the wider availability of ICDs. Unfortunately, the risk of sudden death increases with the severity of heart failure and markers of arrhythmia risk also increase with severity of heart failure and often with the risk of death from pump failure. For most noninvasive markers, strategies using them to select patients for ICDs have not yet been adequately tested in prospective trials.

Syncope
Unexplained syncope is a marker for a high risk of sudden death or sustained VT exceeding 20% per year [28]. A careful arrhythmia evaluation and consideration for ICD is often warranted.

Nonsustained VT
Nonsustained VT and frequent ventricular ectopy are markers of severity of heart failure, increased mortality, and sudden death, but are present in upto 79% of patients [5,29,30]. Nonsustained VT has been associated with a 1.5–1.7-fold increase in mortality and a 2–2.8-fold increase in sudden death, but is not always independent of the severity of ventricular dysfunction [29,30]. Suppression of nonsustained VT by amiodarone therapy did not improve survival in a Veterans Administration (VA) cooperative study [30].

Heart-rate variability

The increase in sympathetic tone in chronic heart failure is associated with diminished heart-rate variability [5]. Diminished heart-rate variability parallels the severity of heart failure and is associated with increased mortality [31]. It has been an independent predictor of sudden death in some, but not all studies [31].

La Rovere *et al.* assessed heart-rate variability from 5 min recordings during controlled breathing, position, and activity (resting supine) to standardize these potentially confounding factors [5]. In 242 patients with a sudden death rate of approximately 3% per year, diminished power in the low frequency band (0.04–0.15 Hz) was associated with approximately a three-fold increased risk of sudden death independent of ventricular function and ventricular ectopy. Use of this method to select patients for ICDs has not been tested.

Abnormalities of repolarization assessed from the QT interval

Vrtovec and coworkers observed that a corrected QT interval >440 ms was associated with increased risk of sudden death in patients with class III or IV heart failure who also had elevated natriuretic peptide levels [32].

The difference in QT intervals in different ECG leads, referred to as QT dispersion, has been proposed as an indicator of ventricular dispersion of recovery, but was not a predictor of outcome in two relatively large heart failure studies [33,34].

T-wave alternans at relatively low heart rates during exercise (e.g. <110 beats/min) is associated with inducible and spontaneous arrhythmias and is a marker for worse heart failure and ventricular dysfunction (Chapter 4) [35,36]. Use will be limited by the inability of some patients to adequately increase heart rate during exercise. Utility for selecting patients for ICDs remains to be established.

Programmed electrical stimulation in patients with coronary artery disease

In patients with coronary artery disease and depressed ventricular function, inducible VT is a marker of sudden death risk that identifies patients who benefit from an ICD (Chapter 15) [37,38]. The Multicenter Unsustained Tachycardia Trial (MUSTT) found inducible sustained VT present in 35% of patients with left ventricular ejection fraction <0.4 and nonsustained VT [37]. Inducible VT was associated with a 9% per year risk of cardiac arrest compared to 6% per year for those without inducible VT [9]. Although treatment with an ICD was not randomized, the patients with inducible VT who received an ICD had a lower 5-year mortality and 5-year risk of sudden death or cardiac arrest of 9% as compared to 37% for patients without ICDs. Thus, the value of both EP studies and ICDs are established in patients with coronary heart disease.

Programmed electrical stimulation in patients with nonischemic cardiomyopathies

Programmed stimulation is not a useful screening test for patients with non-ischemic causes of heart failure. Sustained monomorphic VT is inducible in approximately 7% of patients and those without Inducible VT remain at risk for sudden death.

Prevention of sudden death with pharmacologic therapies

A number of therapies that do not specifically-target arrhythmias reduce sudden death in patients with heart failure [39]. Beneficial effects are likely due to a reductions in the nonarrhythmic causes of sudden death, reducing myocardial ischemia or infarction, and by slowing the progression of heart failure and blunting neurohormonal factors and electrical remodeling that promote arrhythmias.

Beta-adrenergic blockers reduce sudden death in chronic heart failure populations with ischemic and nonischemic causes of heart failure [40,41]. The Metoprolol CR/XL Randomized Intervention Trial (MERIT) randomized 3991 patients with chronic heart failure (class II–IV) and LV ejection fraction of ≤0.40 to sustained-release metoprolol or placebo [42]. After a mean follow-up of 1 year, mortality was lower with metoprolol treatment (7% versus 11%, relative risk reduction 34%, $p = .0062$). Sudden death was reduced from 6.5% to 4% (relative risk reduction 41%, $p = .0002$). The carvedilol prospective randomized cumulative survival trial (COPERNICUS) randomized 2289 patients with functional class III or IV heart failure to carvedilol or placebo [41]. After a mean follow-up of 10 months, sudden death was reduced from 6.1% to 3.9% ($p = .016$). The Cardiac Insufficiency Bisoprolol Study II (CIBIS-II) randomized 2647 patients with class III or IV heart failure and LV ejection fraction of ≤0.35 to bisoprolol or placebo [43]. After a mean follow-up of 1.3 years, bisoprolol reduced mortality from 17.3% to 11.8% (relative risk reduction 34%, $p < .0001$). Sudden death was reduced from 6.3% to 3.6% (relative risk reduction 44%, $p = .0011$).

Antagonism of the renin angiotensin system was found to have a favorable effect on sudden death potential mechanisms including reductions in adrenergic stimulation, aldosterone secretion, electrolyte depletion, ischemic events, and electrical remodeling [39]. Angiotensin converting enzyme inhibitors reduce sudden death in survivors of myocardial infarction [44]. In heart failure trials they reduce mortality, but many trials have not specifically assessed the impact on sudden death [39]. The angiotensin receptor blocking agent valsartan reduced mortality in heart failure patients who were not receiving a concomitant angiotensin converting enzyme inhibitor, with a favorable trend toward a reduction in sudden death with small numbers of patients [45].

Direct aldosterone antagonists spironolactone and eplerenone reduce mortality and sudden death in heart failure, provided precautions are taken to reduce the risk of hyperkalemia [16]. Attention to avoiding hyperkalemia is particularly important when these drugs are combined with other antagonists of the renin angiotensin system, beta-blockers, and potassium supplements. The risk of hyperkalemia is particularly high in patients with increased serum levels of creatinine receiving these combinations. In a randomized trial of 1663 patients with predominantly class III and IV heart failure and LV ejection fraction ≤ 0.35 followed for a mean of 2 years, spironolactone reduced mortality from 46% to 35% (relative reduction 30%, $p < .001$) [16]. Sudden death was reduced from 13% to 10% (relative reduction 29%, $p = .02$). In a randomized trial enrolling 6632 patients with recent myocardial infarction complicated by heart failure, eplerenone reduced mortality from 16.7% to 14.4 % and sudden death from 6% to 4.9% ($p = .03$) during a mean follow-up of 16 months [17].

Lipid lowering hydroxy methyl glutarate-Co (HMG-Co) reductase inhibitors, statins, reduce mortality with favorable trends toward reduction in sudden death in patients with coronary artery disease [39]. In the AVID trial, therapy with a statin was associated with a reduction in recurrences of sustained VT/VF [46]. Benefit may be due to reduction of ischemic episodes, but other antiarrhythmic effects have also been postulated and benefit in heart failure patients without coronary artery disease has also been suggested [47].

Antiarrhythmic drug therapy

Class I antiarrhythmic drugs have negative inotropic effects and proarrhythmic effects that have the potential to increase mortality in patients with depressed ventricular function. Dofetilide is a class III antiarrhythmic drug that blocks the repolarizing potassium current I_{Kr}, prolonging action potential duration. In a randomized trial of 1518 patients who had been hospitalized with class III or IV heart failure dofetilide had no impact on survival [48]. Sotalol blocks the same potassium channel as dofetilide and additionally has nonselective beta-adrenergic blocking activity, but has not been well studied in heart failure. *Torsade de pointes* is an important proarrhythmia concern with sotalol and dofetilide.

Amiodarone is inferior to ICDs in preventing death from arrhythmias, but a meta-analysis of trials in heart failure concluded that amiodarone therapy produced a 17% reduction in mortality and 23% reduction in sudden death compared to no antiarrhythmic therapy [49]. Toxicity is a major problem with 14% more patients discontinuing amiodarone than placebo by 2 years of follow-up. In the Sudden Cardiac Death in Heart Failure Trial (SCD-HeFT), amiodarone did not improve mortality compared to placebo in patients with class II or III heart failure and LV ejection fraction ≤ 0.35 and analysis of the 497 patients with class III symptoms observed an adverse effect on mortality (hazard ratio 1.44, 95% confidence intervals: 1.05–1.97). Amiodarone was maintained at the relatively high dose of 400 mg daily for the first year in the majority of patients; toxicities could be a factor in unfavorable outcomes compared to prior trials.

Implantable defibrillators for primary prevention of sudden death in heart failure

Implantable cardioverter-defibrillators offer the most effective protection from sudden arrhythmic death and reduce mortality by preventing sudden death in selected patients with depressed ventricular function (Chapter 15). Heart failure severity and etiology are important considerations in considering patients for ICD therapy.

In patients with coronary artery disease the Multicenter Automatic Defibrillator Implantation Trial (MADIT) and MUSTT trials demonstrated that ICDs improved survival for patients with depressed LV function, nonsustained VT and inducible VT [37,38,50]. The MADIT II trial demonstrated a survival benefit of ICDs for patients with coronary artery disease and LV ejection fractions of 0.30 or less [50]. The SCD-HeFT trial demonstrated that ICDs improved survival of patients with LV ejection fraction of 0.35 or less, including patients with nonischemic cardiomyopathies [51]. There are important caveats in extrapolating the results of the ICD primary prevention trials to patients with heart failure.

Although the MADIT II and MUSTT trials of primary prevention included only patients with significantly depressed ventricular function, these were not heart failure trials and only 25% of these patients had functional class III symptoms; 75% were functional class I or II. In SCD-HeFT, all patients had symptomatic heart failure, but 70% were functional class II and only 30% had functional class III symptoms; again, class IV patients were excluded. In both MADIT II and SCD-HeFT, a survival benefit did not become apparent until after the first year. In MADIT II, the difference in survival for ICD and no ICD patients was 1% at 1 year. In SCD-HeFT, the curves for placebo and ICD groups do not diverge until approximately 18 months. These trials suggest that ICDs benefit patients who have reasonably preserved functional capacity despite significantly depressed LV function, and who are likely to survive more than 1 year without death from pump failure. The magnitude of the benefit is in the range of a 6–8% absolute increase in survival (relative risk reduction of 28–31%) over follow-up of 20 months for MADIT II and 5 years for SCD-HeFT. Thus, for every 12–16 patients who receive an ICD one life is saved.

It seems likely that ICDs can benefit patients with nonischemic cardiomyopathy, although the magnitude of the benefit may be less than for patients with ischemic cardiomyopathy. Four randomized trials included patients with nonischemic cardiomyopathy. Two relatively small trials, the AMIOdarone Versus Implantable cardioverter-defibrillator Randomized Trial (AMIOVIRT) and the Cardiomyopathy Trial (CAT) found no benefit of an ICD over amiodarone or no antiarrhythmic therapy, respectively [52,53]. The DEFibrillators In NonIschemic cardiomyopathy Treatment Evaluation trial (DEFINITE) found that a third of deaths were sudden, and sudden deaths were reduced by the ICD, but the overall mortality of 7% per year was lower than anticipated and the trend for reduction in mortality did not reach statistical significance [54]. Notably the number of sudden deaths in the DEFINITE trial was low (17 sudden deaths, 14 in the control group versus three in the group with ICDs) and therefore, although statistically significant, the result is not statistically robust. Based on the presented, but yet unpublished data of the SCD-HeFT trial, 48% of the 2521 patients enrolled had nonischemic cardiomyopathy. Subgroup analysis suggests similar benefit for ischemic and nonischemic cardiomyopathy.

Appreciation of the magnitude of benefit and limitiations of ICDs are important considerations in the use of ICDs in heart failure populations. In advanced heart failure, the risk of death from pump failure and options for ventricular assist devices, cardiac transplantation, and potential for benefit from cardiac resynchronization therapy are important considerations. Although patients with severe class IV heart failure are at high risk for sudden death, benefit from an ICD is limited by deaths from pump failure, and an ICD is not appropriate therapy for many. Patients with class IV symptoms have been excluded from all ICD trials. Those patients who are candidates for cardiac transplantation, however, may receive substantial benefit despite severe heart failure if an ICD prevents sudden death while they are on an out-patient list awaiting transplantation [3,4].

Although the risk of ICD implantation is low, occasional patients with advanced heart failure experience deterioration in heart failure following the implantation procedure. In addition, it is important to consider the potential adverse impact that can occur when implantation of an ICD results in right ventricular pacing with consequent change in ventricular activation similar to that of left bundle branch block. This effect likely contributed to the excess mortality observed with dual chamber (DDD) compared to ventricular inhibited (VVI) pacing from ICDs in the Dual Chamber VVI Implantable Defibrillator (DAVID) trial, and to the increase in hospitalizations for heart failure in the ICD group in MADIT II [50,55].

Cardiac resynchronization therapy

Implantation of an ICD with left ventricular pacing is also a reasonable consideration for patients with functional class III or IV heart failure and prolonged QRS duration who may receive hemodynamic benefit from cardiac resynchronization therapy. The COMPANION trial randomized 1520 patients with NYHA functional class III or IV heart failure and QRS duration >120 ms in a 1 : 2 : 2 scheme to medical therapy, a biventricular pacemaker (cardiac resynchronization therapy – CRT) or a biventricular pacer-defibrillators (CRT-D) [56]. After median follow-ups of 15–16 months, mortality in the medical treatment only group was 25% and was reduced to 18% for the CRT-D group (HR = 0.64, $p = .004$). Mortality was 21% in the CRT group (who did not have an ICD); this favorable trend to reduction in mortality did not reach statistical significance. The more than two-fold greater annual mortality in this trial as compared to MADIT II, MUSTT, and SCD-HeFT is consistent with the more advanced heart failure and inclusion of class IV patients as compared to previous ICD trials. Although the impact on sudden death was not reported, the benefit in the ICD groups supports a reduction in arrhythmic death as a likely benefit. CRT has been suggested to have beneficial effects on arrhythmias by improving heart failure and reducing sympathetic tone, but can also potentially have proarrhythmic effects due to the change in ventricular activation induced by LV epicardial pacing [57].

Conclusions

Improvements in medical management of heart failure are reducing both total mortality and sudden death. As therapies that favorably impact on hypertrophy and electrical remodeling evolve, further improvements can be anticipated. ICDs provide protection from arrhythmic sudden death and combining this technology with cardiac resynchronization therapy holds promise for further benefit in patients with advanced heart failure. Substantial costs of device therapy warrant further development of methods to select patients at high risk for arrhythmic sudden death.

References

1. Curtis JP, Sokol SI, Wang Y, *et al.* The association of left ventricular ejection fraction, mortality, and cause of death in stable outpatients with heart failure. *J Am Coll Cardiol* 2003; **42**: 736–742.
2. Uretsky BF, Sheahan RG. Primary prevention of sudden cardiac death in heart failure: will the solution be shocking? *J Am Coll Cardiol* 1997; **30**: 1589–1597.
3. Nagele H, Rodiger W. Sudden death and tailored medical therapy in elective candidates for heart transplantation. *J Heart Lung Transplant* 1999; **18**: 869–876.
4. Sandner SE, Wieselthaler G, Zuckermann A, *et al.* Survival benefit of the implantable cardioverter-defibrillator in patients on the waiting list for cardiac transplantation. *Circulation* 2001; **104**: I171–I176.
5. La Rovere MT, Pinna GD, Maestri R, *et al.* Short-term heart rate variability strongly predicts sudden cardiac death in chronic heart failure patients. *Circulation* 2003; **107**: 565–570.
6. Tapanainen JM, Lindgren KS, Makikallio TH, *et al.* Natriuretic peptides as predictors of non-sudden and sudden cardiac death after acute myocardial infarction in the beta-blocking era. *J Am Coll Cardiol* 2004; **43**: 757–763.
7. Berger R, Huelsman M, Strecker K, *et al.* B-type natriuretic peptide predicts sudden death in patients with chronic heart failure. *Circulation* 2002; **105**: 2392–2397.
8. Baldasseroni S, Opasich C, Gorini M, *et al.* Left bundle-branch block is associated with increased 1-year sudden and total mortality rate in 5517 outpatients with congestive heart failure: a report from the Italian network on congestive heart failure. *Am Heart J* 2002; **143**: 398–405.

9. Buxton AE, Lee KL, DiCarlo L, *et al.* Electrophysiologic testing to identify patients with coronary artery disease who are at risk for sudden death. Multicenter Unsustained Tachycardia Trial Investigators. *N Engl J Med* 2000; **342**: 1937–1945.
10. Delacretaz E, Stevenson WG, Ellison KE, *et al.* Mapping and radiofrequency catheter ablation of the three types of sustained monomorphic ventricular tachycardia in nonischemic heart disease [see comments]. *J Cardiovasc Electrophysiol* 2000; **11**: 11–17.
11. Janse MJ. Electrophysiological changes in heart failure and their relationship to arrhythmogenesis. *Cardiovasc Res* 2004; **61**: 208–217.
12. Studer R, Reinecke H, Bilger J, *et al.* Gene expression of the cardiac Na(+)–Ca^{2+} exchanger in end-stage human heart failure. *Circ Res* 1994; **75**: 443–453.
13. Pastore JM, Rosenbaum DS. Role of structural barriers in the mechanism of alternans-induced reentry. *Circ Res* 2000; **87**: 1157–1163.
14. Uretsky BF, Thygesen K, Armstrong PW, *et al.* Acute coronary findings at autopsy in heart failure patients with sudden death: results from the Assessment of Treatment with Lisinopril and Survival (ATLAS) trial. *Circulation* 2000; **102**: 611–616.
15. Yamada T, Shimonagata T, Fukunami M, *et al.* Comparison of the prognostic value of cardiac iodine-123 metaiodobenzylguanidine imaging and heart rate variability in patients with chronic heart failure: a prospective study. *J Am Coll Cardiol* 2003; **41**: 231–238.
16. Pitt B, Zannad F, Remme WJ, *et al.* The effect of spironolactone on morbidity and mortality in patients with severe heart failure. Randomized Aldactone Evaluation Study Investigators [see comments]. *N Engl J Med* 1999; **341**: 709–717.
17. Pitt B, Remme W, Zannad F, *et al.* Eplerenone, a selective aldosterone blocker, in patients with left ventricular dysfunction after myocardial infarction. *N Engl J Med* 2003; **348**: 1309–1321.
18. Macdonald JE, Struthers AD. What is the optimal serum potassium level in cardiovascular patients? *J Am Coll Cardiol* 2004; **43**: 155–161.
19. Juurlink DN, Mamdani MM, Lee DS, *et al.* Rates of hyperkalemia after publication of the randomized aldactone evaluation study. *N Engl J Med* 2004; **351**: 543–551.
20. Bozkurt B, Agoston I, Knowlton AA. Complications of inappropriate use of spironolactone in heart failure: when an old medicine spirals out of new guidelines. *J Am Coll Cardiol* 2003; **41**: 211–214.
21. Javaheri S. Effects of continuous positive airway pressure on sleep apnea and ventricular irritability in patients with heart failure. *Circulation* 2000; **101**: 392–397.
22. Mansfield D, Kaye DM, Brunner La Rocca H, *et al.* Raised sympathetic nerve activity in heart failure and central sleep apnea is due to heart failure severity. *Circulation* 2003; **107**: 1396–1400.
23. Farwell D, Patel NR, Hall A, *et al.* How many people with heart failure are appropriate for biventricular resynchronization? *Eur Heart J* 2000; **21**: 1246–1250.
24. Schoeller R, Andresen D, Buttner P, *et al.* First- or second-degree atrioventricular block as a risk factor in idiopathic dilated cardiomyopathy. *Am J Cardiol* 1993; **71**: 720–726.
25. Faggiano P, d'Aloia A, Gualeni A, *et al.* Mechanisms and immediate outcome of in-hospital cardiac arrest in patients with advanced heart failure secondary to ischemic or idiopathic dilated cardiomyopathy. *Am J Cardiol* 2001; **87**: 655–657, A10–A11.

26. Grubman EM, Pavri BB, Shipman T, *et al.* Cardiac death and stored electrograms in patients with third-generation implantable cardioverter-defibrillators. *J Am Coll Cardiol* 1998; **32**: 1056–1062.

27. Mitchell LB, Pineda EA, Titus JL, *et al.* Sudden death in patients with implantable cardioverter defibrillators: the importance of post-shock electromechanical dissociation. *J Am Coll Cardiol* 2002; **39**: 1323–1328.

28. Fonarow GC, Feliciano Z, Boyle NG, *et al.* Improved survival in patients with nonischemic advanced heart failure and syncope treated with an implantable cardioverter-defibrillator. *Am J Cardiol* 2000; **85**: 981–985.

29. Teerlink JR, Jalaluddin M, Anderson S, *et al.* Ambulatory ventricular arrhythmias in patients with heart failure do not specifically predict an increased risk of sudden death. PROMISE (Prospective Randomized Milrinone Survival Evaluation) Investigators. *Circulation* 2000; **101**: 40–46.

30. Singh SN, Fisher SG, Carson PE, *et al.* Prevalence and significance of nonsustained ventricular tachycardia in patients with premature ventricular contractions and heart failure treated with vasodilator therapy. Department of Veterans Affairs CHF STAT Investigators. *J Am Coll Cardiol* 1998; **32**: 942–947.

31. Nolan J, Batin PD, Andrews R, *et al.* Prospective study of heart rate variability and mortality in chronic heart failure: results of the United Kingdom heart failure evaluation and assessment of risk trial (UK-heart). *Circulation* 1998; **98**: 1510–1516.

32. Vrtovec B, Delgado R, Zewail A, *et al.* Prolonged QTc interval and high B-type natriuretic peptide levels together predict mortality in patients with advanced heart failure. *Circulation* 2003; **107**: 1764–1769.

33. Gang Y, Ono T, Hnatkova K, *et al.* QT dispersion has no prognostic value in patients with symptomatic heart failure: an ELITE II substudy. *Pacing Clin Electrophysiol* 2003; **26**: 394–400.

34. Brendorp B, Elming H, Jun L, *et al.* QT dispersion has no prognostic information for patients with advanced congestive heart failure and reduced left ventricular systolic function. *Circulation* 2001; **103**: 831–835.

35. Adachi K, Ohnishi Y, Shima T, *et al.* Determinant of microvolt-level T-wave alternans in patients with dilated cardiomyopathy. *J Am Coll Cardiol* 1999; **34**: 374–380.

36. Grimm W, Hoffmann J, Menz V, *et al.* Relation between microvolt level T wave alternans and other potential noninvasive predictors of arrhythmic risk in the Marburg Cardiomyopathy Study. *Pacing Clin Electrophysiol* 2000; **23**: 1960–1964.

37. Buxton AE, Lee KL, Fisher JD, *et al.* A randomized study of the prevention of sudden death in patients with coronary artery disease. Multicenter Unsustained Tachycardia Trial Investigators [see comments]. *N Engl J Med* 1999; **341**: 1882–1890. Erratum appears in *N Engl J Med* 2000; **342**(17): 1300.

38. Moss AJ, Hall WJ, Cannom DS, *et al.* Improved survival with an implanted defibrillator in patients with coronary disease at high risk for ventricular arrhythmia. Multicenter Automatic Defibrillator Implantation Trial Investigators [see comments]. *N Engl J Med* 1996; **335**: 1933–1940.

39. Alberte C, Zipes DP. Use of nonantiarrhythmic drugs for prevention of sudden cardiac death. *J Cardiovasc Electrophysiol* 2003; **14**: S87–S95.

40. Janosi A, Ghali JK, Herlitz J, *et al.* Metoprolol CR/XL in postmyocardial infarction patients with chronic heart failure: experiences from MERIT-HF. *Am Heart J* 2003; **146**: 721–728.

41. Packer M, Fowler MB, Roecker EB, *et al.* Effect of carvedilol on the morbidity of patients with severe chronic heart failure: results of the carvedilol prospective randomized cumulative survival (COPERNICUS) study. *Circulation* 2002; **106**: 2194–2199.

42. Effect of metoprolol CR/XL in chronic heart failure: Metoprolol CR/XL Randomised Intervention Trial in Congestive Heart Failure (MERIT-HF) [see comments]. *Lancet* 1999; **353**: 2001–2007.

43. The Cardiac Insufficiency Bisoprolol Study II (CIBIS-II): a randomised trial [see comments]. *Lancet* 1999; **353**: 9–13.

44. Domanski MJ, Exner DV, Borkowf CB, *et al.* Effect of angiotensin converting enzyme inhibition on sudden cardiac death in patients following acute myocardial infarction. A meta-analysis of randomized clinical trials. *J Am Coll Cardiol* 1999; **33**: 598–604.

45. Maggioni AP, Anand I, Gottlieb SO, *et al.* Effects of valsartan on morbidity and mortality in patients with heart failure not receiving angiotensin-converting enzyme inhibitors. *J Am Coll Cardiol* 2002; **40**: 1414–1421.

46. Mitchell LB, Powell JL, Gillis AM, *et al.* Are lipid-lowering drugs also antiarrhythmic drugs? An analysis of the Antiarrhythmics Versus Implantable Defibrillators (AVID) trial. *J Am Coll Cardiol* 2003; **42**: 81–87.

47. Horwich TB, MacLellan WR, Fonarow GC. Statin therapy is associated with improved survival in ischemic and non-ischemic heart failure. *J Am Coll Cardiol* 2004; **43**: 642–648.

48. Torp-Pedersen C, Moller M, Bloch-Thomsen PE, *et al.* Dofetilide in patients with congestive heart failure and left ventricular dysfunction. Danish Investigations of Arrhythmia and Mortality on Dofetilide Study Group [see comments]. *N Engl J Med* 1999; **341**: 857–865.

49. Effect of prophylactic amiodarone on mortality after acute myocardial infarction and in congestive heart failure: meta-analysis of individual data from 6500 patients in randomised trials. Amiodarone Trials Meta-Analysis Investigators. *Lancet* 1997; **350**: 1417–1424.

50. Moss AJ, Zareba W, Hall WJ, *et al.* Prophylactic implantation of a defibrillator in patients with myocardial infarction and reduced ejection fraction. *N Engl J Med* 2002; **346**: 877–883.

51. Bardy GH, Lee KL, Mark DB, *et al.* for the Sudden Cardiac Death in Heart Failure Trial (SCD-HeFT) Investigators. Amiodatrone or an implantable cardioverter-defibrillator for congestive heart failure. *N Engl J Med* 2005; **352**: 225–37.

52. Strickberger SA, Hummel JD, Bartlett TG, *et al.* Amiodarone Versus Implantable Cardioverter-Defibrillator: randomized trial in patients with nonischemic dilated cardiomyopathy and asymptomatic nonsustained ventricular tachycardia – AMIOVIRT. *J Am Coll Cardiol* 2003; **41**: 1707–1712.

53. Bansch D, Antz M, Boczor S, *et al.* Primary prevention of sudden cardiac death in idiopathic dilated cardiomyopathy: the Cardiomyopathy Trial (CAT). *Circulation* 2002; **105**: 1453–1458.

54. Kadish A, Dyer A, Daubert JP, *et al.* Prophylactic defibrillator implantation in patients with nonischemic dilated cardiomyopathy. *N Engl J Med* 2004; **350**: 2151–2158.

55. Wilkoff BL, Cook JR, Epstein AE, *et al.* Dual-chamber pacing or ventricular backup pacing in patients with an implantable defibrillator: the Dual

Chamber and VVI Implantable Defibrillator (DAVID) trial. *JAMA* 2002; **288**: 3115–3123.

56. Bristow MR, Saxon LA, Boehmer J, *et al.* Cardiac-resynchronization therapy with or without an implantable defibrillator in advanced chronic heart failure. *N Engl J Med* 2004; **350**: 2140–2150.

57. Medina-Ravell VA, Lankipalli RS, Yan GX, *et al.* Effect of epicardial or biventricular pacing to prolong QT interval and increase transmural dispersion of repolarization: does resynchronization therapy pose a risk for patients predisposed to long QT or *torsade de pointes? Circulation* 2003; **107**: 740–746.

CHAPTER 12

Drug-induced sudden death

Dan M. Roden and Milou-Daniel Drici

The notion that drugs can provoke serious arrhythmias is well established in the cardiovascular, general medical, and regulatory communities. Multiple syndromes of proarrhythmia, each with specific clinical characteristics, reasonably well-understood basic electrophysiologic mechanisms, culprit drugs, clinical risk factors (including, in some cases, well recognized genetic predisposition), and approaches to therapy have been described [1–8]. It is not the goal of this chapter to revisit this material in detail; rather, we focus here on features common among these syndromes, and the extent to which they underlie the problem of sudden death in general.

Approaches to identifying drug-induced sudden death

The cases of terfenadine and cisapride-induced *torsades de pointes* highlight this question; the initial reports to the US Food and Drug Administration (FDA) focused on marked QT prolongation and *torsades de pointes*, and included a smaller number of deaths (2/25 and 4/34, respectively), also attributed to the drugs [9,10]; the numbers of cases grew rapidly after these initial publications, and even then likely represent a small fraction of true cases due to underreporting. The cases of these two agents highlight a problem in establishing a clear causal link between drug administration and a generally unwitnessed event such as sudden death. At one end of the spectrum will be cases of otherwise completely healthy individuals who after a dose or two of a culprit drug have witnessed a cardiac arrest and require external DC shock for resuscitation from ventricular fibrillation. At the other end of the spectrum may be a patient with multiple comorbidities and polypharmacy that includes a drug that has been associated with sudden death. When such a patient dies suddenly, a role for recently initiated or even chronic drug therapy may not even be considered as a contributor. Conversely, the death may be attributed to the drug even if some other common cause of sudden death were responsible. Thus, cases of sudden death occurring during therapy even with drugs that are clearly associated with proarrhythmia through well-understood basic electrophysiologic mechanisms may be difficult to interpret.

A second method that has been used to establish drug-induced sudden death is the placebo-controlled trial. The outcome of the Cardiac Arrhythmia

Suppression Trial (CAST) is the best example demonstrating increased mortality during drug therapy [1], but many others have now been presented. CAST-I studied encainide and flecainide, drugs with predominant although not exclusive sodium channel blocking properties [11]. Other trials studied sodium channel blocking drugs (moricizine [12], mexiletine [13], disopyramide [14], and QT-prolonging agents (D-sotalol [15]), and, in heart failure studies, positive inotropic agents (vesnarinone [16], milrinone [17], flosequinan [18], ibopamine [19], and others [20]), and the antihypertensive mibefradil [21]. While the placebo-controlled trial provides inconvertible evidence that a drug increases mortality, assignment of a mechanism is sometimes more difficult. Trials use a variety of definitions of "sudden death" and such definitions often include cases that, even if classified as sudden, may not be directly due to an arrhythmia. Nevertheless, use of standard criteria and adjudication by events committees has lead to the conclusion in these trials that mortality was related, at least in part, to an increase in sudden death.

It is also crucial to recognize that even when a drug can be incontrovertibly associated with a risk of sudden death, the mechanism underlying the risk may not be as obvious as it seems. Thus, although D-sotalol can cause *torsades de pointes* [22], at least one report suggests that other mechanisms may underlie its effect to increase mortality in the survival with oral D-sotalol (SWORD) study [23]. Similarly, although some deaths in CAST were doubtless due to well-recognized syndromes of sodium channel blocker-induced arrhythmia, the possibility of novel or unanticipated mechanisms playing a role cannot be excluded. Keeping an open mind with respect to what is known and what is inferred is a key step to elucidating new mechanisms in disease and drug response.

The major recognized causes of proarrhythmia include cardiac glycosides, QT-prolonging agents, sodium channel blocking drugs, positive inotropic agents, and drugs that cause coronary vasoconstriction and acute myocardial ischemia (Table 12.1). In addition, certain drugs may cause cardiomyopathy that, ultimately, leads to sudden death; anthracyclines used in cancer chemotherapy are an example. These proarrhythmia syndromes share certain common characteristics, discussed here.

Pharmacokinetic risk factors

In most cases, the risk of proarrhythmia rises with increasing drug dosages or plasma concentrations. Indeed, death due to arrhythmias during suicidal ingestion may be an initial clue that the drug, when administered at therapeutic dosages, may have proarrhythmic potential [47–50]. Such proarrhythmic potential may become manifest at usual doses under two groups; patients who happen to be especially sensitive to the electrophysiologic effects of the culprit drug (discussed below; *pharmacodynamic sensitivity*), or patients in whom usual drug dosages nevertheless lead to extreme elevations of plasma concentrations due to pharmacokinetic factors. Occasionally, especially with drugs that have multiple pharmacologic actions, proarrhythmia may be more readily observed at low concentrations, and resolve at higher ones; quinidine seems to be an example [51,52].

Pharmacokinetic sensitivity most commonly occurs when a culprit drug is eliminated by a single metabolizing or excretory pathway, a situation termed "high-risk pharmacokinetics" [53]. If this pathway is inhibited by coadministration of other drugs or by genetic factors, then marked elevation of parent drug concentrations and electrophysiologic toxicity can ensue. This was the case with terfenadine and cisapride, both of which are eliminated to noncardioactive metabolites by the intestinal and hepatic P450 system, CYP3A. While CYP3A activity varies strikingly among individuals, subjects completely lacking activity of this enzyme have not been described. However, many commonly used drugs are potent CYP3A inhibitors; erythromycin, clarithromycin, ketoconazole, itraconazole, certain HIV protease inhibitors (particularly ritonavir), and some calcium-channel blockers, notably mibefradil whose withdrawal after marketing was attributed to CYP3A-based interactions (although a mortality trial in heart failure [21,35] also showed an unfavorable outcome). Indeed, most initial reports to the FDA involving terfenadine or cisapride arose through this mechanism.

Digoxin is eliminated largely by P-glycoprotein mediated efflux in intestine, biliary tract, and kidney. Many commonly used drugs are P-glycoprotein inhibitors and the well recognized effect of drug interactions to elevate digoxin concentrations likely arises through this mechanism [54]; culprit interacters include quinidine, amiodarone, verapamil, erythromycin, itraconazole, and cyclosporine.

In 7% of individuals of Caucasian or African descent, activity of the P450 CYP2D6 is absent [55]. In addition, enzyme activity is inhibited by certain interacting drugs; notably some tricyclic antidepressants, propafenone, and quinidine. In situations in which CYP2D6 is the sole eliminating pathway, individuals with the "poor metabolizer" trait (or those receiving interacting drugs) may display markedly aberrant drug concentrations and responses. Flecainide is a CYP2D6 substrate, but also undergoes renal excretion as the unchanged drug. Hence, the CYP2D6 polymorphism is not usually an important factor in determining toxicity. However, occasional cases of patients with renal dysfunction and lack of CYP2D6 activity have been described [56]. Another CYP2D6 substrate that is well recognized as a cause of proarrhythmia is thioridazine, although data attesting to an increased risk among poor metabolizers have not been definitively generated [57].

Pharmacodynamic sensitivity

A second common feature of all proarrhythmia syndromes is that the incidence of proarrhythmia appears to be higher among patients with multiple

Table 12.1 Mechanisms underlying drug-induced proarrhythmia and sudden death.

Drug Action	Cellular Arrhythmogenic Consequence	Clinical Arrhythmia	Drugs
ATPase inhibition	Intracellular calcium overload-induced delayed afterdepolarizations due to sodium–calcium exchange Vagotonia	Sinus bradycardia; AV block; atrial, junctional, and/or ventricular arrhythmia [24]	Digitalis glycosides, including herbal remedies containing glycosides [25–27]
I_{Kr} block Late I_{Na} enhancement (much rarer) [28]	Action potential prolongation heterogeneous across the ventricular wall Early afterdepolarizations Intramural reentry	*Torsades de pointes*	QT-prolonging antiarrhythmics "Noncardiovascular" drugs that prolong QT [29,30]
Sodium channel block [7,8]	Decreased excitability Conduction slowing Loss of epicardial action potential "dome," with increased dispersion of repolarization	Altered pacing or defibrillation threshold Incessant VT Drug-modified atrial flutter VF risk	Sodium channel blocking, antiarrhythmics Other agents: tricyclic antidepressants [31,32], cocaine [33,34]
Positive inotropic agents	Intracellular calcium overload	Sudden death	Milrinone [17] Others not marketed vesnarinone, flosequinan, ibopamine, and others [16,18–20]

Calcium-channel blocker/CYP3A4 inhibitor		Mortality in heart failure	Mibefradil [21,35]
Activation of atrial K+ current	Shortening of atrial refractoriness	AF, often with rapid ventricular rate	Adenosine [4]
Uncertain		Increased ventricular response during AF in WPW	Digitalis [36]; verapamil [37,38]
Coronary vasospasm and/or acute hypertension	Multiple	Ischemic VF	Cocaine, ecstasy [39] Some anti-cancer drugs [40–43] Anti-migraine agents (triptans) [44] Ephedra [45], phenylpropanolamine [46] (?)
Multiple		Increased mortality during long-term therapy	Many (see text)

Note: AF – atrial fibrillation; VF – ventricular fibrillation; VT – ventricular tachycardia; WPW–Wolff–Parkinson–White syndrome comorbidities. Thus, flecainide is a safe antiarrhythmic in patients with atrial fibrillation and no structural heart disease. However, the same dose of the same drug (attaining the same plasma concentrations) may cause incessant hemodynamically destabilizing ventricular tachycardia when used in a patient with myocardial scarring due to remote myocardial infarction [58]. An analysis of the CAST database provides evidence that recurrent acute myocardial ischemia also potentiated the risk of death related to flecainide [59]. Patients entered CAST after an index myocardial infarction and after a run-in period, were randomly assigned to placebo or drug. In those whose index myocardial infarction was transmural (and hence, in the vernacular of the 1980s, "complete"), drugs increased mortality 1.7-fold. By contrast, those whose index myocardial infarction was a non-Q wave event, a population with a very high incidence of recurrent ischemia, had an 8.7-fold increase in mortality with drug. Thus, these data provide compelling evidence that recurrent ischemia potentiates the proarrhythmic potential of sodium channel blocking agents such as flecainide.

The Danish Investigations of Arrhythmia and Mortality ON Dofetilide (DIAMOND) studies provide evidence from a large trial context that heart failure is a risk factor for drug-induced *torsades de pointes* [60,61]. The two DIAMOND studies, randomized patients with recent acute myocardial infarction or recent hospitalization for heart failure to placebo or to the QT-prolonging agent dofetilide. The potential of dofetilide to cause *torsades de pointes* was well recognized so the drug was initiated with continuous monitoring of cardiac rhythm in in-patients. In the myocardial infarction arm, there were seven cases of *torsades de pointes* among 749 patients randomized to receive drug versus 0/761 who received placebo. By contrast, in the heart failure study, *torsades de pointes* occurred in 25/762 patients on drug (and 0/756 on placebo). In addition, despite continuous cardiac monitoring and prompt initiation of resuscitation, three of the *torsades* patients died. These well-controlled clinical trial data demonstrate that drug-induced proarrhythmia can, indeed, lead to drug-induced sudden death and that recent exacerbation of heart failure appears to be a potent risk factor for the development of *torsades de pointes*. In these trials, under the best controlled clinical situation, the drug caused *torsades de pointes* in over 3% of patients.

This heart failure experience may reflect some fundamental pathophysiology, such as potassium channel down-regulation [62,63] or aberrant intracellular calcium handling [64], that predisposes to arrhythmias when a QT interval prolonging drug is superimposed. Alternatively, therapies used in heart failure may increase risk. The most important example is diuretic therapy; diuretics not only decrease serum potassium, a critical modulator of QT interval and its sensitivity to drugs, but also may directly block potassium channels and potentiate QT prolongation by other drugs through this mechanism [65,66]. Non-potassium-sparing diuretics have been associated with increased mortality in hypertension trials [67,68], suggesting a common mechanism.

Genetic predisposition

Occasionally by patients develop proarrhythmia in the absence of obvious pharmacokinetic or pharmacodynamic explanations. When reasonably healthy people develop such an extreme response to drug therapy, a role for genetic influences is frequently invoked. In some cases, as discussed above, the genetics of drug disposition may play a role. In other cases, administration of a drug may expose a subclinical monogenetic arrhythmia syndrome. Thus, cases of subclinical long-QT syndrome account for a small number of drug-induced *torsades de pointes* [69–71]. Similarly, drugs may expose the Brugada syndrome ECG [72–74], and such exposure during provocative testing is now well recognized to confer a risk for ventricular fibrillation [75,76]. In these monogenetic syndromes, it is clear that penetrance of the electrocardiographic phenotype (QT prolongation or J point elevation) can be highly variable, an effect often attributed to as-yet-unidentified modifier genes [75,77]. It is also possible that sudden death risk in these syndromes is determined by separate loci. Such loci could determine, for example, whether patients with equivalent degrees of QT prolongation have varying risks of *torsades de pointes* [78], or even whether *torsades de pointes* self-terminates or degenerates to ventricular fibrillation.

In addition to cases of drugs exposing disease-associated mutations in individual patients, polymorphisms (relatively common DNA variants) have been identified that may increase risk for drug-associated arrhythmias. For example, approximately 10% of African Americans carry a variant in their sodium channel gene that results in a tyrosine (Y) rather than a serine (S) at position 1103 of the protein [79]. When the variant protein is studied *in vitro*, it appears to confer subtle changes consistent with the sodium channel linked variant of the long-QT syndrome. The frequency of the Y allele was significantly higher in a group of 23 African Americans with a range of arrhythmia symptoms, including sudden death and drug-associated arrhythmias, compared to a group of 100 African American controls. Similarly, the polymorphisms resulting in D85N [80] in the *KCNE1* gene, and in T8A [81] and Q9E [82] (initially reported as a mutation) in the *KCNE2* gene have been associated with unusual *in vitro* characteristics and/or a higher incidence of *torsades de pointes* during drug therapy. The identification of these and other relatively common DNA variants predisposing to drug responses forms the basis of the nascent field of pharmacogenomics [53].

Summary

With the increasing recognition of syndromes of drug-induced proarrhythmia, there seems to be little doubt that some of these cases present as sudden death. However, the proportion of patients with proarrhythmia who present with sudden death, and indeed the extent to which proarrhythmia contributes to the overall problem of sudden death, are unknown. The lessons of the last several decades, notably the terfenadine/cisapride experience and CAST, highlight the potential for drugs to result in unusual, and difficult to detect, adverse effects. The cardiovascular community must remain alert to the possibility that drug therapy may cause sudden death, a particularly difficult entity to recognize, not only through these by now well-recognized mechanisms, but also through other mechanisms that remain to be described.

Acknowledgment

Supported in part by grants from the United States Public Health Service (HL46681, HL49989, HL65962). Dr. Roden is the holder of the William Stokes Chair in Experimental Therapeutics, a gift from the Dai-ichi Corporation.

References

1. The CAST Investigators. Preliminary report: effect of encainide and flecainide on mortality in a randomized trial of arrhythmia suppression after myocardial infarction. *N Engl J Med* 1989; **321**: 406–412.
2. Ben-David J, Zipes DP. *Torsades de pointes* and proarrhythmia. *Lancet* 1993; **341**: 1578–1582.
3. Hohnloser SH, Singh BN. Proarrhythmia with class III antiarrhythmic drugs: definition, electrophysiologic mechanisms, incidence, predisposing factors, and clinical implications. *J Cardiovasc Electrophysiol* 1995; **6**: 920–936.
4. Exner DV, Muzyka T, Gillis AM. Proarrhythmia in patients with the Wolff–Parkinson–White syndrome after standard doses of intravenous adenosine. *Ann Intern Med* 1995; **122**: 351–352.
5. Roden DM. Mechanisms and management of proarrhythmia. *Am J Cardiol* 1998; **82**: 49I–57I.
6. Haverkamp W, Breithardt G, Camm AJ, *et al.* The potential for QT prolongation and proarrhythmia by nonantiarrhythmic drugs: clinical and regulatory implications. Report on a policy conference of the European Society of Cardiology. *Eur Heart J* 2000; **21**: 1216–1231.
7. Naccarelli GV, Wolbrette DL, Luck JC. Proarrhythmia. *Med Clin North Am* 2001; **85**: 503–526, xii.
8. Roden DM, Anderson ME. Proarrhythmia. In: Kass RS & Clancy CE, eds. *Antiarrhythmic Therapy*. Springer-Verlag, Berlin, Germany 2005.
9. Woosley RL, Chen Y, Freiman JP, *et al.* Mechanism of the cardiotoxic actions of terfenadine. *JAMA* 1993; **269**: 1532–1536.
10. Wysowski DK, Bacsanyi J. Cisapride and fatal arrhythmia. *N Engl J Med* 1996; **335**: 290–291.
11. Follmer CH, Colatsky TJ. Block of delayed rectifier potassium current, I_k, by flecainide and E-4031 in cat ventricular myocytes. *Circulation* 1990; **82**: 289–293.
12. The Cardiac Arrhythmia Suppression Trial II Investigators. Effect of the antiarrhythmic agent moricizine on survival after myocardial infarction. *N Engl J Med* 1991; **327**: 227–233.
13. IMPACT Research Group. International mexiletine and placebo antiarrhythmic coronary trial: I. Report on arrhythmia and other findings. *J Am Coll Cardiol* 1984; **4**: 1148–1163.

14. UK Rythmodan Multicentre Study Group. Oral disopyramide after admission to hospital with suspected acute myocardial infarction. *Postgraduate Med J* 1984; **60**: 98–107.

15. Waldo AL, Camm AJ, DeRuyter H, *et al.* Effect of D-sotalol on mortality in patients with left ventricular dysfunction after recent and remote myocardial infarction. *Lancet* 1996; **348**: 7–12.

16. Cohn JN, Goldstein SO, Greenberg BH, *et al.* A dose-dependent increase in mortality with vesnarinone among patients with severe heart failure. Vesnarinone Trial Investigators. *N Engl J Med* 1998; **339**: 1810–1816.

17. Packer M, Carver JR, Rodeheffer RJ, *et al.* Effect of oral milrinone on mortality in severe chronic heart failure. The PROMISE Study Research Group. *N Engl J Med* 1991; **325**: 1468–1475.

18. Packer M, Rouleau J, Swedberg K, *et al.* Effect of flosequinan on survival in chronic heart failure. Preliminary results of the PROFILE study. *Circulation* 1993; **88** Suppl 1: 1–301. abstract

19. Hampton JR, van Veldhuisen DJ, Kleber FX, *et al.* Randomized study of effect of ibopamine on survival in patients with advanced severe heart failure. Second Prospective Randomized Study of Ibopamine on Mortality and Efficacy (PRIME II) Investigators. *Lancet* 1997; **349**: 971–977.

20. van Veldhuisen DJ, Poole-Wilson PA. The underreporting of results and possible mechanisms of "negative" drug trials in patients with chronic heart failure. *Int J Cardiol* 2001; **80**: 19–27.

21. Levine TB, Bernink PJ, Caspi A, *et al.* Effect of mibefradil, a T-type calcium channel blocker, on morbidity and mortality in moderate to severe congestive heart failure: the MACH-1 study. Mortality Assessment in Congestive Heart Failure Trial. *Circulation* 2000; **101**: 758–764.

22. Brachmann J, Schols W, Beyer T, *et al.* Acute and chronic antiarrhythmic efficacy of D-sotalol in patients with sustained ventricular tachyarrhythmias. *Eur Heart J* 1993; **14** (Suppl. H): 85–87.

23. Pratt CM, Camm AJ, Cooper W, *et al.* Mortality in the Survival With ORal D-sotalol (SWORD) trial: why did patients die? *Am J Cardiol* 1998; **81**: 869–876.

24. Antman EM, Smith TW. Digitalis toxicity. *Mod Con Cardiovasc Disease* 1986; **55**: 26–30.

25. Gowda RM, Cohen RA, Khan IA. Toad venom poisoning: resemblance to digoxin toxicity and therapeutic implications. *Heart* 2003; **89**: e14.

26. Eddleston M, Ariaratnam CA, Sjostrom L, *et al.* Acute yellow oleander (*Thevetia peruviana*) poisoning: cardiac arrhythmias, electrolyte disturbances, and serum cardiac glycoside concentrations on presentation to hospital. *Heart* 2000; **83**: 301–306.

27. Bain RJ. Accidental digitalis poisoning due to drinking herbal tea. *Br Med J (Clin Res Ed)* 1985; **290**: 1624.

28. Kuhlkamp V, Mewis C, Bosch R, *et al.* Delayed sodium channel inactivation mimics long-QT syndrome 3. *J Cardiovasc Pharmacol* 2003; **42**: 113–117.

29. Haverkamp W, Breithardt G, Camm AJ, *et al.* The potential for QT prolongation and proarrhythmia by nonantiarrhythmic drugs: clinical and regulatory implications. Report on a Policy Conference of the European Society of Cardiology. *Eur Heart J* 2000; **21**: 1216–1231.

30. Roden DM. Drug-induced prolongation of the QT Interval. *N Engl J Med* 2004; **350**: 1013–1022.

31. Tada H, Sticherling C, Oral H, *et al.* Brugada syndrome mimicked by tricyclic antidepressant overdose. *J Cardiovasc Electrophysiol* 2001; **12**: 275.

32. Boehnert MT, Lovejoy FH. Value of QRS duration versus the serum drug level in predicting seizures and ventricular arrhythmias after an acute overdose of tricyclic antidepressants. *N Engl J Med* 1985; **313**: 474–479.

33. Littmann L, Monroe MH, Svenson RH. Brugada-type electrocardiographic pattern induced by cocaine. *Mayo Clin Proc* 2000; **75**: 845–849.

34. Xu YQ, Crumb WJJ, Clarkson CW. Cocaethylene, a metabolite of cocaine and ethanol, is a potent blocker of cardiac sodium channels. *J Pharmacol Exper Ther* 1994; **271**: 319–325.

35. Mullins ME, Horowitz BZ, Linden DJ, *et al.* Life-threatening interaction of mibefradil and beta-blockers with dihydropyridine calcium channel blockers. *JAMA* 1998; **280**: 157–158.

36. Klein GJ, Bashore TM, Sellers TD, *et al.* Ventricular fibrillation in the Wolff–Parkinson–White Syndrome. *N Engl J Med* 1979; **301**: 1080–1085.

37. Gulamhusein S, Ko P, Carruthers SG, *et al.* Acceleration of the ventricular response during atrial fibrillation in the Wolff–Parkinson–White syndrome after verapamil. *Circulation* 1982; **65**: 348–354.

38. McGovern B, Garan H, Ruskin JN. Precipitation of cardiac arrest by verapamil in patients with Wolff–Parkinson–White syndrome. *Ann Int Med* 1986; **104**: 791–794.

39. Qasim A, Townend J, Davies MK. Ecstasy induced acute myocardial infarction. *Heart* 2001; **85**: E10.

40. Van CE, Hoff PM, Blum JL, *et al.* Incidence of cardiotoxicity with the oral fluoropyrimidine capecitabine is typical of that reported with 5-fluorouracil. *Ann Oncol* 2002; **13**: 484–485.

41. Isetta C, Garaffo R, Bastian G, *et al.* Life-threatening 5-fluorouracil-like cardiac toxicity after treatment with 5-fluorocytosine. *Clin Pharmacol Ther* 2000; **67**: 323–325.

42. Jameson M, Thompson P, Hastie B. 5 Fluorouracil cardiotoxicity. *N Z Med J* 1995; **108**: 21.

43. Schnetzler B, Popova N, Collao LC, *et al.* Coronary spasm induced by capecitabine. *Ann Oncol* 2001; **12**: 723–724.

44. Welch KM, Saiers J, Salonen R. Triptans and coronary spasm. *Clin Pharmacol Ther* 2000; **68**: 337–338.

45. Samenuk D, Link MS, Homoud MK, *et al.* Adverse cardiovascular events temporally associated with ma huang, a herbal source of ephedrine. *Mayo Clin Proc* 2002; **77**: 12–16.

46. Haller CA, Benowitz NL. Adverse cardiovascular and central nervous system events associated with dietary supplements containing ephedra alkaloids. *N Engl J Med* 2000; **343**: 1833–1838.

47. Neuvonen PJ, Elonen E, Vuorenmaa T, *et al.* Prolonged Q-T interval and severe tachyarrhythmias, common features of sotalol intoxication. *Eur J Clin Pharmacol* 1981; **20**: 85–89.

48. Snook J, Boothman-Burrell D, Watkins J *et al. Torsade de pointes* ventricular tachycardia associated with astemizole overdose. *Br J Clin Pract* 1988; **42**: 257–259.

49. Davies AJ, Harindra V, McEwan A, *et al.* Cardiotoxic effect with convulsions in terfenadine overdose. *Br Med J* 1989; **298**: 325.

50. Antman EM, Wenger TL, Butler VPJ, *et al.* Treatment of 150 cases of life-threatening digitalis intoxication with digoxin-specific Fab antibody fragments. Final report of a multicenter study. *Circulation* 1990; **81**: 1744–1752.

51. Yang T, Roden DM. Extracellular potassium modulation of drug block of I_{Kr}: implications for *torsades de pointes* and reverse use-dependence. *Circulation* 1996; **93**: 407–411.

52. Sicouri S, Antzelevitch C. Drug-induced afterdepolarizations and triggered activity occur in a discrete subpopulation of ventricular muscle cells (M cells) in the canine heart: quinidine and digitalis. *J Cardiovasc Electrophysiol* 1993; **4**: 48–58.

53. Roden DM. Cardiovascular pharmacogenomics. *Circulation* 2003; **108**: 3071–3074.

54. Fromm MF, Kim RB, Stein CM, *et al.* Inhibition of P-glycoprotein-mediated drug transport: a unifying mechanism to explain the interaction between digoxin and quinidine. *Circulation* 1999; **99**: 552–557.

55. Meyer UA, Zanger UM. Molecular mechanisms of genetic polymorphisms of drug metabolism. *Annu Rev Pharmacol Toxicol* 1997; **37**: 269–296.

56. Evers J, Eichelbaum M, Kroemer HK. Unpredictability of flecainide plasma concentrations in patients with renal failure: relation to side effects and sudden death? *Ther Drug Monit* 1994; **16**: 349–351.

57. Von Bahr C, Movin G, Nordin C, *et al.* Plasma levels of thioridazine and metabolites are influenced by the debrisoquin hydroxylation phenotype. *Clin Pharmacol Ther* 1991; **49**: 234–240.

58. Oetgen WJ, Tibbits PA, Abt MEO, *et al.* Clinical and electrophysiologic assessment of oral flecainide acetate for recurrent ventricular tachycardia: evidence for exacerbation of electrical instability. *Am J Cardiol* 1983; **52**: 746–750.

59. Akiyama T, Pawitan Y, Greenberg H, *et al.* Increased risk of death and cardiac arrest from encainide and flecainide in patients after non-Q-wave acute myocardial infarction in the Cardiac Arrhythmia Suppression Trial. *Am J Cardiol* 1991; **68**: 1551–1555.

60. Torp-Pedersen C, Moller M, Bloch-Thomsen PE, *et al.* Dofetilide in patients with congestive heart failure and left ventricular dysfunction. Danish Investigations of Arrhythmia and Mortality on Dofetilide Study Group. *N Engl J Med* 1999; **341**: 857–865.

61. Kober L, Bloch Thomsen PE, Moller M, *et al.* Effect of dofetilide in patients with recent myocardial infarction and left-ventricular dysfunction: a randomized trial. Danish Investigations of Arrhythmia and Mortality on Dofetilide (DIAMOND) Study Group. *Lancet* 2000; **356**: 2052–2058.

62. Tomaselli GF, Beuckelmann DJ, Calkins HG, *et al.* Sudden cardiac death in heart failure. The role of abnormal repolarization. *Circulation* 1994; **90**: 2534–2539.

63. Kaab S, Dixon J, Duc J, *et al.* Molecular basis of transient outward potassium current down-regulation in human heart failure: a decrease in Kv4.3 mRNA correlates with a reduction in current density. *Circulation* 1998; **98**: 1383–1393.

64. Pogwizd SM, Schlotthauer K, Li L, *et al.* Arrhythmogenesis and contractile dysfunction in heart failure: roles of sodium-calcium exchange, inward rectifier potassium current, and residual beta-adrenergic responsiveness. *Circ Res* 2001; **88**: 1159–1167.

65. Turgeon J, Daleau P, Bennett PB, *et al.* Block of I_{Ks}, the slow component of the delayed rectifier K^+ current, by the diuretic agent indapamide in guinea pig myocytes. *Circ Res* 1994; **75**: 879–886.

66. Fiset C, Drolet B, Hamelin BA, *et al.* Block of I-Ks by the diuretic agent indapamide modulates cardiac electrophysiological effects of the class III antiarrhythmic drug DL-sotalol. *J Pharmacol Exper Ther* 1997; **283**: 148–156.

67. Siscovick DS, Raghunathan TE, Psaty BM, *et al.* Diuretic therapy for hypertension and the risk of primary cardiac arrest. *N Engl J Med* 1994; **330**: 1852–1857.

68. Bigger JT, Jr. Diuretic therapy, hypertension, and cardiac arrest. *N Engl J Med* 1994; **330**: 1899–1900.
69. Donger C, Denjoy I, Berthet M, *et al*. KVLQT1 C-terminal missense mutation causes a forme fruste long-QT syndrome. *Circulation* 1997; **96**: 2778–2781.
70. Napolitano C, Schwartz PJ, Brown AM, *et al*. Evidence for a cardiac ion channel mutation underlying drug-induced QT prolongation and life-threatening arrhythmias. *J Cardiovasc Electrophysiol* 2000; **11**: 691–696.
71. Yang P, Kanki H, Drolet B, *et al*. Allelic variants in long QT disease genes in patients with drug-associated *torsades de pointes*. *Circulation* 2002; **105**: 1943–1948.
72. Krishnan SC, Josephson ME. ST segment elevation induced by class IC antiarrhythmic agents: underlying electrophysiologic mechanisms and insights into drug-induced proarrhythmia. *J Cardiovasc Electrophysiol* 1998; **9**: 1167–1172.
73. Fujiki A, Usui M, Nagasawa H, *et al*. ST segment elevation in the right precordial leads induced with class IC antiarrhythmic drugs: insight into the mechanism of Brugada syndrome. *J Cardiovasc Electrophysiol* 1999; **10**: 214–218.
74. Roden DM, Wilde AA. Drug-induced J point elevation: a marker for genetic risk of sudden death or ECG curiosity? *J Cardiovasc Electrophysiol* 1999; **10**: 219–223.
75. Alings M, Wilde A. "Brugada" syndrome: clinical data and suggested pathophysiological mechanism. *Circulation* 1999; **99**: 666–673.
76. Wilde AA, Antzelevitch C, Borggrefe M, *et al*. Proposed diagnostic criteria for the Brugada syndrome: consensus report. *Circulation* 2002; **106**: 2514–2519.
77. Priori SG, Napolitano C, Schwartz PJ. Low penetrance in the long-QT syndrome: clinical impact. *Circulation* 1999; **99**: 529–533.
78. Kimbrough JT, Norris K, Kannankeril PJ, *et al*. QT prolongation alone does not predict *torsades de pointes* in patients with drug-induced LQTS. *Heart Rhythm* 2004; **1**: 1S; S83 (257).
79. Splawski I, Timothy KW, Tateyama M, *et al*. Variant of SCN5A sodium channel implicated in risk of cardiac arrhythmia. *Science* 2002; **297**: 1333–1336.
80. Wei J, Yang IC-H, Tapper AR, *et al*. KCNE1 polymorphism confers risk of drug-induced long-QT syndrome by altering kinetic properties of IKs potassium channels. *Circulation* 1999; **100**: Suppl 1: I-495.
81. Sesti F, Abbott GW, Wei J, *et al*. A common polymorphism associated with antibiotic-induced cardiac arrhythmia. *PNAS* 2000; **97**: 10613–10618.
82. Abbott GW, Sesti F, Splawski I, *et al*. MiRP1 forms I_{Kr} potassium channels with HERG and is associated with cardiac arrhythmia. *Cell* 1999; **97**: 175–187.

CHAPTER 13

Sudden death in athletes

Domenico Corrado, Cristina Basso, Mark S. Link,
Gaetano Thiene, and N.A. Mark Estes III

Introduction

The cardiovascular conditions that predispose to the rare but tragic sudden death in the athlete are now known [1–6]. In athletes under 35 years of age hypertrophic cardiomyopathy, arrhythmogenic right ventricular cardiomyopathy/dysplasia, and anomalous coronary arteries are among the most common conditions. In those older than 35 years of age, coronary artery disease is the most common substrate. Although screening strategies have been developed to identify those individuals at risk, only rigorous and expensive programs have sufficient specificity and sensitivity. However, the cost-effectiveness of such programs is too great to warrant widespread implementation. Guidelines for athletic participation have been developed based on the best available information regarding the risks of the underlying cardiovascular condition.

Epidemiological profile of sudden death in athletes

Sudden death in young competitive athletes is an uncommon event. A prospective population-based study in the Veneto region of Italy reported an incidence of sudden death of 2.3 (2.6 in males and 1.1 in females) per 100 000 athletes (age 12–35 years) per year by all causes, and of 2.1 per 100 000 athletes per year by cardiovascular diseases [4]. Previous retrospective studies from the United States reported a lower prevalence of sports-related sudden deaths. Van Camp *et al.* [7] in a nationally based survey estimated the prevalence of sudden death in high school and college athletes in the United States to be 0.4 per 100 000 athletes per year. Maron *et al.* [8] estimated the prevalence of cardiovascular sudden deaths in competitive high school athletes (age 13–19 years, mean 16) from Minnesota to be 0.35 per 100 000 sports participations, and 0.46 per 100 000 individual participants per year (0.77 per 100 000 male athletes). Higher rates of sports-related fatalities (ranging from 1 : 15 000 to 1 : 50 000) have been reported for apparently healthy male joggers or marathon racers. Sudden death in athletes shows a clear gender predilection with striking male predominance (male to female ratio up to 10 : 1). Although predominance of fatal events in male athletes has been related to the higher participation rate of male compared to female athletes in competitive sports,

Table 13.1 Cardiovascular causes of sudden death associated with sports.

Age >35 years
Coronary artery disease
Age <35 years
Hypertrophic cardiomyopathy
Arrhythmogenic right ventricular cardiomyopathy/dysplasia
Congenital anomalies of coronary arteries
Myocarditis
Aortic rupture
Valvular disease
Preexcitation syndromes and conduction diseases
Ion channel disease
Congenital heart disease, operated or unoperated

more recent data suggest that male gender may be in itself a risk factor for sports-related sudden death. This is likely a consequence of the greater prevalence and/or phenotypic expression in young males of cardiac diseases at risk of arrhythmic cardiac arrest such as cardiomyopathies and premature coronary artery disease [4,9].

Causes of sudden death in the athlete

A structural cardiovascular abnormality is found at autopsy in most cases of sudden death in athletes [1,4,5,7,10–12]. The cause of death reflects the age of participants. Atherosclerotic coronary artery disease is by far the most common cause of sudden death in athletes over 35 years of age, whereas in younger athletes a broader spectrum of pathologic conditions, including congenital and inherited cardiovascular diseases, have been reported (Table 13.1).

Hypertrophic cardiomyopathy

Hypertrophic cardiomyopathy is a heart muscle disease, usually genetically transmitted, and characterized by a hypertrophied, nondilated left ventricle in the absence of predisposing diseases [13]. The disease has been implicated as the principal cause of sudden cardiac arrest on the athletic field in the United States, accounting for up to one third of sport-related cardiac fatalities [1,7,10]. Predominant morphofunctional cardiac abnormalities (Figure 13.1(a)) include left ventricular hypertrophy, which usually is "asymmetric" with disproportionate septal thickening, and reduction in left ventricular chamber size with increased myocardial "stiffness," which may critically impair diastolic compliance and intramural coronary blood filling [15]. A "dynamic" left ventricular outflow tract obstruction is also demonstrable in a subset of patients. The histopathologic hallmark of the disease is the so-called "myocardial disarray," which consists in widespread, bizarre, and disordered arrangement of myocytes with associated diffuse interstitial

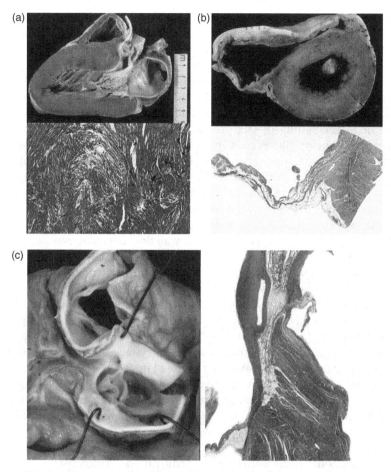

Figure 13.1 Leading causes of sudden cardiovascular death in young competitive athletes. (a) hypertrophic cardiomyopathy: long-axis cut of the heart specimen showing asymmetric septal hypertrophy with subaortic bulging and septal endocardial fibrous plaque (top); histology of the interventricular septum revealing typical myocardial disarray with interstitial fibrosis (Heidenhain trichrome ×47) (bottom). Modified from Reference 12, (b) arrhythmogenic right ventricular cardiomyopathy/dysplasia: cross section of the heart specimen with infundibular and inferior subtricuspidal aneurysms (top); panoramic histological view of the inferior aneurysm showing wall thinning with fibrofatty replacement (bottom) (Azan stain; original magnification, ×2.5). Modified from Reference 14, (c) congenital coronary anomaly: gross view of the aorta showing both left and right coronary arteries arising from the left aortic sinus of Valsalva (left); at histology, the proximal tract of the anomalous right coronary artery runs between the aorta and the pulmonary trunk with an intramural course (right). Modified from Reference 11.

and/or focal fibrosis. Fibrotic changes are an acquired phenomenon, in part related to progressive disease of the intramural coronary arteries that show a dysplasia of the tunica media with or without lumen obstruction ("small vessel disease").

Sudden cardiac arrest in athletes with hypertrophic cardiomyopathy has been attributed to ventricular arrhythmias, most likely arising from the dysplastic myocardium. The observation of acquired myocardial damage, either acute or in the setting of large septal scars, supports the hypothesis that myocardial ischemia intervenes in the natural history of the disease and contributes to the arrhythmogenicity. Other potential mechanisms of syncope and cardiac arrest in hypertrophic cardiomyopathy include paroxysmal supraventricular arrhythmias, hypotension due to inappropriate vasodilator response to exercise, and acute myocardial ischemia [13,15].

Physiologic cardiac adaptation secondary to regular exercise (athlete's heart) may lead to an increase in left ventricular wall thickness that may be difficult to distinguish from pathologic changes of hypertrophic cardiomyopathy. Criteria in favor of hypertrophic cardiomyopathy include a high degree of left ventricular hypertrophy (wall thickness >16 mm) with an unusual distribution (heterogeneous, asymmetric, or sparing the anterior septum); a left ventricular cavity of normal size (<45 mm); the presence of striking ECG abnormalities; and the persistence of hypertrophy after deconditioning [16].

ECG abnormalities such as an increased QRS voltage, pathologic "q" waves, and repolarization changes have been reported in up to 95% of patients with hypertrophic cardiomyopathy. This explains why systematic preparticipation screening of young competitive athletes in Italy by ECG in addition to history and physical examination has allowed the successful identification of athletes with hypertrophic cardiomyopathy [5].

Arrhythmogenic right ventricular cardiomyopathy/dysplasia

Arrhythmogenic right ventricular cardiomyopathy/dysplasia is an inherited heart muscle disorder that is characterized pathologically by fibrofatty replacement of right ventricular myocardium [14,17,18]. The most frequent clinical manifestations consist of ECG depolarization/repolarization changes mostly localized to right precordial leads, global and/or regional morphologic and functional alterations of the right ventricle and arrhythmias of right ventricular origin that can lead to sudden death, especially during physical exercise [19–21]. Arrhythmogenic right ventricular cardiomyopathy/dysplasia has been reported to be the leading cause of sports-related sudden death in the Veneto region of Italy, accounting for one-fourth of cardiovascular sudden death in young competitive athletes [4,5,11]. The most likely explanation of this finding is that systematic preparticipation screening of young competitive athletes has changed the natural prevalence of cardiovascular causes of sports-related sudden death. Hypertrophic cardiomyopathy is the most common underlying anatomic substrate in the US athletes, dying suddenly. By contrast, in Italy fatalities due to hypertrophic cardiomyopathy have been successfully prevented by identification and disqualification of the affected athletes at preparticipation screening. Therefore, other cardiovascular conditions such as arrhythmogenic right ventricular cardiomyopathy/dysplasia have come to account for a greater proportion of all sudden death in Italian athletes.

The heart of young competitive athletes dying suddenly from arrhythmogenic right ventricular cardiomyopathy/dysplasia demonstrates right ventricular dilatation and massive transmural fibrofatty replacement of the right ventricular musculature resulting in aneurysmal dilatations, located in the posterobasal, apical, and outflow tract regions, which are potential sources of life-threatening ventricular arrhythmias (Figure 13.1(b)) [11]. These pathologic features of the right ventricle allows differential diagnosis with training-induced right ventricular changes ("athlete's heart"), usually consisting in global RV enlargement without wall motion abnormalities.

The propensity for sudden arrhythmic death during physical exercise is linked to both hemodynamic and neurohumoral factors [21]. Physical exercise may acutely increase the right ventricular afterload and cavity enlargement, which in turn, may elicit ventricular arrhythmias by stretching the diseased right ventricular musculature. Alternatively, a "denervation supersensitivity" of the right ventricle to catecholamines has been advanced. Finally, in a subgroup of patients with familial arrhythmogenic right ventricular cardiomyopathy/dysplasia (ARVD2) a cardiac ryanodine receptor (RYR2) missense mutation leading to abnormal calcium release from the sarcoplasmic reticulum during effort has been identified (see below).

Early identification of athletes with arrhythmogenic right ventricular cardiomyopathy/dysplasia plays a crucial role in the prevention of sudden death during sport. The disease should be suspected in the presence of inverted T waves in right precordial leads. Diagnosis relies on visualization of morpho-functional right ventricular abnormalities by current imaging techniques, and, in selected cases, by histopathologic demonstration of fibrofatty substitution at endomyocardial biopsy [5,21]. It is noteworthy that more than 80% of athletes of the Veneto region series who died from arrhythmogenic right ventricular cardiomyopathy/dysplasia had had a history of syncope, ECG changes and/or ventricular arrhythmias. Nevertheless, they had not been identified at preparticipation screening because the disease was largely unrecognized. More recently with the increased awareness of clinical findings of arrhythmogenic right ventricular cardiomyopathy/dysplasia, more affected athletes are being detected by screening and protected from the risk of the athletic competition.

Congenital coronary artery anomaly

The anomalous origin of a coronary artery from the "wrong" coronary sinus is a "minor" coronary anomaly with a silent clinical course, which may precipitate sudden and unexpected ischemic cardiac arrest in young competitive athletes [22]. The most frequent anatomic findings consist of both (left and right) coronary arteries arising either from the right or the left coronary sinus.

In both conditions, as the anomalous coronary vessel leaves the aorta, it shows an acute angle with the aortic wall, and, thus, it usually runs between the aorta and the pulmonary trunk, following an early aortic intramural course, with a "slit-like" lumen (Figure 13.1(c)). Fatal myocardial ischemia has been related to exercise-induced aortic root expansion that compresses the anomalous vessel against the pulmonary trunk, increases the acute angulation of the coronary take-off, aggravating the "slit-like" shape of the lumen of the proximal intramural portion of the aberrant coronary vessel. This mechanism of myocardial ischemia is difficult to be reproduced in clinical setting, as shown by the occurrence of false negative ECG exercise testing in young athlete who subsequently died suddenly from the above coronary anomaly [22].

Commotio cordis

Sudden death due to non-penetrating chest wall impact in the absence of structural injury to the ribs, sternum, and heart is known as commotio cordis. Although once considered to be a particularly rare event, it has recently become apparent that these events are more common than previously regarded. Indeed, up to 20% of deaths on the athletic field are due to chest wall impact [23–27]. The Commotio Cordis Registry, in its 7 years of existence, has documented 156 cases of commotio cordis [23]. Cardiac workups and autopsies are notable for the lack of any significant cardiac or thoracic abnormalities. Victims are most often found in ventricular fibrillation; resuscitation is possible with early defibrillation.

An experimental model of commotio cordis has been developed in which anesthetized juvenile swine struck in the chest by a baseball develop ventricular fibrillation (Figure 13.2). Important variables include timing of impact in which only blows occurring in a narrow window of repolarization cause ventricular fibrillation [24]. Energy of the impact object was also found to be critical, with 40 miles/h baseballs more likely to cause ventricular fibrillation than velocities greater or less than 40 miles/h [27]. In addition, more rigid impact objects, and blows directly over the center of the chest were more likely to cause ventricular fibrillation [26]. Peak left ventricular pressure generated by the chest wall blow correlated with the risk of ventricular fibrillation and activation of the K_{ATP}^{+} channel is likely to play a role [25].

Coronary artery disease

Sudden cardiac death in those participating in athletic activity over 35 years of age most commonly occurs due to coronary artery disease [2,28]. For athletes older than 35 years of age, it is recommended that a careful history for coronary risk factors or symptoms of coronary artery disease be taken. If an individual is identified as being at risk for coronary artery disease or if symptoms suggest ischemia, an exercise stress test should be performed. Stress testing is also recommended in males over 40 years or females over 50 years of age in whom coronary artery disease may be present based on the presence of at least two risk factors other than age and gender or one marked abnormal finding [29].

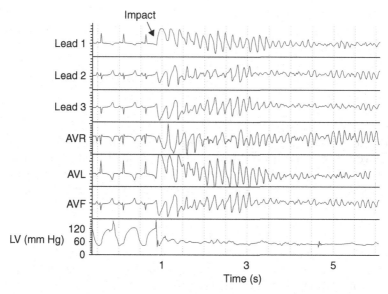

Figure 13.2 Six-lead electrocardiogram showing the electrophysiologic and hemodynamic consequences of an impact to the chest wall by a wooden object at 30 miles/h timed to occur 16 ms before the peak of the T wave in a 9-kg pig. Ventricular fibrillation began within one cardiac cycle after the impact and was associated with immediate loss of left ventricular (LV) pressure. Reproduced from Reference 24, with permission.

In the older athlete with no symptoms of coronary artery disease and no risk factors, the routine use of exercise testing is limited by its low specificity and pretest probability.

Other causes

Myocarditis, either in its acute or healed forms, may provide a myocardial electrical substrate for ventricular arrhythmias and exercise-related sudden death [1,4,12]. Life-threatening ventricular arrhythmias in athletes may be associated with focal myocarditis that is clinically silent and difficult to be detected by endomyocardial biopsy.

Spontaneous laceration or dissection of the ascending aorta with rupture into pericardial cavity and cardiac tamponade is a rare cause of fatal "electromechanical dissociation" during sports [11]. The basic heart defect is an elastic fragmentation of the aortic tunica media with cystic medial necrosis, that may present rarely as isolated histologic feature, but more frequently in association with aortic coarctation and/or bicuspid aortic valve, or in the setting of Marfan syndrome.

Despite its high prevalence in the general population, mitral valve prolapse seems to be a rare cause of sudden death in athletes [4,11]. The pathogenesis of the sudden cardiac arrest is still unknown; fatal coronary embolism

from atrial platelet deposits, and cardiac arrest due to malignant ventricular tachyarrhythmias attributed to "valve friction," have been advanced as
possible mechanisms.

Preexcitation syndrome (Wolff–Parkinson–White (WPW) syndrome) or
progressive cardiac conduction disease (Lenègre disease) may represent an
uncommon substrate of exercise-related sudden death [4].

Ion channel diseases

Five to ten percent of young people and athletes who die suddenly have no
evidence of structural heart diseases and the cause of their cardiac arrest is
in all likelihood related to a primary electrical heart disease such as inherited cardiac ion channel defects (channelopathies) including long-QT syndrome, Brugada syndrome, and cathecholaminergic polymorphic ventricular
tachycardia [30,31].

Brugada syndrome is an inherited ion channel disease characterized by the
peculiar ECG pattern of a right precordial "coved type" ST-segment elevation
(both spontaneous or induced by pharmacologic sodium channel block) in
association with arrhythmia-related symptoms such as syncope/cardiac arrest,
inducibility at programmed ventricular stimulation, or a suggestive familial
history [32]. A cardiac sodium channel gene (*SCN5A*) mutation has been
detected in up to 30% of cases. Ventricular fibrillation leading to sudden
death usually occurs at rest and in many cases at night as a consequence
of an increased vagal stimulation and/or withdrawal of sympathetic activity.
Enhanced adrenergic drive that occurs during sports activity could have an
inhibitory effect and theoretically reduce sudden death risk. On the other
hand, the adaptation of the cardiac autonomic nervous system to systematic
training, which results in increase of resting vagal tone or during the post-
exercise recovery period may enhance the propensity of athletes with Brugada
syndrome to die at rest, during sleep, or immediately after effort [33,34].

Catecholaminergic ventricular tachycardia is an inherited channelopathy
characterized by exercise-induced polymorphic ventricular tachycardia (most
often with the so-called "bidirectional" pattern), which can degenerate in
ventricular fibrillation [35]. Unlike long-QT syndrome and Brugada syndrome, this condition is not associated with abnormalities of basal 12-lead ECG
and remains unrecognized unless the athlete undergoes an ECG stress testing.
A genetically defective ryanodine receptor has been reported to account for an
abnormal calcium release from the sarcoplasmic reticulum. Accordingly, the
potential arrhythmogenic mechanism is triggered activity due to late afterdepolarizations, which are provoked by intracellular calcium overload and
enhanced by adrenergic stimulation such as that during sports exercise.

Drugs and performance enhancing substances

Athletes commonly use drugs and dietary supplements because they are considered to enhance athletic performance [36]. Among these performance
enhancing substances are stimulants, anabolic steroids, and peptide hormones.

Studies assessing the risks and benefits of these substances are limited and clinical observations indicate that some may have serious side effects. The dietary supplement ephedra (ma huang) has been associated with life-threatening toxicity and death resulting on a ban on its sale in the United States and Canada [37]. Anabolic steroids have been associated with premature coronary disease and sudden death. Recreational drugs including cocaine have been associated with fatal myocardial infarctions, sudden death, and strokes. Peptide hormones and analogues such as recombinant erythropoietin (EPO) are used as a pharmacologic alternative to the procedure of "blood doping" or autotransfusion steroids, peptide hormones, and others that may have life-threatening toxicity. Comprehensive lists of prohibited drugs and dietary supplements are available from governing athletic bodies. A rigorous approach to prevent performance enhancing and recreational drug and dietary supplement use should be taken by all athletic bodies. The crucial elements of programs to discourage drug performance enhancing substance include education to the ethical principles inherent in athletic participation.

Screening prior to athletic participation
The AHA recommendations
Preparticipation screening for detection of cardiovascular abnormalities that predispose to sudden cardiac death in the athlete is also recommended in the United States by the American Heart Association and the American College of Cardiology [2,29]. This systematic examination is intended to identify clinically relevant cardiovascular conditions that may increase the risk of athletic competition is recommended, before the initial engagement in organized athletics at the high school or collegiate level. This evaluation should be repeated every 2 years with an interim history obtained in the intervening years. This screening includes personal and family history and physical examination. ECGs and echocardiograms are not recommended routinely but should be selectively used in those with abnormal symptoms, clinical history, and physical examination.

The ECG has a relatively low specificity as a screening test because of a high frequency of changes that occur in association with exercise. It has been estimated that approximately 20–25% of athletes have ECG patterns that are sufficiently abnormal to warrant further evaluation with an echocardiogram. Patterns that might identify individuals at high risk for sudden death include ventricular preexcitation with WPW pattern, long-QT intervals, hypertrophic cardiomyopathy, arrhythmogenic right ventricular cardiomyopathy/dysplasia, and Brugada syndrome [2,29].

The cost-effectiveness, practicality, and utility of the screening process are limited by the uncommon occurrence in the general and athletic population of those cardiovascular conditions that predispose to sudden death. Using the history and physical examination alone, as recommended in the United States, has proven to be of marginal or no value in preventing sudden death. One retrospective study concluded that the history and physical examination were able to detect cardiovascular abnormalities in only 3% of high school and college athletes who ultimately died of cardiovascular disease. ECG and echocardiography have demonstrated a low yield of identifiable cardiovascular conditions that predispose to sudden death. Despite these limitations, the American Heart Association recommended the concept of preparticipation screening for athletes based on medical and ethical considerations [2,29].

The Italian experience

For more than 25 years, a systematic preparticipation screening, predominantly based on 12-lead ECG in addition to history and physical examination, has been in practice in Italy [5,38]. Such a screening strategy has been proven to be effective in identification of athletes with previously undiagnosed hypertrophic cardiomyopathy [5]. Moreover, during a long-term follow-up no deaths were recorded among disqualified athletes with hypertrophic cardiomyopathy, suggesting that identification and disqualification from competition has the potential to improve survival [5]. A subanalysis of Italian data shows that only less than one-fourth of young competitive athletes with hypertrophic cardiomyopathy detected at preparticipation screening had had a positive family history or an abnormal physical examination; thus, the majority of them would not have been identified by a limited screening protocol without 12-lead ECG [5]. Such a three-fold greater number of athletes with hypertrophic cardiomyopathy identified by the Italian screening and disqualified from competitive sports, is expected to result in a corresponding additional number of lives saved compared to other strategy.

In addition, 12-lead ECG offers the potential to detect asymptomatic athletes with other conditions presenting with ECG abnormalities such as arrhythmogenic right ventricular cardiomyopathy/dysplasia, dilated cardiomyopathy, Lenègre conduction disease, WPW syndrome, long- and short-QT syndromes, and Brugada syndrome. Overall, these conditions (including hypertrophic cardiomyopathy) account for up to 60% of sudden death in young competitive athletes [1,4,33]. Of note, most of these conditions have been discovered only recently and the impact on mortality of their detection at preparticipation screening will be assessed only in the future.

A recent consensus document of the study group on sports cardiology of the European Society of Cardiology reinforces the principle of the need of preparticipation medical clearance of all young athletes involved in organized sports programs and recommends the implementation of a common European screening protocol essentially based on 12-lead ECG [39].

Athletic participation

When a definitive cardiovascular condition is identified, the consensus panel recommendations of the thirty-sixth Bethesda Conference provides guidelines for continued participation or disqualification from athletics [28]. Although these recommendation were written for the competitive athlete, as defined by participation in an organized team or individual sport requiring systematic training and regular competition against others while placing a high premium on athletic excellence and achievement, many of the recommendations are relevant to the recreational and non-athletes [2,29].

Updated European guidelines are being elaborated by the Sports Cardiology of the Working Group of Cardiac Rehabilitation and Exercise Physiology of the European Society of Cardiology and are expected with publication planned in the *European Heart Journal* by 2004.

Automated external defibrillators

The concept of public access to defibrillation has received increasing attention as it has become clear that survival of the cardiac arrest victim is more likely to be successful with a system in place to ensure that cardiopulmonary resuscitation and early defibrillation are promptly provided [40–42]. Over the last several years, the automated external defibrillator has played a growing role in improving survival from sudden cardiac death. The current devices require application of pads to the arrest victims chest wall, allowing analysis of the patients cardiac rhythm and, if appropriate, delivery of defibrillator shocks. These devices are approximately the size of a laptop computer, are low maintenance, and have a shelf life for the battery of several years. Use of the device is intuitive and allows both nontraditional responders, including trainers, coaches, police, and untrained responders to respond rapidly in emergency situations. The algorithms for detecting ventricular tachycardia and fibrillation have been shown to be highly sensitive and specific. The success of public access to defibrillation programs using the automated external defibrillator (AED) in improving survival have been demonstrated in many settings. Many athletic organizations now recommend or mandate AED at athletic events [40–42].

Conclusion

Recently, there has been considerable advancement in our knowledge regarding the diagnosis, mechanism, and therapy of sudden death in the athlete. The common cardiovascular conditions that predispose to sudden death are now known. Strategies for predicting and preventing sudden death are being refined to identify those at risk and restrict them from athletic activity. Recommendations regarding screening, evaluation, management, and restriction from athletics are available to assist athletic organizations, trainers, and clinicians. There remains a clear need to refine and assess guidelines for preparticipation screening and athletic restriction with cost-effectiveness studies and tracking of outcomes. Detailed international registries of screening programs and outcomes are needed. Based on the success of public access to defibrillation programs on improving outcomes, strong consideration should be given to developing such programs with the use of AED at athletic events. Finally, athletic organizations, athletes, coaches, educational institutions, coaches trainers, and physicians need to develop strategic partnerships to develop and refine policies regarding the complex issues related to prediction and prevention of sudden death in the athlete.

References

1. Maron, BJ. Sudden death in young athletes. *New Engl J Med* 2003; **349**: 1064–1075.
2. Estes NAM III, Link MS, Cannom D *et al.* NASPE consensus statement report of the NASPE policy conference on arrhythmias and the athlete. *J Cardiovasc Electrophysiol* 2001; **12**: 1208–1219.
3. Link MS, Wang PJ, Estes NAM III. Cardiac arrhythmias and electrophysiologic observations in the athletes. In: Williams RA, ed. *The Athlete and Heart Disease: Diagnosis, Evaluation and Management.* Lippincott Williams & Wilkins: Philadelphia, PA, 1999: 197–216.
4. Corrado D, Basso C, Rizzoli G *et al.* Does sports activity enhance the risk of sudden death in adolescents and young adults? *J Am Coll Cardiol* 2003; **42**: 1959–1963.
5. Corrado D, Basso C, Schiavon M *et al.* Screening for hypertrophic cardiomyopathy in young athletes. *New Engl J Med* 1998; **339**: 364–369.
6. Priori SG, Aliot E, Blomstrom-Lundqvist C *et al.* Task force on sudden cardiac death of the European Society of Cardiology. *Eur Heart J* 2001; **22**(16): 1374–1450.
7. Van Camp SP, Bloor CM, Mueller FO *et al.* Non-traumatic sports death in high school and college athletes. *Med Sci Sports Exerc* 1995; **27**: 641–647.
8. Maron BJ, Gohman TE, Aeppli D. Prevalence of sudden cardiac death during competitive sports activities in Minnesota high school athletes. *J Am Coll Cardiol* 1998; **32**: 1881–1884.
9. Corrado D, Basso C, Poletti A, *et al.* Sudden death in the young: is coronary thrombosis the major precipitating factor? *Circulation* 1994; **90**: 2315–2323.
10. Maron BJ, Roberts WC, McAllister MA *et al.* Sudden death in young athletes. *Circulation* 1980; **62**: 218–229.
11. Corrado D, Thiene G, Nava A, *et al.* Sudden death in young competitive athletes: clinico-pathologic correlations in 22 cases. *Am J Med* 1990; **89**: 588–596.
12. Basso C, Calabrese F, Corrado D *et al.* Postmortem diagnosis in sudden cardiac death victims: macroscopic, microscopic and molecular findings. *Cardiovasc Res* 2001; **50**: 290–300.
13. Maron BJ. Hypertrophic cardiomyopathy: a systematic review. *JAMA* 2002; **237**: 1308–1320.
14. Basso C, Thiene G, Corrado D *et al.* Arrhythmogenic right ventricular cardiomyopathy. Dysplasia, dystrophy, or myocarditis? *Circulation* 1996; **94**: 983–991.
15. Basso C, Thiene G, Corrado D *et al.* Hypertrophic cardiomyopathy and sudden death in the young: pathologic evidence of myocardial ischemia. *Hum Pathol* 2000; **31**: 988–998.
16. Maron BJ, Pelliccia A, Spirito P. Cardiac disease in young trained athletes. Insights into methods for distinguishing athlete's heart from structural heart disease, with particular emphasis on hypertrophic cardiomyopathy. *Circulation* 1995, **91**: 1596–1601.
17. Nava A, Bauce B, Basso C *et al.* Clinical profile and long-term follow-up of 37 families with arrhythmogenic right ventricular cardiomyopathy. *J Am Coll Cardiol* 2000; **36**: 2226–2233.

18. Thiene G, Nava A, Corrado D *et al.* Right ventricular cardiomyopathy and sudden death in young people. *N Engl J Med* 1988; **318**: 129–133.

19. Corrado D, Basso C, Thiene G *et al.* Spectrum of clinicopathologic manifestations of arrhythmogenic right ventricular cardiomyopathy/dysplasia: a multicenter study. *J Am Coll Cardiol* 1997; **30**(6): 1512–1520.

20. Corrado D, Fontaine G, Marcus FI *et al.* Arrhythmogenic right ventricular dysplasia/cardiomyopathy: need for an international registry. *Circulation* 2000; **21**: 101:e101–106.

21. Corrado D, Basso C, Thiene G. Arrhythmogenic right ventricular cardiomyopathy: diagnosis, prognosis, and treatment. *Heart* 2000; **83**: 588–595.

22. Basso C, Maron BJ, Corrado D *et al.* Clinical profile of congenital coronary artery anomalies with origin from the wrong aortic sinus leading to sudden death in young competitive athletes. *J Am Coll Cardiol* 2000; **35**: 1493–1501.

23. Maron BJ, Gohman TE, Kyle SB *et al.* Clinical profile and spectrum of commotio cordis. *JAMA* 2002; **287**: 1142–1146.

24. Link MS, Wang PJ, Pandian NG *et al.* An experimental model of sudden death due to low energy chest wall impact (commotio cordis). *N Engl J Med* 1998; **338**: 1805–1811.

25. Link MS, Wang PJ, VanderBrink BA *et al.* Selective activation of the K^+ATP channel is a mechanism by which sudden death is produced by low-energy chest-wall impact (commotio cordis). *Circulation* 1999; **100**: 413–418.

26. Link MS, Maron BJ, VanderBrink BA *et al.* Impact directly over the cardiac silhouette is necessary to produce ventricular fibrillation in an experimental model of commotio cordis. *J Am Coll Cardiol* 2001; **37**: 649–654.

27. Link MS, Maron BJ, Wang PJ *et al.* Upper and lower limits of vulnerability to sudden arrhythmic death with chest wall impact (commotio cordis). *J Am Coll Cardiol* 2003; **41**: 99–104.

28. Maron BJ, Zipes DP. Eligibility recommendations for competitive athletes with cardiovascular abnormalities-general considerations. *J Am Coll Cardiol.* 2005; **45**(8): 1318–1321.

29. Maron B, Thompson P, Puffer *et al.* Cardiovascular preparticipation screening of competitive athletes: a statement for health professionals from the sudden death committee (clinical cardiology) and congenital cardiac defects committee (cardiovascular disease in the young) American Heart Association. *Circulation* 1996; **94**: 850–856.

30. Corrado D, Basso C, Thiene G. Sudden cardiac death in young people with apparently normal heart. *Cardiovasc Res* 2001; **50**: 399–408.

31. Di Paolo M, Luchini D, Bloise R, *et al.* Postmortem molecular analysis in victims of sudden unexplained death. *Am J Forensic Med Pathol* 2004; **25**(2): 182–184.

32. Wilde AA, Antzelevitch C, Borggrefe M *et al.* Study group on the molecular basis of arrhythmias of the European Society of Cardiology. Proposed diagnostic criteria for the Brugada syndrome: consensus report. *Circulation* 2002; **106**: 2514–2519.

33. Maron BJ, Chaitman BR, Ackerman MJ *et al.* Recommendations for physical activity and recreational sports participation for young patients with genetic cardiovascular diseases. *Circulation* 2004; **109**: 2807–2816.

34. Corrado D, Pelliccia A, Antzelevitch C *et al.* ST segment elevation and sudden death in the athlete. In: Antzelevitch C & Brugada P, eds. *The Brugada Syndrome: From Bench to Bedside.* Blackwell Publishing (in press).

35. Priori SG, Napolitano C, Memmi M *et al.* Clinical and molecular characterization of patients with catecholaminergic polymorphic ventricular tachycardia. *Circulation* 2002; **106**: 69–74.

36. Stout CW, Weinstock J, Homoud MK *et al.* Herbal medicines; beneficial effects, side effects and promising new research in the treatment of arrhythmias. *Curr Cardiol Reports* 2003; **5**: 395–401.

37. Samenuk D, Link MS, Homoud MK *et al.* Adverse cardiovascular events temporally associated with Ma Huang. *Mayo Clinic Proc* 2002; **77**: 12–16.

38. Pelliccia A, Maron BJ. Preparticipation cardiovascular evaluation of the competitive athlete: perspectives from the 30-year Italian experience. *Am J Cardiol* 1995; **75**: 827–829.

39. Corrado D, Pelliccia A, Bjørnstad HH *et al.* Cardiovascular preparticipation screening of young competitive athletes for prevention of sudden death: proposal for a common European protocol. Consensus statement of the Study Group of Sport Cardiology of the Working Group of Cardiac Rehabilitation and Exercise Physiology and the Working Group of Myocardial and Pericardial Diseases of the European Society of Cardiology. *Eur Heart J* 2005; **26**: 1804–1805.

40. Morenco JP, Wang PJ, Link MS *et al.* Improving survival from cardiac arrest: the role of the automated external defibrillator. *JAMA* 2001; **285**: 1193–1200.

41. Hoffman C, Marenco J, Wang P *et al.* Public access defibrillation programs: the role of the automated external defibrillator. *Cardiovascular Reviews & Reports* 2002; **23**: 286–291.

42. Balady GJ, Chaitman B, Foster C *et al.* Automated external defibrillators in health/fitness facilities: supplement to the AHA/ACSM recommendations for cardiovascular screening, staffing and emergency policies at Health/Fitness Facilities. *Circulation* 2002; **105**: 1147–1150.

Section three:
Treatment

CHAPTER 14

Pharmacology of sudden cardiac death

Timothy W. Smith, Michael E. Cain, Günter Breithardt, and Paulus Kirchhof

The implantable cardioverter-defibrillator (ICD) is an effective therapy for the primary and secondary prevention of sudden arrhythmic death. Prescription of ICD therapy for primary prevention is restricted to patients at high risk for developing sustained ventricular tachycardia (VT) or ventricular fibrillation (VF). At present, the medical history and objective clinical findings including the left ventricular ejection fraction and the presence of a myocardial infarct, are utilized to identify high-risk patients who will benefit from ICD therapy. Unfortunately, the majority of sudden arrhythmic deaths do not occur in this high-risk group [1]. Primary prevention of sudden death for patients at intermediate or low risk is based on the use of pharmacological and lifestyle interventions.

The indication for pharmacological therapy to prevent sudden death is to favorably modify the conditions that initiate and maintain sustained VT/VF [2]. These conditions produce electrophysiological derangements that are induced transiently or that develop during the course of healing from injury to ventricular myocardium and persist. Factors known to trigger VT/VF include changes in autonomic nervous system activity, metabolic disturbances, myocardial ischemia, electrolyte abnormalities, acute volume and/or pressure overload of the ventricles, ion channel abnormalities, and proarrhythmic actions of cardiac, and noncardiac drugs. Death of myocardial cells from ischemia, toxins, infectious agents, or chronic pressure/volume overload leads to scar formation, alterations in chamber geometry, and electrical and anatomical remodeling.

Pharmacological agents to prevent sudden death focused initially on drugs that directly affected membrane ion channels. However, adverse effects, proarrhythmia, and low efficacy limit the use of available sodium and potassium channel blocking drugs for primary and secondary prevention of VT/VF. Better drug targets appear to be the prevention of myocardial injury (aspirin, hydroxymethylglutarate CoA reductase inhibitors, beta-blockers), attenuation of the deleterious effects of increased sympathetic tone (beta-blockers), and favorable modification of the proarrhythmic anatomical and electrophysiological remodeling that occurs in response to myocardial injury (angiotensin converting enzyme inhibitors, angiotensin receptor blockers, beta-blockers).

Drugs prescribed to prevent sudden death must favorably alter the electrophysiological derangements that lead to VT/VF and not induce alterations that lead to proarrhythmia. The latter objective is a challenge because drug-induced proarrhythmia is not limited to cardiac drugs and it is difficult to identify patients at risk for this complication. Although VT/VF is the most common rhythm disturbance leading to sudden cardiac death, bradycardia is a cause in some patients. This chapter will focus on: (1) drugs that help prevent sudden cardiac death; and (2) drugs that inadvertently cause sudden death by inducing VT/VF or bradycardia.

Prevention of VT/VF

Patients with acquired structural heart disease
Depressed ventricular function and/or dilatation of the cardiac chambers are used clinically to document structural heart disease in patients. Ischemic heart disease is the most common cause of structural disease and accounts for 75–80% of all sudden cardiac deaths [3]. Electrophysiological derangements that lead to sudden death may occur: (1) transiently during acute ischemia in the absence of myocardial infarction; (2) during the early stages of myocardial injury leading to infarction; or (3) during the healing and remodeling phases that lead to scar formation following acute infarction. Pharmacological therapies that prevent transient ischemia or infarction should have a beneficial impact on the incidence of sudden death. Based on the clinical observation that reduced left ventricular function is by far the best predictor of sudden cardiac death, pharmacological therapies that minimize myocardial injury or the adverse remodeling associated with cardiomyopathies due to conditions other than coronary artery disease would be expected to protect patients from VT/VF.

Amiodarone
In contrast to other sodium and potassium channel blocking agents, amiodarone has consistently been shown to be effective for secondary prevention of VT/VF in patients with ischemic heart disease. The CASCADE trial established the superiority of amiodarone for this purpose compared to therapy with conventional sodium channel blocking drugs. However, the sodium channel blocking drugs used may have had a negative impact on the patient outcomes because of proarrhythmia. The data from CASCADE do not allow conclusions concerning the superiority of amiodarone compared to placebo [4]. Data from other randomized, placebo-controlled trials have shown that amiodarone does not increase mortality in patients with heart failure [5]. Results of randomized secondary prevention studies such as the Amiodarone Versus Implantable Defibrillator (AVID) trial demonstrated a survival benefit of ICD therapy over

amiodarone. However, a subgroup analysis of patients with a measured left ventricular ejection fraction >35%, failed to show superiority of ICD therapy over antiarrhythmic drug therapy (primarily amiodarone) [6]. In patients with ICDs, amiodarone or other antiarrhythmic drugs [7] can be prescribed to reduce the number of delivered ICD therapies.

In patients with remote myocardial infarction, two randomized, placebo-controlled, double-blind trials assessed the impact of amiodarone on prognosis (EMIAT, CAMIAT). Both studies showed that amiodarone significantly reduced sudden death rates, the primary endpoint in CAMIAT and a secondary endpoint in EMIAT [8,9]. Total mortality, however, was not affected, similar to the CHF-STAT study [5] and the SCD-HeFT study [10], among others [2].

Beta-blockers
Beta-blockers are the only proven pharmacological intervention for primary prevention of lethal arrhythmias [11]. They have been shown to have a favorable impact on the incidence of recurrent ischemic events and myocardial infarctions. They are also a key to the treatment strategies for patients with congestive heart failure, even in the presence of severe systolic left ventricular dysfunction. Although most clinical trials assessed the effect of beta-blockers on total mortality rather than sudden death rates, the MERIT-HF trial found a 41% reduction in sudden death rates in patients with NYHA class II–IV heart failure [12]. It is generally accepted that reduction of total mortality by beta-blockers is attributable, at least in part, to an effect on sudden death rates.

Angiotensin converting enzyme inhibitors
Recent attention has focused on slowing or reversing the disease processes that ultimately lead to sudden death. Some therapies prevent sudden death by preventing myocardial infarction, a highly effective approach, since most deadly arrhythmias occur in the setting of coronary plaque rupture with subsequent platelet activation, thrombus formation, and infarction. Angiotensin converting enzyme (ACE) inhibitors have become a mainstay of therapy in patients with depressed left ventricular function. They prevent recurrent infarction and improve overall mortality. ACE inhibitors also prevent progression of ventricular dysfunction and stabilize autonomic activity [2]. Collectively, these salutary actions have the potential to decrease sudden death as well as overall mortality. The results of individual trials regarding reduction in sudden death have been controversial, which can partially be attributed to differences in definition and adjudication of sudden death in individual trials. A meta-analysis of 15 trials that enrolled patients following myocardial infarction suggested that reduction in sudden cardiac death was a significant component of the overall reduction in mortality afforded by ACE inhibition [13].

Angiotensin receptor blockers
Angiotensin receptor blockers (ARBs) lack the anti-kininase activity of ACE inhibitors, an effect that is associated with chronic cough, a clinically relevant

side effect of ACE inhibitors that occurs in up to 10% of patients. Therefore, ARBs are prescribed when ACE inhibitors cannot be administered. In addition, ARBs may at times be used in combination with ACE inhibitors. Based on the results of the CHARM program, ARBs and ACE inhibitors have similar efficacy [14]. Retrospective analysis of key studies suggest that ARBs also reduce sudden death rates [13,15]. Although data acquired from prospective trials are not yet published, it is likely that ARBs have a similar effect on sudden death rates as ACE inhibitors. The mechanisms by which ARBs prevent sudden death are likely related to slowing or reversing of the remodeling processes that form the substrate for VT/VF rather than direct antiarrhythmic effects [15].

Aspirin

The benefit of aspirin in the reduction of platelet aggregation in coronary artery disease is well established. Aspirin administration during the acute and healing phases of myocardial infarction reduces the incidence of recurrent infarction and reduces mortality [16]. There are no clear data concerning the impact on sudden arrhythmic death. As the majority of sudden deaths still occur in the setting of acute ischemic events, it is likely that aspirin reduces sudden death by preventing myocardial ischemia and recurrent infarction. Aspirin is also effective for primary prevention of myocardial infarction, but a decrease in mortality has not been shown [16].

Aldosterone antagonists

Aldosterone has an important role in the pathophysiology of congestive heart failure. Data acquired from a randomized, placebo-controlled trial, demonstrated that spironolactone decreased overall mortality and mortality from cardiac causes, reduced hospitalizations due to heart failure, improved symptoms, and reduced sudden death [17]. Eplerenone is a new selective aldosterone receptor antagonist. In a placebo-controlled randomized trial of patients with heart failure after myocardial infarction, death, and death from cardiovascular cause were reduced in the eplerenone group [18]. Sudden cardiac death was a secondary endpoint in both the spironolactone and eplerenone trials. With this limitation, it is reasonable to assume that aldosterone antagonists prevent sudden cardiac death, either by their effects on ventricular remodeling, by increasing extracellular potassium levels, or by other mechanisms.

Hydroxymethylglutarate CoA reductase inhibitors

There is substantial evidence that hydroxymethylglutarate (HMG) CoA reductase inhibitors, or "statins," reduce serum LDL cholesterol, prevent or slow the progress of atherosclerosis, prevent acute coronary syndromes, and reduce cardiovascular mortality in patients at risk [19]. Sudden cardiac death was rarely an endpoint in the many trials of HMG CoA reductase inhibitors. However, many sudden deaths are associated with plaque rupture and myocardial infarction [3]. Accordingly, it is likely that statins reduce sudden death mainly by preventing acute coronary syndromes and acute myocardial infarctions.

Dietary omega-3 polyunsaturated fatty acids

Polyunsaturated fatty acids (PUFAs) found in fish and fish oil reduce all cause of cardiovascular mortality as well as sudden death [20]. This beneficial effect occurs early in the course of treatment. The mechanism of benefit does not appear to be related to prevention of acute coronary syndromes or myocardial infarction, and may result from a direct antiarrhythmic effect. In an experimental model of sudden arrhythmic death, direct administration of PUFA has been shown to prevent ventricular arrhythmias and sudden death caused by acute coronary artery occlusion [21]. Although not conclusive, some data suggest PUFAs may act on calcium channels, sodium channels, and/or the sarcoplasmic reticulum calcium ATPase (SERCA2A) [22].

The majority of these nontraditional therapies exert their beneficial effect on sudden death by preventing or favorably altering proarrhythmic substrates induced as a consequence of structural heart disease, especially coronary artery disease. It has also been proposed that molecular mechanisms of dyslipidemias are themselves arrhythmogenic and that pharmacological therapies aimed at lipid based pro-thrombotic and pro-inflammatory factors should be a major point of pharmacological interest [23]. In addition to HMG CoA reductase inhibitors, such therapies might in the future include leukotriene pathway antagonists, cyclooxygenase isoenzyme inhibitors, platelet aggregating factor antagonists, and cytokine antagonists.

Patients with inherited arrhythmogenic cardiomyopathies

There are at least three forms of genetically determined diseases that confer structural cardiac abnormalities and predispose to sudden death; familial hypertrophic cardiomyopathy, arrhythmogenic right ventricular cardiomyopathy, and Fabry disease (Chapter 8).

Familial hypertrophic cardiomyopathy

In patients with familial hypertrophic cardiomyopathy (FHC), sudden death is usually due to polymorphic VT/VF. Beta-blockers and calcium-channel antagonists can be effective drugs to ameliorate symptoms associated with obstruction of the left ventricular outflow tract [24]. There is expert opinion that these drugs may reduce the risk for ventricular arrhythmias. The anti-arrhythmic effect of beta-blockers is supported by the fact that ventricular arrhythmias in FHC patients and in experimental models of FHC are usually triggered by catecholaminergic stimulation [25,26]. Whether action potential prolongation is beneficial, for example, by pharmacological potassium channel blockade, is less clear. Amiodarone has some efficacy, but the mechanism of its prevention of arrhythmias in FHC is unclear.

Arrhythmogenic right ventricular cardiomyopathy

Arrhythmogenic right ventricular cardiomyopathy (ARVC) usually manifests as VT with an origin from the right ventricle (i.e. with a left bundle branch pattern in the ECG). Unlike drug treatment for Fabry disease or myectomy/septal alcohol ablation for FHC, there are currently no interventions that can slow or stop the progressive fibrofatty replacement of right ventricular myocardium associated with ARVC. Catheter ablation of tachycardias is often acutely successful, but the natural disease progression creates new arrhythmogenic substrates over time. Beta-blockers can attenuate sympathetic stimulation of the right ventricular myocardium, which is believed to contribute to initiation of VTs and possibly to disease progression. Patients who survived VT/VF are candidates for ICD therapy, but complication rates after implantation are higher than in general ICD patient cohorts, most likely due to loss of right ventricular myocardium and subsequent difficulties with pacing, sensing, and electrode fixation [27]. In addition, VTs are often hemodynamically relatively well tolerated. Therefore, antiarrhythmic drugs may be an alternative even in ARVC patients who already suffered an episode of sustained VT. Sotalol has been used and may be beneficial in some patients, although it remains unclear whether this effect is due to beta-blockade or to prolongation of the action potential prolongation [28]. Amiodarone is also relatively effective. A combination of drug treatment and catheter ablation is effective in some patients with ARVC [29].

An important differential diagnosis to ARVC is a benign form of right ventricular outflow tract tachycardia. Patients with this disease usually suffer from exercise- or catecholamine-induced repetitive monomorphic VT with an ectopic origin. The heart is structurally normal, and the prognosis is good. Treatment is guided by symptoms and may consist of antiarrhythmic drugs (beta-blockers, sotalol, or verapamil) or catheter ablation.

Fabry disease

Fabry disease is due to an inherited lack of alpha-galactosidase and results in renal, facial, and myocardial amyloid deposits [30]. The combination of renal dysfunction, red papulae in the face, and left ventricular hypertrophy with a salt-and-pepper pattern on echocardiography should trigger the clinical suspicion of Fabry disease [30]. The disease can be mistaken for hypertrophic cardiomyopathy [31]. The renal phenotype is often life limiting, but sudden death has been reported. Sudden death can be due to either bradycardia caused by progressive conduction block, sinus nodal dysfunction, or to VT due to the formation of anatomical reentrant circuits [32]. Unlike other inherited arrhythmogenic diseases, there is a specific drug treatment for Fabry disease, that is, substitution of alpha-galactosidase [30]. This treatment can, based on case reports, also revert conduction block and is therefore probably a specific antiarrhythmic treatment option in Fabry disease patients. There are so far, however, no data on the effect of such treatment on arrhythmias.

Inherited arrhythmogenic diseases ("ion channelopathies")

Several syndromes that occur in structurally normal hearts and lead to potentially lethal ventricular arrhythmias and sudden cardiac death have been identified (Chapter 9). Usually, a defect in an ion transporter or ion channel is suspected or identified.

Long-QT syndromes

The congenital long-QT syndrome, which predisposes the affected individual to *torsades de pointes*, has been well characterized. The QT interval is intimately associated with the duration of the ventricular action potential. The action potential duration is determined by the activities of multiple voltage-gated and ligand-gated sarcolemmal ion channels, as well as some ion transporters. The long-QT syndromes have been linked to genetic defects in potassium or sodium channels. There are at least seven different gene defects known to cause long QT (LQT1–LQT7). A relevant portion of patients with long-QT syndrome remains free of arrhythmia recurrences on beta-blockers. Beta-blockers are therefore the first-line therapy for asymptomatic and some symptomatic patients with the long-QT syndrome. Unfortunately, pharmacological prevention of sudden death is imperfect and some genotypes (LQT1 and LQT2) are better protected than others (LQT3) [33]. Some patients require more aggressive treatments, including continuous rapid atrial pacing or ICD therapy, which is recommended in long-QT syndrome patients at high risk of sudden death [34].

There are some clinical data that suggest that drug therapy in long-QT syndromes could be guided by the genetic defect (e.g. mutant potassium or sodium channels) [35]. Sodium channel blockade by flecainide or mexiletine may be useful in LQT3, which is caused by mutated sodium channels with increased late inward current [33,36,37]. Similarly, oral potassium has been proposed as a possible therapy for LQT2, because increased extracellular potassium levels suppress the effect of the mutant I_{Kr} current on the QT interval, and possibly also because arrhythmic events are more likely when extracellular potassium levels are low [38]. Definitive data on genotype-specific treatment are lacking.

Brugada syndrome

The Brugada syndrome is characterized by a right bundle branch block pattern with coved or saddle-type ST segment elevation in the right precordial ECG leads (V_1–V_3) and a predisposition to ventricular arrhythmias and sudden death. Some patients (10–15%) with Brugada syndrome suffer from mutations in the *SCN5A* gene that encodes for the cardiac sodium channel, the same channel that is affected in LQT3. In Brugada syndrome, slowly dissociating sodium channel blockers (flecainide, propafenone, or ajmaline) are contraindicated because they unmask the ECG phenotype and increase the risk for ventricular arrhythmias [34]. Beta-blockers may provoke rather than reduce ventricular arrhythmias in Brugada syndrome. Quinidine, tedisamil, and cilostazol (a phosphodiesterase III inhibitor), all of which inhibit the transient outward potassium current I_{to}, have been suggested as possible therapies for Brugada syndrome [34,39,40]. There is not yet sufficient data concerning safety and efficacy to make recommendations for these gene- or channel-specific agents. ICD therapy is the only established effective treatment to prevent sudden arrhythmic death in high-risk patients.

Short-QT syndrome

The short-QT syndrome is a familial syndrome characterized by a short-QT interval (corrected QT interval <330 ms), frequent palpitations, syncope and sudden death, short atrial and ventricular refractory periods, atrial fibrillation, and inducible ventricular fibrillation [41]. Sudden death occurs in young and otherwise healthy individuals. Data on pharmacological therapy are limited. Data from a small group of patients suggested that quinidine prolongs the QT interval, prolongs the ventricular refractory period, and renders ventricular fibrillation noninducible in affected patients [42].

Catecholaminergic polymorphic ventricular tachycardia

This condition occurs in patients with a structurally normal heart and is characterized by a bidirectional or polymorphic VT triggered by exertion, stress, or catecholamine infusion. It is often inherited in an autosomal-dominant fashion and has been associated with a defect in the ryanodine receptor, which mediates calcium-induced calcium release from the sarcoplasmic reticulum [43]. A defect in the gene encoding calsequestrin may produce a similar syndrome [44]. Beta-blockers provide incomplete protection against sustained ventricular arrhythmias in sudden death survivors, and are used as adjunct treatment to ICD therapy.

Catecholaminergic polymorphic VT may be a subset of idiopathic VF, in which sudden death from a ventricular arrhythmia may occur in the absence of detectable structural heart disease and in the absence of any other marker. ICD therapy is reasonable for survivors. Pharmacological therapy might include beta-blockers, but directed pharmacological therapy is not currently possible in the absence of an understood mechanism.

Further study of some of these syndromes will lead to identification of new therapeutic targets. Cellular calcium handling is one particular aspect of myocardial cell physiology that may deserve continued attention. Many of the syndromes discussed may be related to abnormal calcium handling, including those associated with afterdepolarizations and *torsades de pointes* as well as those associated with altered calcium handling in the sarcoplasmic reticulum. In addition, reentry, the most common mechanism of sustained arrhythmia, may be initiated by extrastimuli that originate with afterdepolarizations or are caused by intracellular "calcium overload." Just as traditional antiarrhythmic drugs are developed to affect specific sarcolemmal ion channels, future drug development may be aimed at agents of intracellular calcium sequestration and release.

Drug-induced ventricular tachycardia/fibrillation

Drug-induced *torsades de pointes*
Torsades de pointes was initially named to describe a specific twisting of the QRS complex in the surface ECG [45], but the term is now usually used for polymorphic VT associated with prolonged QT intervals and provoked by afterdepolarizations. Ever since drug-induced *torsades de pointes* was related to an abnormal prolongation of the QT interval by noncardiovascular drugs, this issue has bothered physicians, pharmaceutical companies, and regulatory bodies [46] (Chapter 12). Drug-induced *torsades de pointes* appears to be a patient-specific phenomenon, that is, there are ambient and genetic factors that are required for *torsades de pointes* to occur [47,48], and the majority of patients will never suffer from such arrhythmias. An association of drug-induced *torsades de pointes* and minimal forms of the long-QT syndromes has been reported [48]. Likewise, minimal forms of other genetically determined arrhythmogenic diseases are likely to contribute to drug-induced proarrhythmia (Figure 14.1) [49]. Cardiac hypertrophy is a common clinical condition known to both prolong the QT interval and to predispose to sudden arrhythmic death, and is found in many patients that suffer from drug-induced *torsade de pointes*. Any combination of such factors will additionally reduce the amount of repolarizing currents available in the myocardium (the "repolarization reserve") and thereby prolong the action potential and the QT interval [50].

The list of drugs that convey such a risk is continuously expanding and includes antibiotics, antipsychotic drugs, and antihistaminic compounds [51,52]. Knowledge of the clinical characteristics that identify patients at increased risk for drug-induced *torsades de pointes* (a combination of female gender, longer-than-average QT interval, left ventricular hypertrophy, bradycardia, and/or hypokalemia) and of the drugs known to provoke such arrhythmias (www.torsades.org) can help to prevent the occurrence of drug-induced proarrhythmia.

Mechanism of drug-induced *torsades de pointes*
Almost all drugs that have been associated with drug-induced proarrhythmia inhibit the rapid component of the delayed cardiac rectifier current (I_{Kr}), although the specific function of this current for drug-induced proarrhythmia is still not fully understood. The available experimental and clinical data suggest that action potential prolongation in combination with other factors such as bradycardia, hypokalemia, and intracellular calcium overload provokes early afterdepolarizations during the prolonged repolarization phase of the action potential. These afterdepolarizations produce triggered activity that in turn causes functional reentry. Functional reentry is believed to be possible due to regional (e.g. transmural) and temporal variations in local action potential duration and refractoriness. The combination of afterdepolarizations (i.e. the trigger for *torsades de pointes*) and a substrate for functional reentry (i.e. local

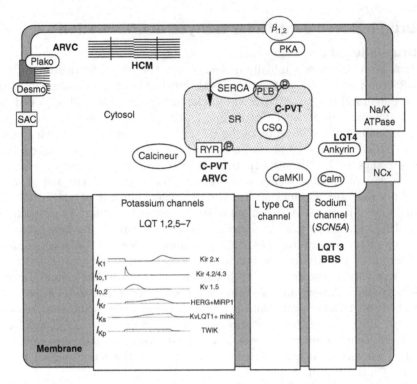

Figure 14.1 Molecular mechanisms of sudden arrhythmic death. ARVC denotes arrhythmogenic right ventricular cardiomyopathy; HCM, hypertrophic cardiomyopathy; CPVT, catecholaminergic polymorphic ventricular tachycardia; LQT, long-QT syndrome; BBS, Brugada syndrome; SR, sarcoplasmic reticulum; SAC, stretch-activated channel; Calm, calmodulin; CaMKI, calmodulin kinase II; NCx, sodium calcium exchanger; PKA, protein kinase A; RYR, ryanodine receptor; CSQ, calsequestrin. (Adapted from Reference 49, with permission from Springer.)

conduction block due to inhomogeneities in repolarization) can initiate and sustain *torsades de pointes*.

QT prolongation

Similar to the changes in QT interval in the congenital long-QT syndromes, drug-induced prolongation of the QT interval is a sensitive, but not specific marker for the potential of certain drugs to provoke *torsades de pointes* in susceptible patients. There is evidence that blockade of the rapid component of the inward rectifier (I_{Kr}) is necessary for *torsades de pointes* to occur [46]. Indeed, patients who suffered from drug-induced *torsades de pointes* have a super-normal prolongation of the QT interval in response to the I_{Kr} blocker sotalol [47]. Drug-induced QT-interval prolongation *per se*, however, is often found without *torsades de pointes*.

Other contributing factors

A variety of other factors adds to the risk of *torsades de pointes*. Some are genetically determined, that is, female gender or subclinical forms of long-QT syndrome mutations [48]. Others are acquired and partially reversible structural alterations, that is, left ventricular hypertrophy, which is known to prolong the ventricular action potential and predisposes to early afterdepolarizations, possibly via activating specific intracellular signaling pathways [53,54]. In addition, there are transient factors such as hypokalemia, which can be drug- or food-induced, that is, by consumption of liquorice, grapefruit juice, or large quantities of alcohol, or bradycardia, which can also be secondary to bradycardia-inducing drugs (see below). Avoidance of such transient factors should be attempted whenever QT-prolonging drugs are used.

Digitalis

The digitalis investigation group (DIG) trial has established that digoxin treatment does not affect mortality in patients with heart failure who are in sinus rhythm, but that such treatment can reduce hospitalizations when compared to placebo [55]. A much-debated *post hoc* subanalysis identified excessive sudden deaths in the digoxin group. Indeed, an increased intracellular calcium content of the myocardial cell could in theory provoke afterdepolarizations and trigger ventricular arrhythmias, but there are only limited data to support a potential proarrhythmic effect of digitalis preparations in heart failure, while there appears to be a net benefit in terms of heart failure-related morbidity, at least in the DIG trial.

Antiarrhythmic agents in patients with reduced ejection fraction

Sodium channel blocking agents effectively suppress ventricular and atrial ectopy. The CAST trial has, however, shown that these compounds increase mortality when myocardial infarction and decreased left ventricular function are present [56]. This is probably due to the excessive risk for VT associated with conduction slowing after myocardial infarctions. A similar increase in mortality was found associated with sotalol in the survival with oral D-sotalol (SWORD) trial [57]. The use of these drugs, which may be helpful in the treatment of atrial fibrillation, should therefore be limited to patients without coronary heart disease and with a reasonably preserved left ventricular function.

Preventing sudden death due to bradyarrhythmias

The single most effective treatment to prevent sudden bradyarrhythmic death is implantation of a permanent pacemaker. Drugs can, however, be used to increase heart-rate transiently, for example, in clinical situations where placement of a transient pacemaker is not feasible. In such situations, beta-adrenoreceptor agonists such as orciprenaline and/or parasympatholytic agents such as atropine can increase heart rate and prevent circulatory failure,

usually until the patient receives a pacemaker. Definitive data on the safety
of this form of treatment are not available.

Sudden death due to drug-induced bradyarrhythmias

A variety of cardiac drugs can provoke bradycardia and AV nodal block
[58]. The best-known drug groups are beta-blockers, digitalis, and calcium-
channel antagonists of the verapamil type. Most antiarrhythmic agents,
especially sodium channel blockers, but also amiodarone and potassium channel blocking drugs, can also provoke profound bradycardia, and at times
(mostly infra-Hisian) AV nodal block, especially in structurally altered hearts.
Drug-induced bradycardia and/or AV nodal block can usually be treated
with withdrawal of the drug, or reduction of its dose. In urgent cases, specific antibodies (e.g. for digoxin) or extracorporal filtration techniques, for
example, by ultrafiltration or plasmapheresis, are available to speed up elimination of the drug. At times, the beneficial effects of drugs with bradycardic
side effects (e.g. beta-blockers) may warrant implantation of a pacemaker to
correct drug-induced bradycardia. Continuous right ventricular pacing may,
however, have adverse effects on the progression of heart failure [59]. Such
effects need to be carefully weighed against the continuation of a beneficial,
bradycardia-inducing drug in individual patients.

References

1. Priori SG, Aliot E, Blomstrom-Lundqvist C, et al. Task force on sudden cardiac death
   of the European Society of Cardiology. Eur Heart J 2001; 22: 1374–1450.
2. Zipes DP, Wellens HJJ. Sudden cardiac death. Circulation 1998; 98: 2334–2351.
3. Myerburg RJ, Interian A Jr, Simmons J, et al. Sudden cardiac death. In: Zipes DP
   & Jalife J, eds. Cardiac Electrophysiology: From Cell to Bedside, 4th edn. Saunders:
   Philadelphia, PA 2004; 720–731.
4. Myerburg RJ, Mitrani R, Interian A Jr, et al. Interpretation of outcomes of antiarrhythmic clinical trials: design features and population impact. Circulation 1998;
   97: 1514–1521.
5. Singh SN, Fletcher RD, Fisher SG, et al. Amiodarone in patients with congestive heart failure and asymptomatic ventricular arrhythmia. Survival trial of
   antiarrhythmic therapy in congestive heart failure. N Engl J Med 1995; 333: 77–82.
6. Domanski MJ, Sakseena S, Epstein AE, et al. Relative effectiveness of the implantable cardioverter-defibrillator and antiarrhythmic drugs in patients with varying
   degrees of left ventricular dysfunction who have survived malignant ventricular
   arrhythmias. J Am Coll Cardiol 1999; 34: 1090–1095.
7. Dorian P, Borggrefe M, Al-Khalidi H, et al. Placebo-controlled, randomized clinical
   trial of azimilide for prevention of ventricular tachyarrhythmias in patients with
   an implantable cardioverter-defibrillator. Circulation 2004; 110: 3646–3654.
8. Julian DG, Camm AJ, Frangin G, et al. Randomised trial of effect of amiodarone
   on mortality in patients with left-ventricular dysfunction after recent myocardial
   infarction: EMIAT. European Myocardial Infarct Amiodarone Trial Investigators.
   Lancet 1997; 349: 667–674.

9. Cairns JA, Connolly SJ, Roberts R, *et al.* Randomised trial of outcome after myocardial infarction in patients with frequent or repetitive ventricular premature depolarisations: CAMIAT. Canadian Amiodarone Myocardial Infarction Arrhythmia Trial. *Lancet* 1997; **349**: 667–674.

10. Bardy G. SCD-HeFT: The Sudden Cardiac Death in Heart Failure Trial. *American College of Cardiology Annual Scientific Sessions*, New Orleans, LA, 2004.

11. Huikuri HV, Castellanos A, Myerburg RJ. Sudden death due to cardiac arrhythmias. *N Engl J Med* 2001; **345**: 1473–1482.

12. MERIT-HF Study Group. Effect of Metoprolol CR/XL in Chronic Heart Failure: Metoprolol CR/XL Randomised Intervention Trial in Congestive Heart Failure (MERIT-HF). *Lancet* 1999; **353**: 2001–2007.

13. Domanski MJ, Exner DV, Borkowf CB, *et al.* Effect of angiotensin converting enzyme inhibition on sudden cardiac death in patients following acute myocardial infarction: a meta-analysis of randomized controlled trials. *J Am Coll Cardiol* 1999; **33**: 598–604.

14. Granger CB, McMurray JJ, Yusuf S, *et al.* Effects of candesartan in patients with chronic heart failure and reduced left-ventricular systolic function intolerant to angiotensin-converting-enzyme inhibitors: the CHARM-alternative trial. *Lancet* 2003; **362**: 772–776.

15. Gavras I, Gavras H. The antiarrhythmic potential of angiotensin II antagonism: experience with losartan. *Am J Hypertens* 2000; **13**: 512–517.

16. Awtry EH, Loscalzo J. Aspirin. *Circulation* 2000; **101**: 1206–1218.

17. Pitt B, Zannad F, Remme WJ, *et al.* The effect of spironolactone on morbidity and mortality in patients with severe heart failure. *N Engl J Med* 1999; **341**: 709–717.

18. Pitt B, Remme WJ, Zannad F, *et al.* Eplerenone, a selective aldosterone blocker, in patients with left ventricular dysfunction after myocardial infarction. *N Engl J Med* 2003; **348**: 1309–1321.

19. Grundy SM, Cleeman JI, Merz CNB, *et al.* Implications of recent clinical trials for the national cholesterol education program adult treatment panel III guidelines. *J Am Coll Cardiol* 2004; **44**: 720–732.

20. Marchioli R, Barzi F, Bomba E, *et al.* Early protection against sudden death by n-3 polyunsaturated fatty acids after myocardial infarction: time course analysis of the results of the Gruppo Italiano per lo Studio della Sopravvivenza nell'Infarto Miocardico (GISSI)-Prevenzione. *Circulation* 2002; **105**: 1897–1903.

21. Billman GE, Kang JX, Leaf A. Prevention of sudden cardiac death by dietary pure omega-3 polyunsaturated fatty acids in dogs. *Circulation* 1999; **99**: 2452–2457.

22. Leaf A, Kang JX, Xiao Y-F, *et al.* The antiarrhythmic and anticonvulsant effects of dietary n-3 fatty acids. *J Membr Biol* 1999; **172**: 1–11.

23. Henry PD, Pacifico A. Altering molecular mechanisms to prevent sudden cardiac death. *Lancet* 1998; **351**: 1276–1278.

24. Elliott P, McKenna WJ. Hypertrophic cardiomyopathy. *Lancet* 2004; **363**: 1881–1891.

25. Knollmann BC, Kirchhof P, Sirenko SG, *et al.* Familial hypertrophic cardiomyopathy-linked mutant troponin T causes stress-induced ventricular tachycardia and Ca^{2+}-dependent action potential remodeling. *Circ Res* 2003; **92**: 428–436.

26. Maass AH, Ikeda K, Oberdorf-Maass S, *et al.* Hypertrophy, fibrosis, and sudden cardiac death in response to pathological stimuli in mice with mutations in cardiac troponin T. *Circulation* 2004; **110**: 2102–2109.

27. Wichter T, Paul M, Wollmann C, *et al.* Implantable cardioverter/defibrillator therapy in arrhythmogenic right ventricular cardiomyopathy: single-center experience of long-term follow-up and complications in 60 patients. *Circulation* 2004; **109**: 1503–1508.

28. Wichter T, Borggrefe M, Haverkamp W, *et al.* Efficacy of antiarrhythmic drugs in patients with arrhythmogenic right ventricular disease. Results in patients with inducible and noninducible ventricular tachycardia. *Circulation* 1992; **86**: 29–37.

29. Marchlinski FE, Zado E, Dixit S, *et al.* Electroanatomic substrate and outcome of catheter ablative therapy for ventricular tachycardia in setting of right ventricular cardiomyopathy. *Circulation* 2004; **110**: 2293–2298.

30. Desnick RJ, Brady R, Barranger J, *et al.* Fabry disease, an under-recognized multisystemic disorder: expert recommendations for diagnosis, management, and enzyme replacement therapy. *Ann Intern Med* 2003; **138**: 338–346.

31. Chimenti C, Pieroni M, Morgante E, *et al.* Prevalence of Fabry disease in female patients with late-onset hypertrophic cardiomyopathy. *Circulation* 2004; **110**: 1047–1053.

32. Sachdev B, Takenaka T, Teraguchi H, *et al.* Prevalence of Anderson-Fabry disease in male patients with late onset hypertrophic cardiomyopathy. *Circulation* 2002; **105**: 1407–1411.

33. Moss AJ. Long-QT syndrome. *JAMA* 2003; **289**: 2041–2044.

34. Antzelovich C, Brugada P, Brugada J, *et al.* Brugada syndrome – 1992–2002: a historical perspective. *J Am Coll Cardiol* 2003; **41**: 1665–1671.

35. Priori SG, Schwartz PJ, Napolitano C, *et al.* Risk stratification in the long-QT syndrome. *N Engl J Med* 2003; **348**: 1866–1874.

36. Benhorin J, Taub R, Goldmit M, *et al.* Effects of flecainide in patients with new *SCN5A* mutation: mutation-specific therapy for long-QT syndrome? *Circulation* 2000; **101**: 1698–1706.

37. Windle JR, Geletka RC, Moss AJ, *et al.* Normalization of ventricular repolarization with flecainide in long-QT syndrome patients with *SCN5A*: *DeltaKPQ* mutation. *Ann Noninvasive Electrocardiography* 2001; **6**: 153–158.

38. Etheridge SP, Compton SJ, Tirstani-Firouzi M, *et al.* A new oral therapy for long-QT syndrome: long term oral potassium improves repolarization in patients with *HERG* mutations. *J Am Coll Cardiol* 2003; **42**: 1777–1782.

39. Belhassen B, Viskin S, Antzelovich C. The Brugada syndrome: is an implantable cardiovertor defibrillator the only therapeutic option. *Pacing Clin Electrophysiol* 2002; **25**: 1634–1640.

40. Hermida JS, Denjoy I, Clerc J, *et al.* Hydroquinidine therapy in Brugada syndrome. *J Am Coll Cardiol* 2004; **43**: 1853–1860.

41. Gaita F, Giustetto C, Bianchi F, *et al.* Short QT syndrome: a familial cause of sudden death. *Circulation* 2003; **108**: 965–970.

42. Gaita F, Giustetto C, Bianchi F, *et al.* Short QT syndrome: pharmacological treatment. *J Am Coll Cardiol* 2004; **43**: 1494–1499.

43. Wehrens XHT, Lenhart SE, Huang F, *et al.* FKBP12.6 deficiency and defective calcium release channel (ryanodine receptor) function linked to exercise-induced sudden cardiac death. *Cell* 2003; **113**: 829–840.

44. Lahat H, Pras E, Olender T, *et al.* A missense mutation in a highly conserved region of *CASQ2* is associated with autosomal recessive catecholamine-induced polymorphic VT in Bedouin families from Israel. *Am J Hum Genet* 2001; **69**: 1378–1384.

45. Dessertenne F. Ventricular tachycardia with 2 variable opposing foci. *Arch Mal Coeur* 1966; **59**: 263–272.
46. Haverkamp W, Breithardt G, Camm J, *et al.* The potential for QT prolongation and proarrhythmia by nonantiarrhythmic drugs: clinical and regulatory implications. Report on a policy conference of the European Society of Cardiology. *Cardiovasc Res* 2000; **47**: 219–233.
47. Kääb S, Hinterseer M, Näbauer M, *et al.* Sotalol testing unmasks altered repolarization in patients with suspected acquired long-QT-syndrome–a case–control pilot study using i.v. sotalol. *Eur Heart J* 2003; **24**: 649–657.
48. Paulussen AD, Gilissen RA, Armstrong M, *et al.* Genetic variations of *KCNQ1*, *KCNH2*, *SCN5A*, *KCNE1*, and *KCNE2* in drug-induced long-QT syndrome patients. *J Mol Med* 2004; **82**: 182–188.
49. Kirchhof P, Breithardt G. Molekulare mechanismen des plotzlichen herztods und ihre klinische bedeutung. *Zeitschr Elektrophysiol Schrittmacherth* 2003; **14**: 168–179.
50. Roden DM. Taking the "idio" out of "idiosyncratic": predicting *torsades de pointes*. *Pacing Clin Electrophysiol* 1998; **21**: 1029–1034.
51. Ray W, Murray K, Meredith S, *et al.* Oral erythromycin and the risk of sudden death from cardiac causes. *N Engl J Med* 2004; **351**: 1089–1096.
52. Haverkamp W, Breithardt G, Camm AJ, *et al.* The potential for QT prolongation and proarrhythmia by nonantiarrhythmic drugs: clinical and regulatory implications. Report on a policy conference of the European Society of Cardiology. *Eur Heart J* 2000; **21**: 1216–1231.
53. Kirchhof P, Fabritz L, Begrow F, *et al.* Ventricular arrhythmias, increased cardiac calmodulin kinase II expression, and altered repolarization kinetics in ANP-receptor deficient mice. *J Mol Cell Cardiol* 2004; **36**: 691–700.
54. Wu Y, Temple J, Zhang R, *et al.* Calmodulin kinase II and arrhythmias in a mouse model of cardiac hypertrophy. *Circulation* 2002; **106**: 1288–1293.
55. The Digitalis Investigation Group. The effect of digoxin on mortality and morbidity in patients with heart failure. *N Engl J Med* 1997; **336**: 525–533.
56. Echt DS, Liebson PR, Mitchell LB, *et al.* Mortality and morbidity in patients receiving encainide, flecainide, or placebo: the cardiac arrhythmia suppression trial. *N Engl J Med* 1991; **324**: 781–788.
57. Waldo AL, Camm AJ, Deruyter H, *et al.* Effect of D-sotalol on mortality in patients with left ventricular dysfunction after recent and remote myocardial infarction. *Lancet* 1996; **348**: 7–12.
58. Ovsyshcher IE, Barold SS. Drug induced bradycardia: to pace or not to pace? *Pacing Clin Electrophysiol* 2004; **27**: 1144–1147.
59. Wilkoff BL, Cook JR, Epstein AE, *et al.* Dual-chamber pacing or ventricular backup pacing in patients with an implantable defibrillator: the Dual Chamber and VVI Implantable Defibrillator (DAVID) Trial. *JAMA* 2002; **288**: 3115–3123.

CHAPTER 15
Implantable devices

A. John Camm and Arthur J. Moss

Pacemakers

Introduction

The original indication for the cardiac pacemaker was to improve survival in patients with prolonged asystole. The first human pacemaker implantation was undertaken in 1958 by Elmqvist and Senning [1]. However, there is surprisingly little concrete trial evidence to support the use of pacemakers in order to reduce overall mortality, let alone sudden death. Individual case reports [2] and small series [3] documenting survival in patients with refractory life-threatening syncope due to refractory asystole were striking. Early results comparing the survival of patients with complete heart block and Morgagni–Stokes–Adams seizures with anticipated death rates in the normal population were so convincing [4,5] and the relief of severe symptoms such as syncope was so great that pacemakers were immediately assumed to be life saving. It was presumed that the mechanism behind the therapeutic success was the prevention of severe bradycardia, asystole, or ventricular tachyarrhythmias related to underlying extreme bradycardia or asystole.

Disorders of impulse generation and conduction

The life-saving value of pacemakers in patients with asymptomatic acquired complete heart block and in sick-sinus syndrome, even when associated with symptoms is still less well documented. However, it is increasingly assumed that patients with acquired complete heart block, irrespective of associated symptoms, should be treated by pacemaker implantation in order to improve survival [6]. There is a relatively high mortality in patients with sick-sinus syndrome usually related to underlying cardiovascular disorders. There is little evidence that asymptomatic cases should receive pacemakers for improvement of prognosis [7], although when symptoms related to bradycardia are present, a pacemaker will clearly offer symptom relief [8]. There is a small likelihood (2% each year) of the development of complete atrioventricular (AV) block although this is much more likely if there is also evidence of associated intraventricular (IV) conduction disturbances. However, patients treated with atrial pacing have a similar prognosis to a general population matched for age, gender, and major cardiovascular risk [9].

There is a strong suggestion that young adult patients with complete congenital heart block will eventually need a pacemaker [10] to prevent severe symptoms including sudden death, although this is only documented in relatively small registries and not by randomized trials [11,12]. Most clinicians recommend pacing therapy for adolescents and young adults with either symptomatic or asymptomatic congenital heart block [13]. There is clear value in pacemaker treatment for children with symptoms related to congenital complete heart block but there is still considerable confusion about the value of pacemaker therapy in asymptomatic children with complete heart block [14,15] particularly since pacing in young children is not without significant complications [16]. Those with a marked prolongation of the QRS or QT interval [17,18], ventricular dysfunction and congenital anomalies [19], severe bradycardia (<50 bpm) [20] or asystolic episodes [21], associated ventricular arrhythmias, including a high density of ventricular extrasystoles, or a failure to increase the heart rate on exercise usually receive a pacemaker ostensibly to reduce the likelihood of sudden death.

Patients with lesser degrees of AV block, congenital or acquired, are generally not paced, although mortality is generally increased in such patients [22]. However, Mobitz type II AV block, high grade AV block with AV ratios of 3 : 1 and above, and trifascicular block (bifascicular block with first degree AV block, alternating bundle branch block, right bundle branch block with alternating left fascicular block, or IV conduction disturbances associated with intra-His (His potential width >50 ms) or infra-His delay [23] (His-ventricular (HV) interval longer than 80–100 ms) are at risk of progressing to transient or permanent complete heart block [24,25] with a presumed possibility of sudden cardiac death [26]. For this reason, pacemakers are often used prophylactically to reduce the likelihood of sudden death [27–30].

Other pathologies
Long-QT syndrome
The primary therapy for asymptomatic children or young adults at risk of sudden death due to the long-QT syndrome is beta-blockade, but many patients need additional therapy. Pacemaker treatment is advocated especially when there is significant bradycardia induced by beta-blockade or when *torsades de pointes* (TdP) is induced by long-short sequences [31–32]. In general bradycardia increases the amplitude of early afterdepolarizations and produces abnormal repolarization, thus increasing the risk of TdP. There is a strong correlation between the preceding RR interval and the amplitude of the early afterdepolarizations [33].

Pacing therapy results in a shorter absolute QT interval and the prevention of pauses that may be crucial for the initiation of the arrhythmia. Atrial pacing is preferred to single chamber ventricular pacing since the latter is necessarily associated with a longer measured QT interval. However, the influence of beta-blockade and the association of the long-QT syndrome with structural cardiac abnormalities and AV/IV conduction disturbances generally require that a dual chamber pacemaker is needed. Pacing therapy has been shown to reduce the number of critical cardiac events such as syncope and sudden death [34], but it rarely eliminates the problem [35]. Pacemaker therapy is particularly effective in conjunction with beta-blockade [36], and the added value of the pacemaker to beta-blockade has been well demonstrated by matched cohort studies (Schwartz PJ, personal communication). Pacemaker therapy may be most effective in the LQT3 variant of the syndrome in which the arrhythmia often occurs during sleep and in association with bradycardia. An increase of heart-rate substantially shortens the QT interval in this genotype as opposed to LQT1 and LQT2 [37]. More often, however, patients with long-QT syndrome and life-threatening ventricular arrhythmias refractory to beta-blockade, irrespective of the genotype are treated by implantation of a cardioverter defibrillator, which will not only prevent some serious ventricular arrhythmias but will also cardiovert those that do occur [38].

Hypertrophic obstructive cardiomyopathy

Syncope and sudden death occur in patients with hypertrophic cardiomyopathy. A variety of mechanisms, including electrical instability due to bradycardia, acquired long-QT syndrome associated with hypertrophy and with cardioactive drugs, and outflow tract obstruction leading to reduced cardiac output and myocardial ischemia, are potentially responsible. Pacemaker therapy may reduce bradycardia-dependent electrical instability. Right ventricular pacing has also been demonstrated to reduce outflow tract obstruction by producing septal preexcitation and uncoordinated contraction of the left ventricle. Pacing therapy may also be of critical value in patients who have undergone surgical or nonsurgical (alcohol ablation) resection of the septal muscle and have developed infra-His conduction disturbances [39,40].

Carefully optimized dual chamber pacing can reduce outflow tract obstruction to a modest degree [41]. Pacing is associated with some symptomatic relief and improved exercise capacity although some of this improvement may be due to a placebo effect [42]. Pacing may also be effective in reducing symptoms and extending exercise tolerance in patients with left ventricular cavity obliteration associated with ventricular hypertrophy due to hypertension [43]. There is no evidence that sudden cardiac death or cardiovascular mortality can be favorably impacted by pacemaker therapy [44,45].

Congestive cardiac failure

Abnormal coordination of left ventricular contraction in patients with heart failures and a wide QRS complex impairs cardiac efficiency and results in reduced cardiac output, decreased exercise tolerance, and aggravation of associated symptoms. Left ventricular pacing or the combination of both left and right ventricular pacing may restore a more normal contraction sequence and improve hemodynamics, exercise tolerance, and quality of life and eventually improve survival.

Furthermore since biventricular pacing, compared with right ventricular pacing is associated with a decrease of ambient ventricular extrasystoles, a reduction of inducibility of ventricular tachycardia [46] and less frequent implantable cardioverter-defibrillator (ICD) shocks, in patients also fitted with an ICD [47], it might be expected that sudden cardiac death might also decline. However, in the MIRACLE ICD trial, cardiac resynchronization therapy did not reduce the incidence of spontaneously occurring ventricular tachyarrhythmias, although the short (6 months) follow-up should be acknowledged [48]. On the other hand, easier provocation of ventricular arrhythmias [49] and greater transmyocardial dispersion [50] have also been documented in association with biventricular pacing.

A very thorough systematic review and metaanalysis of the four major biventricular pacing studies in patients with heart failure, reduced ejection fraction, and prolonged ventricular depolarization demonstrated a definite trend towards reduction of all-cause mortality (hazard ratio: 0.77) but this just failed to be significant [51]. Recently a much larger single randomized study (Comparison of Medical Therapy, Pacing, and Defibrillation in Heart Failure – COMPANION) has compared heart failure patients treated optimally with medical therapy with similarly treated patients who in addition had biventricular pacing or biventricular pacing plus an ICD. The secondary endpoint of death from any cause was reduced by 24% in the patients treated with biventricular pacing when compared to optimally medically treated patients, but this was not quite statistically significant [52]. A recently published metaanalysis that incorporated the preliminary results of COMPANION in addition to those from the trials included in the previous metaanalysis (1133 patients in all) did show a statistically significant reduction of all-cause mortality associated with biventricular pacing (hazard ratio: 0.74, 95% CI: 0.56–0.97) (Figure 15.1) [53]. The reduced mortality is almost certainly related predominantly to a decrease of deaths due to failing pump function rather than deaths related to arrhythmia [54]. Combined ICD and biventricular pacing will probably be advocated for significant heart failure associated with reduced ejection fraction, and abnormally coordinated ventricular contraction. The Cardiac

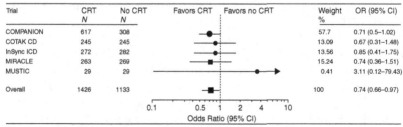

Trial	CRT N	No CRT N	Favors CRT	Favors no CRT	Weight %	OR (95% CI)
COMPANION	617	308			57.7	0.71 (0.5–1.02)
COTAK CD	245	245			13.09	0.67 (0.31–1.48)
InSync ICD	272	282			13.56	0.85 (0.41–1.75)
MIRACLE	263	269			15.24	0.74 (0.36–1.51)
MUSTIC	29	29			0.41	3.11 (0.12–79.43)
Overall	1426	1133			100	0.74 (0.66–0.97)

0.1   0.5   1   2   4   10
Odds Ratio (95% CI)

Odds ratios (OR) of all-cause mortality among patients randomized to cardiac resynchronziation therapy (CRT or no CRT. Confidence interval, CI: Comparison of medical therapy, pacing, and defibrillation in heart failure, COMPANION: Multicenter InSync Randomized Clinical Evaluation, MIRACLE: Multisite Stimulation in Cardiomyopathies, MUSTIC.

Figure 15.1 Metaanalysis of biventricular pacing studies. Reproduced from Reference 51 with permission.

Resynchronization-Heart Failure (CARE-HF) trial [55] demonstrated that cardiac resynchronization therapy improves survival in patients with advanced congestive heart failure. This trial enrolled patients with New York Heart Association (NYHA) class III or IV heart failure and an ejection fraction of ≤35%. Patients were randomly assigned to either standard medical therapy with or without cardiac resynchronization. Resynchronization therapy significantly reduced the occurrence of the primary endpoint (the time to death or hospitalization for a major cardiovascular event). Interestingly all-cause mortality was reduced from 30% in the medical-therapy group to 20% in the resynchronization group (hazard ratio, 0.64; $p < .002$). In agreement with the results of the previous trials, cardiac resynchronization improved indexes of left ventricular function, symptoms, and quality of life.

Post His bundle ablation
After His bundle ablation spontaneous ventricular activation is dependent on a ventricular pacemaker that usually discharges too slowly to maintain an adequate cardiac output. Artificial ventricular pacing is therefore essential. Recently, it has been suggested that right ventricular pacing may be associated with a deleterious outcome because of progressive impairment of ventricular function. It has been suggested that this may be alleviated by biventricular pacing. Improved hemodynamics and less deterioration of left ventricular function have been noted with left ventricular pacing [56] and biventricular pacing rather than right ventricular pacing [57,58]. The Post AtrioVentricular node ablation Evaluation trial (PAVE) randomized 184 patients treated with AV node ablation to either biventricular pacing or conventional right ventricular pacing and followed them for 6 months. Patients who were assigned to biventricular pacing benefited from a significant improvement in functional capacity over conventional pacing as measured by the 6-min walk test, peak VO_2 and exercise duration, which was sustained over time and resulted in better quality of life. The left ventricular ejection fraction was maintained from baseline in the biventricular paced group, but declined from 44.9% to 40.7% in the conventionally paced group. A small reduction in mortality was observed in this study but a large prospective study in a diverse population of patients with conventional indications for pacing is now underway (BioPace).

Sleep apnea
Sleep apnea is associated with cardiac arrhythmias most of which are benign [59]. However this condition, which is common in patients with hypertension and congestive cardiac failure [60], is also associated independently with a high risk of cardiovascular events, including cardiovascular death [61]. In patients with an ICD there was no difference in the discharge frequency in those with and without sleep apnea [62]. Significant bradyarrhythmias are relatively common [63]. Cardiac pacemaker therapy will directly prevent life-threatening bradycardia and asystole, but may also relieve mild to moderate

sleep apnea and improve cardiac hemodynamics [64]. As yet there is no evidence that sudden cardiac death related to sleep apnea can be prevented by cardiac pacing.

Mode of pacing

In patients with sick-sinus syndrome, single-chamber atrial pacing has been reported, in retrospective studies, to be associated with lower mortality than in ventricular pacing [65]. Recent important randomized controlled trials of pacemaker therapy have focused predominantly on the choice of pacing mode in patients with sick-sinus syndrome and complete or incomplete AV block. In general physiological pacing (atrial of AV rather than ventricular) has been associated with improved hemodynamics, better exercise tolerance, less pacemaker syndrome, less atrial fibrillation, and/or stroke. However, only one of these trials has shown a statistically significant reduction of mortality related to mode selection. In the Danish trial of DDD versus AAI pacing for the treatment of sick-sinus syndrome a report after an extended follow-up of 5.5 years demonstrated that all-cause mortality was reduced [66,67]. However, it is not clear whether there was any decrease in sudden cardiac death.

Conclusions

There is very little evidence that pacemaker treatment reduces sudden cardiac death except in the setting of severe bradyarrhythmias. In this situation the benefit of pacing is largely presumed from clinical observations and from early observational studies. The therapeutic success in this setting is probably striking but in other circumstances pacing has only been tenuously associated with an improvement of survival, but its exact value in preventing sudden cardiac death is not known.

Implantable cardioverter-defibrillators

Introduction

The automatic implantable defibrillator was introduced into clinical medicine in 1980, when Mirowski reported the successful termination of life-threatening ventricular tachyarrhythmias with the implanted device in three patients with organic heart disease [68]. Between 1980 and 1995, there were numerous descriptive reports of the efficacy of the implantable defibrillator in saving lives in individual patients, with termination of ventricular fibrillation automatically by the device. During the evolving use of the automatic implantable defibrillator, the device became coupled with antitachycardia pacing and with a variety of technological improvements including transvenous leads, better rhythm detection algorithms, pacing capability, enhanced data storage and interrogation, augmented programmability, extended battery life, and size reduction. With these features, the device became known as the ICD.

A series of randomized ICD trials was initiated in the early 1990s, and since 1996 nine major randomized clinical trials have reported on the safety and efficacy of ICD therapy in a spectrum of at-risk cardiac patients. Seven of the trials were primary prevention trials in that the ICD was initiated as prophylactic therapy in cardiac patients who were at risk for experiencing life-threatening ventricular arrhythmias, but had not yet experienced such an arrhythmia. Two of the trials were secondary-prevention trials and involved patients who had survived an aborted cardiac arrest or experienced a documented or suspect life-threatening ventricular tachyarrhythmia. The 7714 patients who have been randomized in these nine trials have, for the most part, reduced ventricular systolic cardiac function due to coronary heart disease. Patients with nonischemic cardiomyopathy have been included in a few of the recently reported primary preventions trials. Patients with a spectrum of different cardiac disorders are included in the two secondary prevention trials.

Randomized primary prevention ICD trials

The clinical and design characteristics of the seven primary prevention ICD trials are presented in Table 15.1 [52,69–74]. Four of the trials involved patients with coronary heart disease, two trials involved patients with ischemic and nonischemic cardiomyopathy, and one trial studied only patients with nonischemic cardiomyopathy. The hazard ratios and 95% confidence intervals (CIs) for death from any cause in the ICD-treated patients compared with those not receiving ICD therapy in the seven primary prevention trials are presented in Figure 15.2. The overall pooled hazard ratio of 0.72 ($p < .01$) indicates a 38% reduction in the risk of death in the ICD versus the non-ICD-treated patients. Two trials showed no benefit from the ICD: (1) the Coronary Artery Bypass Graft (CABG)-Patch trial that involved implantation of ICDs at the time of thoracotomy during coronary bypass graft surgery; and (2) the DINAMIT trial in which ICD therapy was initiated between 6 and 40 days after acute myocardial infarction in patients with reduced ejection fraction.

In a secondary analysis of the Multicenter Automatic Defibrillator Implantation Trial (MADIT) II trial [75], mortality events were subcategorized into the suspected mechanism of cardiac death. Kaplan–Meier estimates of the cumulative probability of sudden and nonsudden cardiac death in the groups assigned to ICD and conventional medical therapy are presented in Figure 15.2. The rate of sudden cardiac death was significantly reduced by ICD therapy (Figure 15.3(a)). The hazard ratio for sudden cardiac death was 0.33 ($p < .0001$) indicating a 67% reduction in the risk of sudden cardiac death when compared with patients in the conventional therapy group. The nonsudden cardiac death rates were similar in the two treatment arms (Figure 15.3(b)).

Randomized secondary prevention trials

The clinical and design characteristics of the two secondary prevention ICD trials are presented in Table 15.2 [76,77]. The eligibility for enrolment in

Table 15.1 Randomized primary prevention ICD trials.

Trial	Date started; date published	No. of patients	Eligibility	Average follow-up (months)	Reference
MADIT (ICD versus Conv.)	12/27/1990; 12/27/1996	196	Prior MI, EF ≤ 0.35, NSVT, EPS+	27	70
CABG-Patch (ICD versus Conv.)	08/14/1990; 11/27/1997	900	CAD, abn. SAECG, CABG surgery	32	71
MADIT II (ICD versus Conv.)	07/11/1997; 03/21/2002	1232	Prior MI, EF ≤ 0.30	20	72
COMPANION (CRT-D versus OPT)[a]	01/20/2000; 05/10/2004	903	I and NICM, NYHA III or IV, EF ≤ 0.35, QRS ≥ 0.12 s,	16	53
DEFINITE (ICD versus conv.)	07/09/1998; 05/10/2004	458	NICM, EF ≤ 0.35, NSVT or >10 PVC/24 h	29	73
SCD-HeFT (ICD versus placebo)[b]	09/16/2001; 03/08/2004	1676	I and NICM, EF ≤ 0.35	48	74
DINAMIT (ICD versus Conv.)	04/01/1998; 12/09/2004	674	Within 6–40 days of acute MI, EF ≤ 0.35, HRV (SDNN) ≤ 70 ms	30	75

Notes: CABG = coronary artery bypass graft; CAD = coronary artery disease; Conv. = conventional medical therapy; CRT-D = cardiac-resynchronization therapy with pacemaker-defibrillator; EF = ejection fraction; I and NICM = ischemic and nonischemic cardiomyopathy; HRV = heart-rate variability; MI = myocardial infarction; NYHA = New York Heart Association; NSVT = nonsustained ventricular tachycardia; OPT = optimal pharmacologic therapy; PVC = premature ventricular contraction; SDNN = standard deviation of normal heart beat intervals.
[a] Three-arm trial (CRT-D, CRT, and OPT), but comparison in this analysis is only for CRT-D versus optimal pharmacologic therapy.
[b] Three-arm trial (ICD, amiodarone, and placebo), but comparison in this analysis is only for ICD versus placebo.

these two trials involved patients with documented or suspect life-threatening ventricular tachyarrhythmias including patients who were resuscitated from ventricular fibrillation, those with rapid ventricular tachycardia culminating in syncope or severe hemodynamic compromise, and those with unmonitored syncope in whom further workup suggested that the cause of the loss

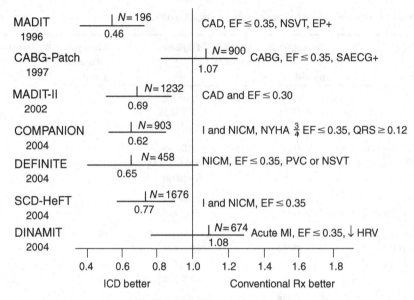

Figure 15.2 Hazard ratio and 95% CIs (horizontal lines) for death from any cause in the ICD group as compared with the group receiving conventional medical therapy in each of the seven randomized primary prevention ICD trials. The number below each trial name is the year of publication or presentation at a national meeting (SCD-HeFT and DINAMIT). The point estimate of the hazard ratio is denoted by the short vertical line with the value of the hazard ratio below the vertical line. N denotes the number of subjects in each clinical trial. Abbreviations as in Tables 15.1 and 15.2. The overall pooled hazard ratio is 0.72 ($p < .01$).

of consciousness was due to a ventricular tachyarrhythmias. The patients in these two trials had ejection fractions in the range of 0.31–0.34, values considerably higher than in the primary prevention trials. The efficacy of ICD therapy in these two trials was compared against antiarrhythmic drugs, mostly amiodarone. The hazard ratios and 95% CIs for death from any cause for the ICD-treated patients compared with those receiving antiarrhythmic therapy are presented in Figure 15.4. The overall pooled hazard ratio of 0.69 ($p < .01$) indicates a 31% reduction in the risk of death in the ICD versus the antiarrhythmic-treated patients. In secondary analyses from the CIDS trial, there was a 33% relative reduction in arrhythmic death.

Comments regarding ICD therapy

The overall findings from these nine randomized ICD trials clearly demonstrate the survival benefit of ICD therapy over conventional therapy in patients at high risk for sudden cardiac death. The mortality reduction with ICD therapy is quite considerable, in the range of approximately 30% during a 2-year follow-up, with the life-saving benefit clearly due to reduction in sudden cardiac death. This benefit is on top of optimal pharmacologic therapy for ventricular

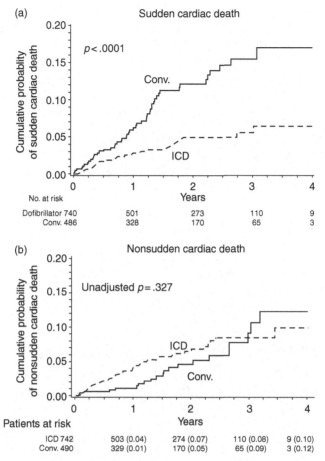

Figure 15.3 Kaplan–Meier estimates of the cumulative probability of (a) sudden and (b) nonsudden cardiac death in the MADIT II trial by randomized treatment to ICD and conventional medical therapy (Conv.). Reprinted from Reference 75 with permission from Elsevier.

dysfunction. The consistency of the ICD benefit in patients with ischemic and nonischemic cardiomyopathy and in various prespecified subgroups within each clinical trial provides strong and convincing support for the life-saving benefit of ICD therapy in appropriate at-risk patients. All of the reported trials were powered to detect a prespecified gradient reduction in all-cause mortality, so it is inappropriate to use *post hoc* secondary analyses to identify and select subgroups of patients from within the reported trials who should or should not receive ICD therapy. This issue has surfaced regarding QRS duration in MADIT II, with the recommendation that patients with QRS durations >0.12 s are the ones who obtain the major benefit from ICD therapy, and ICD therapy should be restricted to this subgroup [78]. This conclusion is simply

Table 15.2 Randomized secondary prevention ICD trials.

Trial	Date started; date published	No. of patients	Eligibility	Average follow-up (mo.)	Reference
AVID (ICD versus AAD)	06/01/1993; 11/27/1997	1016	Near-fatal VF, VT with syncope or hemodynamic compromise	18	77
CIDS (ICD versus amiodarone)	10/01/1990; 03/21/2000	659	Near-fatal VF, VT with syncope or hemodynamic compromise, unmonitored syncope thought to be due to VT	36	78

Notes: AAD = antiarrhythmic drugs; VF = ventricular fibrillation; VT = ventricular tachycardia.

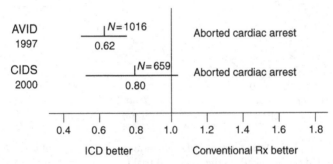

Figure 15.4 Hazard ratio and 95% CIs for death from any cause in the ICD group as compared with the group receiving conventional medical therapy in each of the two randomized primary prevention ICD trials. The overall pooled hazard ratio is 0.69 ($p < .01$).

wrong, with a serious Type I error associated with *post hoc* retrospective data analysis.

Potential complications and adverse reactions related to the ICD should be appreciated. As with any implanted device, special care must be taken to avoid infection. Lead fracture is an infrequent occurrence, but lead malposition or instability may give rise to inappropriate shocks. Although ICD algorithms have been developed to better detect supraventricular tachycardias and rapid ventricular response to atrial fibrillation, inappropriate ICD therapy for these nonventricular tachyarrhythmias can be a problem.

It has recently been shown that ventricular pacing in ICD-treated patients with left ventricular dysfunction may be detrimental for it can contribute to dys-synchronous ventricular contraction with increased risk for death and heart failure [79]. In ICD-treated patients without an indication for bradycardia support, every effort should be made to avoid unnecessary ventricular pacing by programming the pacing component of the ICD to a slow, ventricular-demand, back-up pacing rate of approximately 40 ppm.

Routine patient follow-up with device interrogation and reprogramming as necessary should be carried out every 4 months. At the present time, generator replacement for battery depletion is required at approximately 5-year intervals.

Conclusions

A substantial number of patients with ischemic and nonischemic cardiomyopathy have now been studied in randomized clinical trials in which the ICD has been compared with conventional medical therapy. The vast majority of these patients have compromised left ventricular systolic function as manifested by an ejection fraction below 0.36. ICD is effective and safe therapy for improving survival through the reduction of sudden cardiac death, with overall reduction in mortality in the range of 30% during an average follow-up of approximated 2 years. As a general rule, the sicker patients achieve greater benefit from ICD therapy.

References

1. Elmqvist R, Senning A. Implantable pacemaker for the heart. In: Smyth CN, ed. *Medical Electronics*. Proceedings of the Second International Conference on Medical Electronics, Paris, June 24–27, Tliffe and Sons, London, UK, 1959, 1960: 253–254.
2. Roe BB, Katz HJ. Complete heart block with intractable asystole and recurrent ventricular fibrillation with survival. *Am J Cardiol* 1965; **15**: 401–403.
3. Lawrence GH, King RL, Paine RM, Spencer MP, Hughes ML. Complete heart block. Patient selection and response to implantation of electronic pacemaker. *JAMA* 1964; **190**: 1093–1098.
4. Edhag O, Swahn A. Prognosis of patients with complete heart block or arrhythmic syncope who were not treated with artificial pacemakers. A long-term follow-up study of 101 patients. *Acta Med Scand* 1976; **200**(6): 457–463.
5. Hansen JF, Meibom J. The prognosis for patients with complete heart block treated with permanent pacemaker. *Acta Med Scand* 1974; **195**(5): 385–389.
6. Gregoratos G, Abrams J, Epstein AE, *et al*. American College of Cardiology/American Heart Association Task Force on Practice Guidelines American College of Cardiology/American Heart Association/North American Society for Pacing and Electrophysiology Committee. ACC/AHA/NASPE 2002 guideline update for implantation of cardiac pacemakers and antiarrhythmia devices: summary article. A report of the American College of Cardiology/American Heart Association Task Force on Practice Guidelines (ACC/AHA/NASPE Committee to Update the 1998 Pacemaker Guidelines). *J Cardiovasc Electrophysiol* 2002; **13**(11): 1183–1199.

7. Lichstein E, Aithal H, Jonas S, *et al.* Natural history of severe sinus bradycardia discovered by 24 hour Holter monitoring. *Pacing Clin Electrophysiol* 1982; **5**(2): 185–189.

8. Shaw DB, Holman RR, Gowers JI. Survival in sinoatrial disorder (sick-sinus syndrome). *Br Med J* 1980; **280**(6208): 139–141.

9. Brandt J, Anderson H, Fahraeus T, Schuller H. Natural history of sinus node disease treated with atrial pacing in 213 patients: implications for selection of stimulation mode. *J Am Coll Cardiol* 1992; **20**(3): 633–639.

10. Michaelsson M, Engle MA. Congenital complete heart block: an international study of the natural history. *Cardiovasc Clin* 1972; **4**(3): 85–101.

11. Michaelsson M, Jonzon A, Riesenfeld T. Isolated congenital complete atrioventricular block in adult life. A prospective study. *Circulation* 1995; **92**(3): 442–449.

12. Eronen M. Long-term outcome of children with complete heart block diagnosed after the newborn period. *Pediatr Cardiol* 2001; **22**(2): 133–137.

13. Odemuyiwa O, Camm AJ. Prophylactic pacing for prevention of sudden death in congenital complete heart block? *Pacing Clin Electrophysiol* 1992; **15**(10 Pt 1): 1526–1530.

14. Celiker A, Cicek S, Ozme S. Long-term results of patients with congenital complete atrioventricular block. *Turk J Pediatr* 1993; **35**(2): 93–98.

15. Pordon CM, Moodie DS. Adults with congenital complete heart block: 25-year follow-up. *Cleve Clin J Med* 1992; **59**(6): 587–590.

16. Walsh CA, McAlister HF, Andrews CA, Steeg CN, Eisenberg R, Furman S. Pacemaker implantation in children: a 21-year experience. *Pacing Clin Electrophysiol* 1988; **11**(11 Pt 2): 1940–1944.

17. Esscher E, Michaelsson M. Q–T interval in congenital complete heart block. *Pediatr Cardiol* 1983; **4**(2): 121–124.

18. Solti F, Szatmary L, Vecsey T, Renyi-Vamos F Jr, Bodor E. Congenital complete heart block associated with QT prolongation. *Eur Heart J* 1992; **13**(8): 1080–1083.

19. Pinsky WW, Gillette PC, Garson A Jr, McNamara DG. Diagnosis, management, and long-term results of patients with congenital complete atrioventricular block. *Pediatrics* 1982; **69**(6): 728–733.

20. Dewey RC, Capeless MA, Levy AM. Use of ambulatory electrocardiographic monitoring to identify high-risk patients with congenital complete heart block. *N Engl J Med* 1987; **316**(14): 835–839.

21. Nagashima M, Nakashima T, Asai T, *et al.* Study on congenital complete heart block in children by 24-hour ambulatory electrocardiographic monitoring. *Jpn Heart J* 1987; **28**(3): 323–332.

22. Shaw DB, Kekwick CA, Veale D, Gowers J, Whistance T. Survival in second degree atrioventricular block. *Br Heart J* 1985; **53**(6): 587–593.

23. McAnulty JH, Murphy E, Rahimtoola SH. Prospective evaluation of intrahisian conduction delay. *Circulation* 1979; **59**(5): 1035–1039.

24. Sobrino JA, Sotillo JF, del Rio A, Sobrino N, Mate I. Fascicular block within the His bundle. *Chest* 1978; **74**(2): 215–218.

25. Ranganathan N, Dhurandhar R, Phillips JH, Wigle ED. His bundle electrogram in bundle-branch block. *Circulation* 1972; **45**(2): 282–294.

26. Bergfeldt L, Edvardsson N, Rosenqvist M, Vallin H, Edhag O. Atrioventricular block progression in patients with bifascicular block assessed by repeated

electrocardiography and a bradycardia-detecting pacemaker. *Am J Cardiol* 1994; **74**(11): 1129–1132.

27. Denes P, Dhingra RC, Wu D, Wyndham CR, Amat-y-Leon F, Rosen KM. Sudden death in patients with chronic bifascicular block. *Arch Intern Med* 1977; **137**(8): 1005–1010.

28. Dhingra RC, Wyndham C, Bauernfeind R, *et al*. Significance of block distal to the His bundle induced by atrial pacing in patients with chronic bifascicular block. *Circulation* 1979; **60**(7): 1455–1464.

29. Dhingra RC, Denes P, Wu D, *et al*. Prospective observations in patients with chronic bundle branch block and marked H–V prolongation. *Circulation* 1976; **53**(4): 600–604.

30. Denes P, Dhingra RC, Wu D, *et al*. H–V interval in patients with bifascicular block (right bundle branch block and left anterior hemiblock). Clinical, electrocardiographic and electrophysiologic correlations. *Am J Cardiol* 1975; **35**(1): 23–29.

31. Viskin S, Fish R, Roth A, Copperman Y. Prevention of *torsade de pointes* in the congenital long QT syndrome: use of a pause prevention pacing algorithm. *Heart* 1998; **79**(4): 417–419.

32. Dorostkar PC, Eldar M, Belhassen B, Scheinman MM. Long-term follow-up of patients with long-QT syndrome treated with beta-blockers and continuous pacing. *Circulation* 1999; **100**(24): 2431–2436.

33. Shimizu W, Tanaka K, Suenaga K, Wakamoto A. Bradycardia-dependent early afterdepolarizations in a patient with QTU prolongation and *torsade de pointes* in association with marked bradycardia and hypokalemia. *Pacing Clin Electrophysiol* 1991; **14**(7): 1105–1111.

34. Viskin S, Fish R. Prevention of ventricular arrhythmias in the congenital long QT syndrome. *Curr Cardiol Rep* 2000; **2**(6): 492–497.

35. Moss AJ, Liu JE, Gottlieb S, Locati EH, Schwartz PJ, Robinson JL. Efficacy of permanent pacing in the management of high-risk patients with long QT syndrome. *Circulation* 1991; **84**(4): 1524–1529.

36. Eldar M, Griffin JC, Van Hare GF, *et al*. Combined use of beta-adrenergic blocking agents and long-term cardiac pacing for patients with the long QT syndrome. *J Am Coll Cardiol* 1992; **20**(4): 830–837.

37. Schwartz PJ, Priori SG, Locati EH, *et al*. Long QT syndrome patients with mutations of the *SCN5A* and *HERG* genes have differential responses to Na+ channel blockade and to increases in heart rate. Implications for gene-specific therapy. *Circulation* 1995; **92**(12): 3381–3386.

38. Zareba W, Moss AJ, Daubert JP, Hall WJ, Robinson JL, Andrews M. Implantable cardioverter defibrillator in high-risk long QT syndrome patients. *J Cardiovasc Electrophysiol* 2003; **14**(4): 337–341.

39. Chang SM, Nagueh SF, Spencer WH III, Lakkis NM. Complete heart block: determinants and clinical impact in patients with hypertrophic obstructive cardiomyopathy undergoing nonsurgical septal reduction therapy. *J Am Coll Cardiol* 2003; **42**(2): 296–300.

40. Reinhard W, Ten Cate FJ, Scholten M, De Laat LE, Vos J. Permanent pacing for complete atrioventricular block after nonsurgical (alcohol) septal reduction in patients with obstructive hypertrophic cardiomyopathy. *Am J Cardiol* 2004; **93**(8): 1064–1066.

41. Nishimura RA, Trusty JM, Hayes DL, *et al*. Dual-chamber pacing for hypertrophic cardiomyopathy: a randomized, double-blind, crossover trial. *J Am Coll Cardiol* 1997; **29**(2): 435–441.
42. Linde C, Gadler F, Kappenberger L, Ryden L. Placebo effect of pacemaker implantation in obstructive hypertrophic cardiomyopathy. PIC Study Group. Pacing in Cardiomyopathy. *Am J Cardiol* 1999; **83**(6): 903–907.
43. Kass DA, Chen CH, Talbot MW, *et al*. Ventricular pacing with premature excitation for treatment of hypertensive-cardiac hypertrophy with cavity-obliteration. *Circulation* 1999; **100**(8): 807–812.
44. Fananapazir L, Epstein ND, Curiel RV, Panza JA, Tripodi D, McAreavey D. Long-term results of dual-chamber (DDD) pacing in obstructive hypertrophic cardiomyopathy. Evidence for progressive symptomatic and hemodynamic improvement and reduction of left ventricular hypertrophy. *Circulation* 1994; **90**(6): 2731–2742.
45. Maron BJ, Nishimura RA, McKenna WJ, *et al*. Assessment of permanent dual-chamber pacing as a treatment for drug-refractory symptomatic patients with obstructive hypertrophic cardiomyopathy. A randomized, double-blind, crossover study (M-PATHY). *Circulation* 1999; **99**(22): 2927–2933.
46. Zagrodzky JD, Ramaswamy K, Page RL, *et al*. Biventricular pacing decreases the inducibility of ventricular tachycardia in patients with ischemic cardiomyopathy. *Am J Cardiol* 2001; **87**(10): 1208–1210; A7.
47. Higgins SL, Yong P, Sheck D, *et al*. Biventricular pacing diminishes the need for implantable cardioverter defibrillator therapy. Ventak CHF Investigators. *J Am Coll Cardiol* 2000; **36**(3): 824–827.
48. Leon AR, Young JB, Abraham WT (for the MIRACLE ICD Investigators). Resynchronization does not change the incidence of ventricular arrhythmias. *J Am Coll Cardiol* 2003; **41**(6 Suppl. A).
49. Garrigue S, Reuter S, Efimov IR *et al*. Optical mapping technique applied to biventricular pacing: potential mechanisms of ventricular arrhythmias occurrence. *Pacing Clin Electrophysiol* 2003; **26**(1 Pt 2): 197–205.
50. Medina-Ravell VA, Lankipalli RS, Yan GX, *et al*. Effect of epicardial or biventricular pacing to prolong QT interval and increase transmural dispersion of repolarization: does resynchronization therapy pose a risk for patients predisposed to long QT or *torsade de pointes*? *Circulation* 2003; **107**(5): 740–746.
51. Salukhe TV, Dimopoulos K, Francis D. Cardiac resynchronisation may reduce all-cause mortality: meta-analysis of preliminary COMPANION data with CONTAK-CD, InSync ICD, MIRACLE and MUSTIC. *Int J Cardiol* 2004; **93**(2–3): 101–103.
52. Bristow MR, Saxon LA, Boehmer J, *et al*. Cardiac-resynchronization therapy with or without an implantable defibrillator in advanced chronic heart failure. *N Engl J Med* 2004; **350**(21): 2140–2150.
53. Bradley DJ, Bradley EA, Baughman KL, *et al*. Cardiac resynchronization and death from progressive heart failure: a meta-analysis of randomized controlled trials. *JAMA* 2003; **289**(6): 730–740.
54. Carson P, Anand I, O'Connor CM, *et al*. Relation of cardiac device therapy to mode of death in advanced heart failure – COMPANION trial. *Circulation* 2003; **108**(17 Suppl.): IV–628.
55. Cleland JGF, Daubert J-C, Erdmann E, *et al*. The effect of cardiac resynchronization on morbidity and mortality in heart failure. *N Engl J Med* 2005; **352**: 1539–1549.

56. Puggioni E, Brignole M, Gammage M, *et al*. Acute comparative effect of right and left ventricular pacing in patients with permanent atrial fibrillation. *J Am Coll Cardiol* 2004; **43**(2): 234–238.
57. Garrigue S, Bordachar P, Reuter S, *et al*. Comparison of permanent left ventricular and biventricular pacing in patients with heart failure and chronic atrial fibrillation: prospective haemodynamic study. *Heart* 2002; **87**(6): 529–534.
58. Brignole M, Gammage M, Puggioni E, *et al*. Comparative assessment of right, left, and biventricular pacing in patients with permanent atrial fibrillation. *Eur Heart J* 2005; **26**: 712–722.
59. Guilleminault C, Connolly SJ, Winkle RA. Cardiac arrhythmia and conduction disturbances during sleep in 400 patients with sleep apnea syndrome. *Am J Cardiol* 1983; **52**(5): 490–494.
60. Javaheri S, Parker TJ, Liming JD, *et al*. Sleep apnea in 81 ambulatory male patients with stable heart failure. Types and their prevalences, consequences, and presentations. *Circulation* 1998; **97**(21): 2154–2159.
61. Hu FB, Willett WC, Manson JE, *et al*. Snoring and risk of cardiovascular disease in women. *J Am Coll Cardiol* 2000; **35**(2): 308–313.
62. Grimm W, Hoffmann JJ, Muller HH, Maisch B. Implantable defibrillator event rates in patients with idiopathic dilated cardiomyopathy, nonsustained ventricular tachycardia on Holter and a left ventricular ejection fraction below 30%. *J Am Coll Cardiol* 2002; **39**(5): 780–787.
63. Simantirakis EN, Schiza SI, Marketou ME, *et al*. Severe bradyarrhythmias in patients with sleep apnoea: the effect of continuous positive airway pressure treatment: a long-term evaluation using an insertable loop recorder. *Eur Heart J* 2004; **25**(12): 1070–1076.
64. Garrigue S, Bordier P, Jais P, *et al*. Benefit of atrial pacing in sleep apnea syndrome. *N Engl J Med* 2002; **346**(6): 404–412. Erratum in: *N Engl J Med* 2002; **346**(11): 872.
65. Connolly SJ, Kerr C, Gent M, Yusuf S. Dual-chamber versus ventricular pacing: critical appraisal of current data. *Circulation* 1996; **94**(3): 578–583.
66. Andersen HR, Thuesen L, Bagger JP, Vesterlund T, Thomsen PE. Prospective randomised trial of atrial versus ventricular pacing in sick-sinus syndrome. *Lancet* 1994; **344**(8936): 1523–1528.
67. Andersen HR, Nielsen JC, Thomsen PE, *et al*. Long-term follow-up of patients from a randomised trial of atrial versus ventricular pacing for sick-sinus syndrome. *Lancet* 1997; **350**(9086): 1210–1216.
68. Mirowski M, Reid PR, Mower MM, *et al*. Termination of malignant ventricular arrhythmias with an implanted automatic defibrillator in human beings. *N Engl J Med* 1980; **303**: 322–324.
69. Moss AJ, Hall WJ, Cannom DS, *et al*. Improved survival with an implanted defibrillator in patients with coronary disease at high risk for ventricular arrhythmia. Multicenter Automatic Defibrillator Implantation Trial Investigators. *N Engl J Med* 1996; **335**: 1933–1940.
70. Bigger JT Jr. Prophylactic use of implanted cardiac defibrillators in patients at high risk for ventricular arrhythmias after coronary-artery bypass graft surgery. Coronary Artery Bypass Graft (CABG) Patch Trial Investigators. *N Engl J Med* 1997; **337**: 1569–1575.
71. Moss AJ, Zareba W, Hall WJ, *et al*. Prophylactic implantation of a defibrillator in patients with myocardial infarction and reduced ejection fraction. *N Engl J Med* 2002; **346**: 877–883.

72. Kadish A, Dyer A, Daubert JP, *et al.* Prophylactic defibrillator implantation in patients with nonischemic dilated cardiomyopathy. *N Engl J Med* 2004; **350**: 2151–2158.
73. Bardy GH, Lee KL, Mark DB, *et al.* Amiodarone or an implantable cardioverter-defibrillator for congestive heart failure. *N Engl J Med* 2005; **352**: 225–237.
74. Hohnloser SH, Kuck KH, Dorian P, *et al.* Prophylactic use of an implantable cardioverter-defibrillator after acute myocardial infarction. *N Engl J Med* 2004; **351**: 2481–2488.
75. Greenberg H, Case RB, Moss AJ, Brown MW, Carroll ER, Andrews ML. Analysis of mortality events in the Multicenter Automatic Defibrillator Implantation Trial (MADIT-II). *J Am Coll Cardiol* 2004; **43**: 1459–1465.
76. A comparison of antiarrhythmic-drug therapy with implantable defibrillators in patients resuscitated from near-fatal ventricular arrhythmias. The Antiarrhythmics Versus Implantable Defibrillators (AVID) Investigators. *N Engl J Med* 1997; **337**: 1576–1583.
77. Connolly SJ, Gent M, Roberts RS, *et al.* Canadian implantable defibrillator study (CIDS): a randomized trial of the implantable cardioverter defibrillator against amiodarone. *Circulation* 2000; **101**: 1297–1302.
78. Centers for Medicare and Medicaid Services. National coverage analysis: implantable cardioverter defibrillators (#CAG-00157N). Tracking sheet. Available at: http://www.cms.hhs.gov/ncdr/trackingsheet.asp?id=39. Assessed September 5, 2003.
79. Wilkoff BL, Cook JR, Epstein AE, *et al.* Dual-chamber pacing or ventricular backup pacing in patients with an implantable defibrillator: the Dual Chamber and VVI Implantable Defibrillator (DAVID) Trial. *JAMA* 2002; **288**: 3115–3123.

CHAPTER 16

Sudden cardiac death: ablation

Prashanthan Sanders, John M. Miller, Mélèze Hocini,
Pierre Jaïs, and Michel Haïssaguerre

Background

The most prevalent cause of sudden cardiac death (SCD) remains ventricular fibrillation (VF) [1]. VF can occur either as a primary arrhythmia or by degeneration of ventricular tachycardia (VT). Among survivors of SCD, there is abundant evidence that the implantable cardioverter-defibrillator (ICD) prolongs life in a variety of patient subsets, including those with as well as without structural heart disease. ICD therapy is thus the default treatment for SCD survivors. However, such therapy remains restricted in many countries mainly associated with a prohibitive cost to the community, and may be a cause of significant morbidity in patients with frequent episodes or storms of arrhythmia. In addition, occasionally patients present for medical care for very frequent episodes of polymorphic (PM) VT or VF. While drug therapy successfully quells many of these episodes of so-called arrhythmia storm, there is an increasing body of data showing that catheter ablation of initiating premature complexes that appear to trigger these life-threatening arrhythmias can prevent recurrent episodes. In this chapter, we will consider techniques of catheter ablation of VT and the elimination of the triggers of PMVT and VF.

Ventricular fibrillation

Catheter mapping and ablation of PMVT and VF have not been considered feasible, not only because both the ECG and myocardial activation sequence change from beat to beat, but also due to hemodynamic instability. However, the recognition of the importance of triggers to the initiation of VF has led to catheter ablation techniques targeting this arrhythmia. In addition to the obvious clinical benefit of this strategy, catheter ablation of VF has provided some important insights into the mechanisms of these arrhythmias in humans.

Catheter ablation

Potential targets for the ablation of VF could theoretically be either the triggers and/or substrate of the arrhythmia. However, thus far, reports have only targeted the triggers, perhaps reflecting our poor understanding of the substrate maintaining VF and the large mass of ventricular myocardium involved) [2–10]. Whether ablation of triggers also has a role in modifying the substrate of VF remains to be determined.

Idiopathic VF

Although VF is frequently the mode of death in patients with abnormal substrates, it has been described in patients with structurally normal hearts; 5–10% surviving SCD. Several different terminologies have been used to describe this clinical entity but it is perhaps best described as "idiopathic VF." Recently we presented the results of mapping and ablation of the trigger initiating VF in patients with arrhythmic storm [3,4].

Patient selection

Thirty-two patients with recurrent episodes of resuscitated idiopathic VF have been studied. These patients were aged 41 ± 14 years with an equal representation of both genders. Six had a family history of sudden cardiac death. All patients were studied in the immediate aftermath of recurrent episodes of VF, having 9 ± 13 (range 1–50) episodes of VF despite therapy with 3 ± 2 antiarrhythmics. In most, VF was associated with activities of daily living; however, in some this occurred during sleep. Importantly, none had arrhythmia during exertion. All patients had apparently normal hearts based on established criteria, including normal physical examination, electrocardiogram, echocardiography, coronary angiography, endomyocardial biopsy (n = 6), ergonovine provocation (n = 5), exercise stress testing or isoproterenol challenge, class IC drug challenge, and SCN5A/HERG screens (n = 12).

While this series represents consecutive patients undergoing mapping and ablation of VF, all patients were observed to have frequent ventricular premature beats (VPB) in the immediate aftermath of VF. These patients were observed to have 2 ± 1 (range 1–5) different VPB morphologies with the VPB initiating VF demonstrating a coupling interval to the preceding ventricular complex of 297 ± 42 ms. Importantly, the morphology of VPB triggering VF was observed independent of the episodes of the VF.

Radio frequency ablation

Mapping and ablation was performed opportunistically within days of VF to enable localization of the origin of spontaneous VPBs. Mapping used two to four catheters introduced percutaneously via the femoral vessels. The intracardiac electrograms were filtered at 30–500 Hz after sampling at 1 or 10 KHz, the latter being better-suited for the detection of Purkinje potentials. In addition, high amplification was used (1 mm = 0.1 mV) to facilitate recognition of Purkinje potentials. The origin of the VPBs was localized to the earliest site of activity or using pace mapping.

The peripheral Purkinje network was identified by the presence of an initial sharp spike potential (<10 ms duration) that preceded the local ventricular

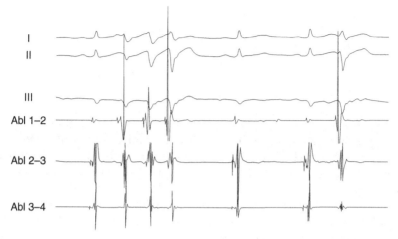

Figure 16.1 Repetitive burst of VPBs in a patient with idiopathic VF. On the ablation electrograms, each VPB is seen to be preceded by a sharp spike potential (Purkinje potential) that is also seen during sinus rhythm on the more proximal electrodes. Ablation at this site resulted in elimination of the local Purkinje potential and VPBs.

activation during sinus rhythm by <15 ms, while longer durations were considered to represent more proximal fascicular sites. Such a potential preceding ventricular activation during VPB defined a Purkinje origin of these beats (Figure 16.1), while its absence indicated a ventricular origin. The site of origin of these VPBs was further confirmed by their acute elimination by ablation. Radio frequency energy was delivered in the temperature controlled mode with a target temperature of 55–60°C and a maximum power of 45 W using a conventional 4 mm-tip ablation catheter. In cases where the maximum power delivery was limited, externally irrigated ablation was used (maximum power 45 W, irrigation 5–20 mL/min).

The VPBs that occurred in these patients and that were observed to trigger VF had characteristic morphological features. Most patients demonstrated a positive VPB morphology in V1, suggesting a left ventricular origin but with significant morphological variations in the limb leads (in 66%). In 27 patients, VPBs were mapped to the left or right Purkinje network, while in five these were found to be of right ventricular outflow tract (RVOT) origin. The Purkinje sources were localized to the anterior right ventricle or in a wider region of the lower half of the septum in the left ventricle; from ramifications of the anterior and posterior fascicles resulting in an inferior and superior axis respectively, and from the intervening region in intermediate morphologies. VPBs of Purkinje origin demonstrated significantly narrower QRS durations compared with those from the RVOT (128 ± 18 ms versus 145 ± 13 ms).

At the site of successful ablation, endocardial activity preceded the QRS activation on ECG by 130 ± 19 ms. Ablation resulted in temporary exacerbation of VPBs that, in some cases, were associated with the induction of VF.

VPBs of different morphology were progressively eliminated using 13 ± 7 radiofrequency energy applications. Electrograms recorded after ablation demonstrated the abolition of the local Purkinje potential and slight delay in the local ventricular electrogram. The fluoroscopic and procedural durations were 51 ± 68 min and 189 ± 78 min respectively. Two patients had recurrent VPBs during their hospital stay and required re-ablation.

Follow-up
Follow-up was performed both clinically and by interrogation of the defibrillator memory after ablation and the cessation of antiarrhythmic therapy. One patient had recurrence of VF and one had a single episode of pre-syncope due to polymorphic ventricular tachycardia lasting 6 s without defibrillator discharge; they did not undergo a repeat procedure. In other patients, Holter recordings showed no or few (28 ± 49; range 0–145) isolated VPBs per 24 h. During 22 ± 28 months, there was no sudden death, syncope, or recurrence of VF in 28 (88%) patients.

VF in abnormal repolarization syndromes (long-QT/Brugada syndrome)
The long-QT syndrome (LQTS) and Brugada syndrome are established causes of sudden cardiac death. Current observations suggest an important role for VPBs of right ventricular origin in the Brugada syndrome (Figure 16.2). Chinushi *et al.* [11] described recurrent episodes of VF in a patient with Brugada syndrome initiated by monomorphic VPBs with left bundle branch blood (LBBB) morphology. This was corroborated by Morita *et al.* [12] who observed VPBs in nine out of 45 patients studied; of 11 VPB morphologies in these nine patients, 10 were of right ventricular origin.

While the management of VF in these conditions has been centered on implantation of a defibrillator, we have recently evaluated the role of trigger elimination by ablation in patients with LQT or Brugada syndromes [7].

Patient selection
We have studied four patients with LQTS (two male; age 37 ± 8 years) and four patients with Brugada syndrome (three male; age 36 ± 8 years). These patients presented with documented episodes of PMVT or VF (1–21 episodes), three with a family history of sudden death. While patients with the Brugada syndrome had 12 ± 9 episodes of VF, those with LQTS had 6 ± 4 episodes of VF or syncope prior to mapping. Medical treatment in patients with LQTS included beta-blockers alone or combined with class IC drugs ($n = 3$), verapamil ($n = 2$), and amiodarone ($n = 1$). No drug therapy had been attempted in three patients with Brugada syndrome while quinidine failed in one.

The LQTS was diagnosed in four patients based on established criteria with a corrected QT interval of >460 ms; KCNQ1, SCN5A, and HERG channelopathies were excluded. The Brugada syndrome was diagnosed by abnormal QRST complexes in leads V1 and V2 with a coved ST segment elevation in

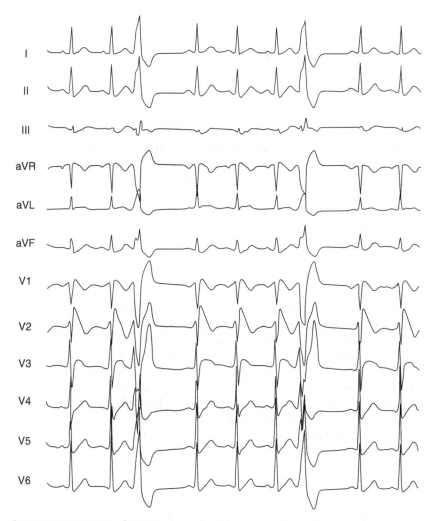

Figure 16.2 Monomorphic VPBs from the right ventricular outflow tract in a patient with the Brugada syndrome. While this ectopy was observed to occur in isolation, the same ectopy was also responsible for the initiation of VF in this patient.

four patients of which one had a familial SCN5A channelopathy (2850delT). No patient had evidence of structural heart disease based on physical examination, echocardiography, and right/left ventricular ejection fraction. Exercise testing in all and coronary angiography in four patients excluded myocardial ischemia. While the LQTS was diagnosed at the time of ventricular arrhythmia, the Brugada syndrome had been diagnosed 9 months and 3 years prior to the clinical episodes of VF in two patients.

All patients were studied within 2 weeks of their arrhythmic storm and were documented to have frequent VPBs. The triggering role of VPBs in the initiation of VF was observed by ambulatory monitoring or stored electrograms of the defibrillator. VPBs in the LQTS had a coupling interval of 503 ± 29 ms, they were monomorphic in two patients (one with LBBB-inferior axis typical of RVOT and one with right bundle branch blood (RBBB)-superior axis), and polymorphic and repetitive (sometimes bidirectional) with a positive morphology in lead V1 in two patients; the latter had varying cycle lengths of 280–420 ms with repetitive beats lasting 3–45 beats, which were well tolerated during hospitalization. VPBs in the Brugada syndrome were monomorphic in all, with a RVOT morphology (coupling interval of 343 ± 59 ms) in three patients and with LBBB-superior axis in one (coupling interval 278 ± 29 ms). The monomorphic VPBs were first observed at the time of VF in two patients whereas in another two they had been documented (with a normal QRS/QT in sinus rhythm) 14 and 11 years before they triggered VF, following development of abnormal QRST. Exercise testing and isoproterenol infusion eliminated all VPBs, excluding catecholaminergic PMVT.

Radiofrequency ablation
Mapping and ablation was performed as previously described in patients with idiopathic VF. In the LQTS, one patient had VPBs originating from the RVOT that was ablated by 6 min of radio frequency energy application. Two patients had polymorphic VPBs that originated from the peripheral Purkinje arborization in the left ventricle, including the ramifications of anterior or posterior fascicles, and from the intervening regions. In one patient, premature beats originated from the posterior fascicle. During premature beats, the earliest Purkinje potential preceded the local endocardial muscle activation by a conduction interval of 34 ± 17 ms. Repetitive beats were also preceded by Purkinje activity with a variable delay ranging from 20–110 ms (52 ± 24).

In the Brugada syndrome, the three patients having RVOT triggers (Fig. 16.2), VPBs were eliminated by 7–10 min of radiofrequency energy applications at the earliest site of activity. In the fourth patient, the VPBs were found to originate from the anterior right ventricular Purkinje network. Ten minutes of radiofrequency energy application eliminated all VPBs in this patient. Noteworthy is that VF inducibility was modified after ablation.

Follow-up
There has been no recurrence of VF, syncope, or sudden cardiac death in any patient, 24 ± 20 months after ablation in patients with LQTS and 9 ± 8 months in those with Brugada syndrome. One patient with LQTS was maintained on a beta-blocker. Another had a late recurrence of VPBs but refused further procedures.

VF and PMVT after myocardial infarction
Ventricular fibrillation is most frequently associated with structural heart disease such as myocardial infarction (MI) or ischemia. While episodes are frequently short lived and managed with the use of beta-blockers with/without

amiodarone, occasionally patients present with arrhythmic storms that cannot be managed medically. The Purkinje network is subendocardial and therefore seems to survive transmural myocardial infarction. We and others have recently evaluated the role of such trigger elimination in the management of VF storms after MI [6,8,9].

We have studied three male patients (age 66 ± 2 years) with VF storm resistant to antiarrhythmics (including beta-blockers/amiodarone). These patients presented 13 ± 2 days after anterior MI with significant left ventricular dysfunction (left ventricular ejection fraction $31 \pm 13\%$) and persistent arrhythmia despite coronary revascularization. These patients were in critical care requiring mechanical ventilation after 23 ± 10 cardioversions for VF. They had frequent PM VPBs that triggered VF. Mapping and ablation progressively targeted the most frequent VPB morphology, in all cases localizing the origin of these to the Purkinje network bordering the infarct zone, with a coupling interval to the preceding sinus Purkinje activation of 379 ± 56 ms. Significant variation in Purkinje-muscle (P-M) activation was observed associated with change in VPB morphology. Ablation was performed at one to three regions in the infarct border zone for 27 ± 7 min that abolished all VPBs. One patient died with worsening heart failure and two remained arrhythmia-free at 1 and 9 months after ablation.

We have recently observed a similar origin of triggers from the Purkinje network initiating PMVT after MI [13]. In these patients, Purkinje triggers were observed to originate from the border-zone of the MI. In addition, some of these patients presented months after the initial infarction.

Bänsch et al. [8] studied patients with VF storm after MI. Of 2340 patients managed for acute MI at this centre, four presented with VF storm or recurrent PMVT resistant to revascularization and antiarrhythmic therapy, and required an attempt at ablation. These patients (three male, aged 66 ± 8 years) had inferior or anterior MIs with left ventricular ejection fraction of $32 \pm 5\%$. Interestingly, all episodes of ventricular arrhythmias were triggered by monomorphic VPBs with RBBB morphology. Mapping of the earliest site of activation during VPB demonstrated that ventricular activation at these sites was preceded by Purkinje potentials (126–160 ms earlier). Around 6–30 applications of radio frequency energy was required to eliminate VPBs and resulted in arrhythmia suppression at 13 ± 13 months follow-up. Likewise, Marrouche et al. [9] have presented a multicenter case series of patients undergoing ablation Purkinje triggers of VF after MI.

VF in valvular heart disease

Other structural heart disease can also be associated with VF. Recently, catheter ablation of VF occurring after aortic valve repair has been successfully performed [10]. The VF episodes were triggered by VPBs of Purkinje origin, which were mapped to the anteroseptal and inferoseptal areas of the left ventricle. During short-term follow-up of 2 months, there had been no VF recurrence. Similarly, we have recently performed mapping and successful ablation of VF initiated by VPBs originating from the left ventricular Purkinje system in a patient who had aortic valve replacement.

Ventricular tachycardia

Therapy for VT as a cause of SCD has evolved in the last several decades from antiarrhythmic drugs to surgical therapies, to the ICD, which remains the default therapy for VT in the setting of structural heart disease. Although recent developments have provided an ablation option for some patients with VF, it is paradoxical that catheter ablation of VT – at least, in principle, a more easily ablated arrhythmia than VF – is rarely used for prevention of SCD. There are several reasons for this as will be noted below.

Unlike ablatable forms of VF, most VT that causes SCD is due to reentry that most often involves a portion of the superficial endocardial layers as an essential component in the reentrant circuit (subepicardial layers may also be involved in some cases). Clinical settings include healed MI, dilated cardiomyopathy, right ventricular dysplasia, sarcoid heart disease, and a variety of less common disorders. The principles of mapping and ablation of sustained VT in this setting are generally the same as for VT that is more hemodynamically stable. These include searching for sites from which isolated, non-dissociable mid-diastolic potentials can be recorded during VT and at which overdrive pacing during VT yields entrainment with concealed fusion with a stimulus-QRS interval similar to the electrogram-QRS interval during VT [14–16]. However, in the patient population in which VT episodes have resulted in hemodynamic collapse or sudden death, VT that is induced in the electrophysiology laboratory commonly causes a precipitous fall in cardiac output such that mapping for extended periods of time is impractical. A variety of methods have been used to facilitate mapping during VT episodes in the face of hemodynamic instability, including those that stabilize hemodynamics (intravenous inotropic and pressor agents, intra-aortic balloon counter-pulsation, ventricular assist device support, and antiarrhythmic agents), or speed the process of mapping (use of multielectrode arrays and catheters to quickly map and interpolate activation data from large areas during just 1–5 VT complexes) [17]. Other methods avoid activation mapping during VT altogether by using electroanatomic voltage mapping to locate and ablate presumed critical portions of the VT substrate (transecting essential diastolic "corridors" with lines of RF applications bridging between zones of low voltage or scar) [18]. Although these methods have reported success rates of 75–90% in eliminating the target VT, other morphologies of sustained VT are often inducible. During follow-up, although the majority of patients are free of recurrence of the targeted/ablated VT(s), upto 5% suffer sudden death despite a good initial result [19–22]. The same has held true with surgical procedures to treat VT [23]. Even patients who present with hemodynamically stable VT are at risk of subsequent sudden death episodes due to other ventricular tachyarrhythmias [24]. Thus, ablation is not uniformly reliable in preventing recurrent ventricular tachyarrhythmias in these patients, whose risk of sudden death is best addressed with the ICD. Ablation methods are generally reserved for treatment of patients with frequent episodes of VT resulting in ICD discharges, syncope, or symptoms of severe light-headedness or dyspnea [21].

There are no firm indications for attempting catheter ablation of VT in patients for prevention of sudden death. The following are situations in which ablation could be considered as an option for this indication.

Incessant VT prior to ICD therapy

Incessant VT (VT as the predominant rhythm for a 24 h period, or nearly immediate recurrence of VT after pacing termination or cardioversion) is a contraindication to ICD implantation [25–30]. Patients with incessant VT have either already experienced or are at the risk of experiencing sudden death; ablation therapy is an excellent option for controlling the arrhythmia. Ablation can eliminate the VT morphology responsible for incessant episodes in up to 90% of patients. However, it is important to note that these patients often have other morphologies of VT induced even after successful ablation of the target VT and a high enough recurrence rate that eventual ICD therapy is warranted. Patients must often be stabilized hemodynamically prior to and during the ablation procedure to facilitate mapping and ablation; active ischemia should be considered and treated if present. Finally, exclusion of an intracavitary left ventricular thrombus is necessary prior to placing catheters in the left ventricle for ablation.

Bundle branch reentrant VT

Reentry involving the bundle branches can produce very rapid VT rates that can in turn result in hemodynamic collapse and/or degeneration to VF [31,32]. Patients with this disorder typically have valvular or other types of cardiomyopathy with at least mild heart failure. Most have either block or delay in the left bundle branch and the typical VT circuit consists of anterograde right bundle branch propagation and transseptal conduction then retrograde propagation in the left bundle branch. Once the diagnosis is established at electrophysiology study, catheter ablation of either the right or left bundle branches can be performed relatively easily. Ablation of the right bundle branch results in either complete heart block or preserved conduction in the left bundle branch with very long His-Ventricular (HV) intervals, both requiring permanent ventricular pacing. Ablation of the left bundle branch, though technically more difficult, may obviate the need for permanent pacing [33]. Controversy remains as to whether ICD therapy is needed in all patients with bundle branch reentry, especially those in whom no other ventricular tachyarrhythmias can be initiated following ablation. Since most patients with this disorder have significant structural heart disease with an increased risk of sudden death, many investigators favor ICD therapy even after successful ablation of bundle branch reentry. This is certainly true in patients in whom other, myocardial-based VTs can be induced [32].

Primary therapy for patients with VT who are not candidates for, or refuse ICD therapy

Within this small group are patients in whom an ICD is contraindicated or those who decline defibrillator implantation due to personal reasons. Contraindications to ICD therapy include uncontrollable systemic infection, technical inability to place an endocardial or epicardial defibrillating system, or other systemic illness that limits lifespan to <6 months [30]. Other options, such as automatic external or vest defibrillators, are also available in these situations.

Expense

In some settings, economic considerations (cost or availability of ICDs) may favor ablation as a less-expensive primary treatment alternative for patients who would ordinarily have an ICD indication.

Summary

In general, patients with VT in the setting of structural heart disease, who are at increased risk for sudden death, should receive ICD therapy. Except in a very small subset of patients, the major role of catheter ablation is palliative (i.e. to decrease the frequency of ICD activations) rather than as primary therapy.

Conclusion

The concept that apparently disorganized polymorphic tachycardias or fibrillation could have a focal origin is relatively new. Originally described in atrial fibrillation, focal initiators were at first considered rare but are now believed to account for the majority of cases in this arrhythmia. Extension of the concept of focal initiators to ventricular arrhythmias such as PMVT and VF has occurred in just the last few years. Emerging evidence from a number of groups demonstrates the feasibility of catheter ablation techniques for the treatment of recurrent VF in a variety of clinical situations. These studies have demonstrated the important role of focal triggers from the Purkinje system and RVOT in the initiation of VF. Reducing the incidence of VF with localized ablation may reduce defibrillation requirement and replacement and improve the patients' quality of life. With the development of new catheter designs and mapping technologies, and greater physician experience, catheter ablation of VF, with the ultimate aim of curing such patients at risk of SCD, may not be an unrealistic goal in the future.

References

1. Zipes DP, Wellens HJ. Sudden cardiac death. *Circulation* 1998; **98**: 2334–2351.
2. Takatsuki S, Mitamura H, Ogawa S. Catheter ablation of a monfocal premature ventricular complex triggering idiopathic ventricular fibrillation. *Heart* 2001; **86**: e3.

3. Haissaguerre M, Shah DC, Jais P, *et al*. Role of Purkinje conducting system in triggering of idiopathic ventricular fibrillation. *Lancet* 2002; **359**: 677–678.
4. Haissaguerre M, Shoda M, Jais P *et al*. Mapping and ablation of idiopathic ventricular fibrillation. *Circulation* 2002; **106**: 962–967.
5. Paul T, Laohakunakorn P, Long B, Saul JP. Complete elimination of incessant polymorphic ventricular tachycardia in an infant with MIDAS syndrome: use of endocardial mapping and radiofrequency catheter ablation. *J Cardiovasc Electrophysiol* 2002; **13**: 612–615.
6. Haissaguerre M, Weerasooriya R, Walczak F, *et al*. Catheter ablation of polymorphic VT or VF in multiple substrates. In: Santini M, ed. *Non Pharmacological Treatment of Sudden Death*. Bologna, Arianna Editrice, 2003: 237–253.
7. Haissaguerre M, Extramiana F, Hocini M. Mapping and ablation of ventricular fibrillation associated with long-QT and Brugada syndromes. *Circulation* 2003; **108**: 925–928.
8. Bansch D, Oyang F, Antz M, *et al*. Successful catheter ablation of electrical storm after myocardial infarction. *Circulation* 2003; **108**: 3011–3016.
9. Marrouche NF, Verma A, Wazni O. Mode of initiation and ablation of ventricular fibrillation storms in patients with ischemic cardiomyopathy. *J Am Coll Cardiol* 2004; **43**: 1715–1720.
10. Li YG, Gronefeld G, Israel C, Hohnloser S. Catheter ablation of frequently recurring ventricular fibrillation in a patient after aortic valve repair. *J Cardiovasc Electrophysiol* 2004; **15**: 90–93.
11. Chinushi M, Washizuka T, Chinushi Y, Higuchi K, Toida T, Aizawa Y. Induction of ventricular fibrillation in Brugada syndrome by site-specific right ventricular premature depolarization. *Pacing Clin Electrophysiol* 2002; **25**: 1649–1651.
12. Morita H, Fukushima-Kusano K, Nagase S, *et al*. Site-specific arrhythmogenesis in patients with Brugada syndrome. *J Cardiovasc Electrophysiol* 2003; **14**: 373–379.
13. Szumowski L, Sanders P, Walczak F, *et al*. Mapping and ablation of polymorphic ventricular tachycardia after myocardial infarction. *J Am Coll Cardiol* 2004; **44**: 1700–6.
14. Stevenson WG, Friedman PL, Kocovic D, Sager PT, Saxon LA, Pavri B. Radiofrequency catheter ablation of ventricular tachycardia after myocardial infarction. *Circulation* 1998; **98**: 308–314.
15. El Shalakany A, Hadjis T, Papageorgiou P, Monahan K, Epstein L, Josephson ME. Entrainment/mapping criteria for the prediction of termination of ventricular tachycardia by single radiofrequency lesion in patients with coronary artery disease. *Circulation* 1999; **99**: 2283–2289.
16. Bogun F, Knight B, Goyal R, Strickberger A, Hohnloser SH, Morady F. Clinical value of the postpacing interval for mapping of ventricular tachycardia in patients with prior myocardial infarction. *J Cardiovasc Electrophysiol* 1999; **10**: 43–51.
17. Strickberger A, Knight BP, Michaud GF, Pelosi F, Morady F. Mapping and ablation of ventricular tachycardia guided by virtual electrograms using a noncontact, computerized mapping system. *J Am Coll Cardiol* 2000; **35**: 414–421.
18. Marchlinski FE, Callans DJ, Gottlieb CD, Zado E. Linear ablation lesions for control of unmappable ventricular tachycardia in patients with ischemic and nonischemic cardiomyopathy. *Circulation* 2000; **101**: 1288–1296.
19. Rothman SA, Hsia HH, Cossu SF, Chmielewski IL, Buxton AE, Miller JM. Radiofrequency catheter ablation of postinfarction ventricular tachycardia: long-term success and the significance of inducible nonclinical arrhythmias. *Circulation* 1997; **96**: 3499–3508.

20. Stevenson WG, Friedman PL, Ganz LI. Radiofrequency catheter ablation of ventricular tachycardia late after myocardial infarction. *J Cardiovasc Electrophysiol* 1997; **8**: 1309–1319.
21. Strickberger SA, Man KC, Daoud EG, et al. A prospective evaluation of catheter ablation of ventricular tachycardia as adjuvant therapy in patients with coronary artery disease and an implantable cardioverter-defibrillator. *Circulation* 1997; **96**: 1525–1531.
22. O'Callaghan PA, Poloniecki J, Sosa-Suarez G, Ruskin JN, McGovern BA, Garan H. Long-term clinical outcome of patients with prior myocardial infarction after palliative radiofrequency catheter ablation for frequent ventricular tachycardia. *Am J Cardiol* 2001; **87**: 975–979.
23. Miller JM, Kienzle MG, Harken AH, Josephson ME. Subendocardial resection for ventricular tachycardia: predictors of surgical success. *Circulation* 1984; **70**: 624–631.
24. Sarter BH, Finkle JK, Gerszten RE, Buxton AE. What is the risk of sudden cardiac death in patients presenting with hemodynamically stable sustained ventricular tachycardia after myocardial infarction? *J Am Coll Cardiol* 1996; **28**: 122–129.
25. Belhassen B, Miller HI, Laniado S. Catheter ablation of incessant ventricular tachycardia refractory to external cardioversions. *Am J Cardiol* 1985; **55**: 1637–1639.
26. Jordaens L, Vertongen P, Provenier F. Radiofrequency ablation of incessant ventricular tachycardia to prevent multiple defibrillator shocks. *Int J Cardiol* 1992; **37**: 117–120.
27. Trappe HJ, Klein H, Wenzlaff P, Lichtlen PR. Early and long-term results of catheter ablation in patients with incessant ventricular tachycardia. *J Interv Cardiol* 1992; **5**: 163–170.
28. Borggrefe M. Catheter ablation of incessant ventricular tachycardia. *Isr J Med Sci* 1996; **32**: 868–871.
29. Cao K, Gonska BD. Catheter ablation of incessant ventricular tachycardia: acute and long-term results. *Eur Heart J* 1996; **17**: 756–763.
30. Gregoratos G, Abrams J, Epstein AE et al. ACC/AHA/NASPE 2002 guideline update for implantation of cardiac pacemakers and antiarrhythmia devices: summary article: a report of the American College of Cardiology/American Heart Association task force on practice guidelines (ACC/AHA/NASPE committee to update the 1998 pacemaker guidelines). *Circulation* 2002; **106**: 2145–2161.
31. Caceres J, Jazayeri M, McKinnie J, et al. Sustained bundle branch reentry as a mechanism of clinical tachycardia. *Circulation* 1989; **79**: 256–270.
32. Blanck Z, Dhala A, Deshpande S, Sra J, Jazayeri M, Akhtar M. Bundle branch reentrant ventricular tachycardia: cumulative experience in 48 patients. *J Cardiovasc Electrophysiol* 1993; **4**: 253–262.
33. Blanck Z, Deshpande S, Jazayeri MR, Akhtar M. Catheter ablation of the left bundle branch for the treatment of sustained bundle branch reentrant ventricular tachycardia. *J Cardiovasc Electrophysiol* 1995; **6**: 40–43.

CHAPTER 17

External automated defibrillators

M.A. Peberdy, K.A. Ellenbogen, and D.A. Chamberlain

The development of automated external defibrillators

History

The potential of defibrillation for prehospital cardiac arrest will not be achieved without widespread use of strategies to limit the critical delay from the onset of lethal tachyarrhythmias to shock delivery, or unless better ways are found of widening the window of opportunity for a successful outcome. Automated external defibrillators (AEDs) offer an opportunity to meet the first of these requirements. Their value was limited initially by the belief that defibrillation is a procedure calling for considerable expertise, and should therefore be limited to healthcare professionals. Incredibly, laws in some parts of Europe mandated that only physicians may defibrillate, a situation that has been changing only over the past decade. By 1975, however, Diack had already realized that electronic pattern recognition of the waveforms of ventricular fibrillation (VF) could be used in the logic of a defibrillator to permit or withhold the electrical discharge [1]. The human role could therefore be reduced to the simple task of recognizing the possible need for defibrillation, applying electrodes, and activating the machine. The first automated unit was used successfully by paramedics in Brighton in 1980 [2], and the first successful randomized trial of their efficacy was published from Seattle in 1989 [3].

Current variations

All AEDs have built-in algorithms that can detect whether a heart rhythm needs a shock and require minimal knowledge and participation by the operator. But other important properties vary to suit requirements for use in diverse environments. The first commercial AED was fully automatic [1] in that once the machine was switched on and the electrodes placed, no further action was needed to initiate shock delivery. Most subsequent units have incorporated an additional button that must be pushed for the charge to be delivered, and these are appropriately designated as semi-automatic or "automated" devices. Involvement in decision-making increases operator responsibility and slows shock delivery but adds to the confidence that inappropriate shocks will not be given. Concerns have lessened with increasing reliability of analysis, and fully automatic units are again available. Most, however, retain the need for operator interaction.

Operator participation need not be limited to shock decision; some AEDs also incorporate a screen that can be used either for written guidance or for visual presentation of the electrocardiogram. This was of limited value while AEDs were used only for existing cardiac arrest but a monitoring role is now accepted for some models. An option also exists for subsequent downloading of electrocardiograms recorded during AED use, in association with coincident voice prompts. Both can be seen on the screen and printed out in hard copy; they may be important for quality control, audit, research, and training. The electronic presentation may or may not be associated with an audio channel recorded in real time during the emergency. Some AEDs can be switched to manual mode, with the diagnostic function disabled. Such units may also have other sophisticated modalities for expert use so that they can be used either by professional healthcare workers or by those with modest training. The penalty of increased complexity, weight, and cost is not disadvantageous in some settings. Other models have the simplest possible design; some are small enough to fit into an average pocket for situations in which miniaturization may be advantageous.

The debate on relative advantages of monophasic or biphasic waveform is no longer valid because the advantages of the latter are universally accepted. Considerable variation exists, however, in the precise characteristics of the biphasic waveform. Ideally, each should be tested in a clinical setting against a gold standard – a goal that is unlikely ever to be practicable. The possible advantage of escalating energy for treating fibrillation that has proved refractory to an initial shock or shock sequence also remains controversial, but the debate is of only limited importance because of the high first shock success rate of most biphasic units.

No "best-buy" can be selected for AEDs. The large variety of units that are available commercially reflect at least in part the diverse needs in different environments and the range of skills of those with the responsibility of using them. It is important, therefore, to consider very carefully the properties that are most suited to any intended use. Two possible types of use are relevant to choice. AEDs may be intended for transport to victims elsewhere in response to emergency calls, or be placed in fixed locations for events expected to occur on site, either because it is at high risk for the occurrence of sudden cardiac death, or because it is not readily accessible to conventional rescue systems.

Within any selected specification there is still likely to be choice that may require considerations of availability, price, reputed reliability, support, ergonomics, robustness, and even aesthetics.

First responders: healthcare professionals

Experience in hospitals

Survival from cardiac arrest in the hospital has remained nearly constant for the past 30 years despite significant advances in resuscitation technology and science. Overall survival typically ranges from 3 to 27% depending on the inclusion criteria and outcome definitions [4,5]. Even though many communities and public locations have reported improved survival from cardiac arrest using AEDs in public access defibrillation (PAD) systems, hospitals have been slow to adopt the concept of having first responders deliver lifesaving defibrillation. Inside the intensive care unit (ICU), nurses provide defibrillation often using their own rhythm recognition and standing orders. In other areas, nurses and other employees perform cardiopulmonary resuscitation (CPR) but usually must wait for a physician to provide defibrillation.

Use of AEDs in the hospital was first described by Kaye *et al.* in 1995 [6]. Warwick *et al.* [7] and Destro *et al.* [8] showed that non-ICU nurses can be trained to use AEDs and can function as first responders. Unfortunately, nearly a decade later, the majority of hospitals do not have AED capability and many still lack an appropriate response to victims of cardiac arrest. The limited data that are available have been reviewed by Kenward *et al.* [9] and give an indication of the potential of the strategy. Nevertheless, in the United States only 33% of hospitals participating in the National Registry of Cardiopulmonary Resuscitation database have AEDs anywhere in their institution [10]. Hospitals must strengthen the in-hospital chain of survival if improved outcomes are ever to be achieved. This requires multidisciplinary support from both administrative and clinical personnel; inappropriate bias from physicians, nurses, and administrators are often based solely on the lack of familiarity with the benefit of early defibrillation and the technology available to provide it safely. A strong commitment is needed to education, training, and continuous quality improvement, as well as finance to acquire and maintain the necessary equipment.

Experience in primary care

In most healthcare systems, primary care physicians have an appreciable chance of seeing several cases of acute myocardial infarction each year, and at least some patients will arrest in their presence. Possession of, and expertise in, the use of a defibrillator should therefore be the norm, but this seems not to be the case in any country. Few studies have been published. In the United Kingdom, the British Heart Foundation – a leading charity – has had a policy since 1985 of contributing to the cost of defibrillators for general medical practitioners. In return, the physicians are expected to provide data on attempted resuscitations. In 2002, Colquhoun [11] published the results of a questionnaire to all who had been supported in this way. In all, 259 events were disclosed from 1045 donated units – a majority of which were AEDs.

A physician was present in 110 of these and was close-by in 29 others. In this group, who were treated within an estimated 4 min, 83% of those with a monitored rhythm had VF, and 62% of the 139 survived to hospital discharge. The survival was 13% for the remaining 120 cases who were treated only after a longer delay. Although these are only observational data, they offer powerful evidence that VF remains the dominant *initial* rhythm of cardiac arrest with symptomatic coronary disease, that prompt treatment is highly effective, and that defibrillators should be standard equipment in all primary care settings that may include the initial management of acute coronary disease.

First responders: non healthcare professionals

Experience of law enforcement agencies

Law enforcement personnel trained and equipped to use AEDs provide one strategy for providing early defibrillation in the community. The concept of police as first responders seems intuitive, given that there are many more law enforcement officers than traditional emergency medical services personnel in most communities. In the United States, 81% of police agencies respond to medical emergencies and 50% provide some medical care. Police often arrive at the scene of a medical emergency before emergency medical services (EMS) personnel. Adding defibrillation with AEDs to police first responder duties should theoretically improve survival from out of hospital cardiac arrest by reducing the time from collapse to first shock. White and Vokov [12] tested the use of AEDs by police officers in 1994 and several cities throughout the world have reported their experience since then. Results have varied, depending on factors such as the efficiency of control systems, distance traveled in rural areas, absence of a medical response culture, unease with acting as a medical care provider, variable medical direction, and frequency of refresher training. Groh *et al.* [13] surveyed over 1000 law enforcement officers in Indiana and found that most officers have very limited knowledge regarding cardiac arrest. Only 35% stated that they would feel comfortable using an AED.

Negative attitudes and limited knowledge may impact on the success of law enforcement AED programs. Not all programs have achieved a shortened collapse to first shock time interval and thereby improved survival [14]. Even within the square mile of the city of London, the average response time over a 3-year period achieved by police was a little over the modest target of 8 min [15]. In a controlled study comparing areas with and without the facility, van Alem *et al.* [16] found that although police and firefighters use of AEDs in the Netherlands improved return of spontaneous circulation and admission to the hospital, survival to discharge was not improved. On the other hand, a program developed in Piacenza, Italy, placed AEDs throughout an entire community in ambulances, police cars, and public places, and tripled neurologically intact survival to hospital discharge [17]. The goal however, should be early defibrillation by whatever mechanism is most successful in a given community, not specifically police defibrillation.

Box 17.1 Ten Attributes of Successful Law Enforcement Defibrillation Programs

1 Ability to respond quickly and reliably.
2 Supportive medical response culture.
3 Strong champions to serve as program advocates.
4 Integration with the EMS system.
5 Effective, coordinated dispatch system.
6 A proactive medical director.
7 Designated program coordinator.
8 Effective, competency-based, initial and refresher training.
9 Familiarity with laws, regulations, and liability.
10 Effective continuous quality improvement program.

The position statement on Law Enforcement Agency Defibrillation published in 2002 by the US National Center for Early Defibrillation lists 10 attributes of successful law enforcement defibrillation programs (Box 17.1) [14].

Experience in airlines

Aircraft provide an example of fixed site AEDs that reflects the concept of equity in the provision of care. The "population of the sky" has a lower than average risk, in that the very elderly and the sick tend not to be represented. A review of in-flight deaths reported to the International Air Transport Association from 1977 to 1984, suggested an incidence of approximately one case per three million passengers [18]. Most were sudden and unexpected and more than half were believed to have a cardiac cause. These figures were felt to support the strategy of carrying AEDs in passenger aircraft. They may, however, underestimate the incidence because reporting of events has not been mandatory. An influential special report in the *Chicago Tribune* [19] underscored the need for better data. Public concern in the United States was no doubt influential in prompting the recent Federal Aviation Administration ruling that all commercial aircraft regulated by the Federal Aviation Authority traveling with at least one flight attendant must carry an AED by after April 2004 [20].

The first airline to carry AEDs was British Caledonian in 1986, but this experience was short-lived because they were removed when the airline was taken over only 2 weeks later. But others followed, and by early 2001 no less than 76 operators were known to have equipped some or all of their aircraft. Published experience, however, is limited. QANTAS were the first to report their experience [21], followed by American Airlines [22], Virgin [23], Varig [24], and Air France [25]. QANTAS had almost one cardiac arrest per million passengers, supporting the belief that previous official figures represented an under-estimate of risk. But their data also highlights the difficulties that occur on long flights; 11 of 27 cardiac arrests were unwitnessed and 21 had non-shockable rhythms recorded by the first electrocardiogram. There were only two long-term successes. American Airlines has more short-haul flights so that immediate detection of cardiac arrest is more likely. Of 29 cases of cardiac arrest that occurred in the air during the 2 years of the survey, 11 were shocked for VF and 6 (55%) survived – about three times the success rate of QANTAS, probably reflecting the different times and duration of flights.

An airline that does not carry defibrillators may find such a decision hard to justify in court. Previous concerns raised particularly in the United States about the liability of medical practitioners called upon to assist in an attempted resuscitation have largely been allayed by provisions such as the Aviation Medical Assistance Act [26]. Another consideration is the problem of diversions for patients with possible cardiac pain that have in the past been relatively common, very inconvenient, and hugely expensive. Some evidence already exists that they may become less frequent with increasing use of AEDs [21,22]. Modern technology also permits transmission of both clinical data and ECG records to specialized centers on the ground; this may provide the most reliable method to limit diversions [27]. Whatever future experience may show, it is inconceivable that airlines will give up the use of AEDs; the practice will surely become universal.

Experience in casinos

Valenzuela *et al.* [28] trained security officers in US casinos to perform CPR and use an AED. AEDs were placed at 3-min intervals for retrieval and return to the victim. In their report, 105 patients who suffered a VF cardiac arrest had an overall survival to discharge of 53%. Eighty-six percent of patients had a witnessed arrest. Of those who were witnessed, the mean time interval from collapse to attachment of the defibrillator was 3.5 ± 2.9 min, from collapse to first shock was 4.4 ± 2.9 min, and from collapse to arrival of EMS was 9.8 ± 4.3 min, demonstrating first shock delivery long before EMS arrival. Survival was related to time to first shock with a 74% survival when this was achieved within 3 min after a witnessed collapse. This was one of the first large-scale studies of non-traditional first responders improving survival with on site, early layperson defibrillation.

In the Greater Windsor study from Ontario, Fedoruk *et al.* [29] compared survival rates of cardiac arrest victims from a similar casino program with contemporaneous survival in the surrounding community. Of the 23 casino cases, all were witnessed and 91% had VF/VT, whereas in the main study area only 55% were witnessed and 34% were found with a shockable rhythm. Overall survival was 65% in the casino but only 5.5% in the non-AED equipped surrounding areas, providing further evidence of the effectiveness of early on-site defibrillation in large public venues.

Experience in airports and railway stations

Airports and railway stations share one characteristic with casinos. They generate anxiety and thus promote adrenergic drive that may trigger arrhythmias in vulnerable subjects. It is reasonable speculation that this provides a favorable substrate for defibrillation, with an opportunity for successful treatment if devices can be available within a few minutes walk-time from large numbers of people. The policy of high density distribution of AEDs in such areas was introduced at O'Hare International airport in Chicago [30] where 59 units were placed no more than 90 s walk-time apart. All but 17 were in glass-faced cabinets accessible to the public, and frequent public service announcements indicated their availability. Eighty million passengers pass through the airport annually. In 2 years, 21 individuals had a nontraumatic cardiac arrest with ventricular fibrillation in 18 of them. Successful resuscitation was achieved in 11; all but one was alive and neurologically intact a year later. Of the 11 rescuers, 6 had no training or experience in the use of automated defibrillators, indicating the potential of public access defibrillation in suitable circumstances.

The English Department of Health defibrillation program, for placing devices in public places, included 300 AEDs in 23 airports by 2002 [31]. The same program also included 254 units at 63 busy railway stations. Overall in the program, 92 (73%) of 126 individuals with cardiac arrest on site were found in shockable rhythms, and 22 (24%) of these survived to hospital discharge. These data, in association with those from O'Hara airport, indicate that the policy of placing AEDs in busy transport terminals can be successful. The best method of implementing such a program in a cost-effective manner must depend on local circumstances.

Experience in sports stadia

Although similar considerations apply to sports stadia as to busy travel terminals – on-site units with large numbers of previously healthy but excited or stressed individuals – there is an important caveat. In stadia, crowds are densely packed, full recognition of an emergency will be delayed, and access will be difficult. These problems may account for the dearth of publications on the use of AEDs in this situation. The most promising report involved a cricket ground where crowd density is a lesser problem [32]. This gave an incidence of cardiac arrest of 1 : 500 000 admissions, and in all 20 of 28 individuals (71%) survived; but both regular manual defibrillators and on-site AEDs were used. This paper also provides earlier references on manual defibrillation at sports stadia. They provide additional evidence that defibrillation can have a useful role in these situations.

Experience of public access and home defibrillation

The Public Access Defibrillation (PAD) Trial was a prospective, community based, multicenter trial that randomized public and multifamily residential places from 24 cities in the United States and Canada to have lay, on-site volunteers trained in CPR alone versus CPR plusan an AED [33]. Over 20 000 volunteer responders from 993 community units were trained to perform CPR and to access EMS with additional training in the use of an AED in the units randomized to this intervention. The AED arm of the trial involved 1600 units, at a density to achieve retrieval and return to the victim within 3 min. Eighty four percent of study units were in public places with the remainder being residential. There were 526 presumed cardiac arrests that occurred during the trial data collection. After blinded review, there were 235 definite cardiac arrest cases, yielding one event per unit every 7.4 years. Survival was achieved in 31 cases in the CPR + AED arm and 16 in the CPR-alone arm (RR = 2.0, CI = 1.07–3.77). There was only one survivor in each treatment arm from the multi-unit residential sites, despite these locations accounting for 28% of the presumed cardiac arrests in the trial. Delay in diagnosis and mobilization of volunteer responders is a likely explanation for the low survival. Adverse events were rare and comprised mostly transient emotional distress for the volunteer responder. There were no inappropriate shocks and no failures to shock when indicated. No patient or volunteer was harmed by the AED. These data demonstrate that widespread AED use in public places by trained lay volunteers is safe and effective.

Evidence from the PAD trial can be generalized only with caution. The sites chosen to participate in the trial had a significant percentage of their population over the age of 55 and were therefore at a higher risk of having an event. The event rate in the trial was lower than expected, suggesting that there may be some difficulty in identifying public sites where cardiac arrest is most likely to occur prospectively. The survival rate and safety profile in this study are based on trained volunteers. Extrapolation should not be made for programs with untrained first responders. The impact of community-wide PAD implementation must also be put into perspective. If nationwide achievement of lay-based PAD programs resulted in a similar doubling of survival, an additional 2000 to 4000 lives per year would be saved in the United States. Although this would represent a notable achievement, the impact would be relatively small on the 450 000 deaths that occur annually. Several studies have documented that approximately 80% of out-of-hospital cardiac arrests occur in the home [34,35]. PAD trial results achieved 29.9% survival in public locations compared with 0.6% survival in multifamily residential units. We must develop better strategies for early defibrillation and improved resuscitation practices in the home to obtain an appreciable impact on overall survival.

The National Institutes of Health (NIH) is currently sponsoring the Home AED Trial (HAT). HAT is an international, randomized, controlled, un-blinded study evaluating the effects of home AED placement on survival in patients at increased risk for sudden death. Eligible patients must have had a previous anterior wall myocardial infarction and must be living with a spouse or companion who is willing to learn to use an AED. This trial does not mandate CPR training as was the case for PAD, but provides video instruction on AED use rather than a conventional "hands-on" educational program. Enrolment is scheduled to occur through 2005. Information from this important trial will help determine whether early defibrillation in the home setting will have a significant impact on survival and will also provide safety and effectiveness data on AED use without traditional "hands-on" training.

AED use in children

VF and pulseless ventricular tachycardia are a much less common cause of cardiac arrest in children than in adults. It is estimated that approximately 10% of children have VF as a presenting rhythm and up to 25% demonstrate VF at some time during their arrest. The prevalence of VF is exceedingly rare in young infants and increases with increasing age. However, survival from VF arrest in the pediatric population remains dependent on timely defibrillation as it is in adults.

Several issues have been evaluated recently to assess the safety and effectiveness of AED use in infants and children. The rhythm analyses used by AEDs are derived from adult shockable and nonshockable rhythms. Maximum sensitivity and specificity are derived solely from a library of adult arrhythmias; it was not known whether or not these rhythm analysis programs could differentiate as precisely in children. Recent data suggest, however, that these algorithms are highly specific and reasonably sensitive as they are in adults. Children typically require less energy for successful defibrillation than adults. There is a possibility of increased myocardial damage if excessive energy is used. Both monophasic and biphasic AEDs deliver nonweight-based energy greater than is needed or optimal for children. Some AED manufacturers have developed pediatric pad and cable systems that can be used on adult AEDs to reduce the energy delivered to children under 8 years of age.

The growing numbers of AEDs in public places available to nontraditional first responders increases the likelihood that the devices will be used on children. The International Liaison Committee on Resuscitation published an updated Advisory Statement in 2003, after evaluating and summarizing the data on AED use in children [36]. They conclude that AEDs are safe and appropriate for defibrillation in children aged 1–8. Further investigation is needed to develop diagnostic algorithms specific to infants and children, and more data are needed on appropriate energy doses. Box 17.2 outlines the summary recommendations for pediatric AED use.

Box 17.2 Key Facts for AED Use in Children

1 Defibrillation is recommended for documented VF/pulseless VT (class I).
2 AEDs may be used for children 1–8 years of age who have no signs of circulation (class IIb).
3 Pediatric pads and cables should be used when available.
4 There is insufficient evidence to support the use of AEDs in children less than 1 year of age.

Cost implications

There is little direct information regarding the cost effectiveness of AED place-ment, but several large NIH studies are prospectively collecting or analyzing this information. In the OPALS (Ontario Prehospital Advanced Life Support) study performed at 19 urban and suburban communities with populations ranging from 16 000 to 750 000, the cost for establishing the rapid defibrillation program was estimated at $46 900 and the annual cost of maintaining the pro-gram per life saved was $2400 [37]. Forrer *et al.* [38] estimated the cost of a 7 year police AED program in four suburban communities to vary from $23 542 to $70 342 for each life saved (including subsequent Advanced Cardiac Life Support (ACLS) care) or $1582 to $16 060 per year of life. This was a ret-rospective analysis that used estimated costs of the AED program from the police agency, sensitivity analysis for estimating potential benefit of improved survival based on decreased response times, and literature-based estimates of life expectancy after cardiac arrest survival.

Cost effectiveness of the airline AED program was analyzed by simulation of the costs associated with the airline program and found to compare favorably to that of other widely accepted medical interventions [39]. Addition of AED's to passenger aircraft with more than 200 passengers would cost $35 300 per quality-adjusted life-year (QALY) gained. Additional AED's on aircraft carry-ing between 100 and 200 persons would result in a $40 800 cost per added QALY compared with deployment on large capacity aircraft only, and full deployment on all passenger aircraft would cost an additional $94 700 per QALY gained compared to limited deployment on larger aircraft only.

Public access defibrillation by community responders was associated with a cost of $44 000 per QALY (interquartile range: $29 000–68 900). In compar-ison, public access defibrillation by police had a cost of $27 000 (interquartile range: $15 700–47 800) [40]. Casinos with standard EMS and first responder defibrillation had a median cost of $14 100 per cardiac arrest (interquartile range: $8600–21 900), and early defibrillation by security guards was associ-ated with an increment in cost of a median of $56 700 (interquartile range: $44 100–77 200) [41]. These studies highlight the fact that costs vary widely according to the strategy and location of AED deployment; fixed sites in vul-nerable areas may involve high unit density with relatively low use per AED but high success rate – as opposed to transported AEDs involving fewer units used more frequently but with lower success rates. Costs are also related to the overall health of the target population. Public access defibrillation is generally more expensive than standard EMS, but may be economically acceptable [41].

Current limitations and future developments

Limitations
Even with increasing use of AEDs, community survival from resuscitation is still unsatisfactory. The evidence is clear that a watershed exists in the prospect

for survival at around 4 min, an interval that is only slightly prolonged by current methods of CPR. The EMS system is still seen as the primary provider of resuscitation but only in a few locations can response times offer defibrillation within the required time frame. The community itself should provide the primary response, but major problems of motivation, cost, and organization must be overcome to make this a reality. The major role of the EMS is ideally the provision of skilled assistance to follow the first aid measures of both CPR and defibrillation. But here too there are limitations at present. Current guidelines with short compression sequences, relatively long analysis times of AEDs, and user hesitancy all conspire to cause excessive hands-off time; the number of compressions actually given tends to fall far short of that which can provide sufficient forward flow to sustain life.

The knowledge that for any delayed defibrillation, good preliminary compressions are of considerable importance was initially related only to maintaining coronary and cerebral perfusion pressure [42], but now are believed to relate also to the flow of blood from the arterial to the venous circulation during cardiac arrest – known to physiologists for 40 years but only recently stressed in the field of resuscitation [43]. This causes serious ventricular interaction that can be relieved only briefly by chest compressions. It follows that long delays to shock for the purposes of analysis – as long as 25 s even without operator delay – are unacceptable.

Future developments

The design of AEDs continues to evolve. Some features comply with guidelines that at present may not be optimal, but these could be changed by software updates. Long analysis times will be overcome. Increasingly, modern equipment is able to perform an analysis with less than 10 s of "hands-off" time; this facility will quickly be matched by all manufacturers. The algorithms for arrhythmia detection and analysis are already well developed and have specificity and sensitivity that are generally satisfactory, leaving scope for only possible marginal improvements. In one important respect, however, progress seems likely; sophisticated analysis of fibrillatory waveforms can now predict the likelihood of successful defibrillation [44]. In future, AEDs might well advise against shock if it is likely to be unsuccessful without additional CPR or other appropriate treatment.

Units that are designed primarily for healthcare professionals will continue to offer features not appropriate for the simple devices needed by lay first responders, but the latter will increasingly be able to offer more audio and/or visual support for correct performance of Basic Cardiac Life Support (BLS) either by a sensor under the compressing hands or by analysis of the electrical consequences of compression rate and depth. The importance of maintaining sufficient good quality compressions is likely to increase the popularity of mechanical devices; a combination of mechanical compression and defibrillation into a single device is an obvious development. The uniformity of mechanical compression offers the opportunity to filter electrically the resulting artifact. The desirability of achieving reliable filtering with manual compressions to permit detailed assessment of fibrillation waveforms offers a more difficult challenge.

Both procedures and devices will continue to evolve. AEDs will play an ever-increasing role in reducing community mortality from coronary disease.

References

1. Diack AW, Welborn WS, Rullman RG, Walter CW, Wayne MA. An automatic cardiac resuscitator for emergency treatment of cardiac arrest. *Med Instrum* 1979; **13**: 78–83.
2. Jaggarao NSV, Heber M, Grainger R, Vencent R, Chamberlain DA, Aronson AL. Use of an automated external defibrillator-pacemaker by ambulance staff. *Lancet* 1982; **ii**: 73–75.
3. Cummins RO, Eisenberg MS, Litwin PE, Graves JR, Hearne TR, Hallstrom AP. Automatic external defibrillators used by emergency medical technicians. A controlled clinical trial. *J Am Med Assoc* 1987; **257**: 1605–1610.
4. Patrick A, Rankin N. The in-hospital Utstein style: use in reporting outcome from cardiac arrest in Middlemore Hospital 1995–1996. *Resuscitation* 1998; **36**: 91–94.
5. Skogvoll E, Isern E, Sangolt GK, Gisvold SE. In-hospital cardiopulmonary resuscitation: 5 years' incidence and survival according to the Utstein template. *Acta Anaesthesiol Scand* 1999; **43**: 177–184.
6. Kaye W, Mancini ME, Richards N. Organizing and implementing a hospital-wide first responder automated external defibrillation program: strengthening the in-hospital chain of survival. *Resuscitation* 1995; **30**: 151–156.
7. Warwick JP, Mackie K, Spencer I. Towards early defibrillation. *Resuscitation* 1995; **30**: 231–235.
8. Destro A, Marzaloni M, Sermasi S, Rossi F. Automatic external defibrillators in the hospital as well? *Resuscitation* 1996; **31**: 39–44.
9. Kenward G, Castle N, Hodgetts TJ. Should ward nurses be using automatic external defibrillators as first responders to improve the outcome from cardiac arrest?: a systematic review of the primary research. *Resuscitation* 2002; **52**: 31–37.
10. Peberdy MA, Kaye W, Ornato JP *et al.* Cardiopulmonary resuscitation of adults in the hospital. *Resuscitation* 2003; **58**: 298–308.
11. Colquhoun MC. Defibrillation by general practitioners. *Resuscitation* 2002; **52**: 143–148.
12. White RD, Vokov LF. Early defibrillation by police: initial experience with measurement of critical time intervals and patient outcomes. *Ann Emerg Med* 1994; **23**(5): 1009–1013.
13. Groh WJ, Lowe MR, Overgaard AD, Neal JM, Fishburn WC, Zipes DP. Attitudes of law enforcement officers regarding automated external defibrillators. *Acad Emerg Med* 2002; **9**(7): 751–753.
14. Mosesso VN, Newman MM, Ornato JP *et al.* Law enforcement agency defibrillation (LEA-D): Proceedings of the National Center for Early Defibrillation Police AED Issues Forum. *Prehosp Emerg Care* 2002; **6**: 273–282.

15. Ross P, Nolan J, Hill E, Dawson J, Whimster F, Skinner D. The use of AEDs by police officers in the City of London. *Resuscitation* 2001; **50**: 141–146.
16. van Alem AP, Vrenken RH, de Vos R, Tijssen JG, Koster RW. Use of automated external defibrillator by first responders in out of hospital cardiac arrest: prospective controlled trial. *Br Med J* 2003; **327**: 1312.
17. Capucci A, Aschieri D, Piepoli MF, Bardy GH, Iconomu E, Arvedi M. Tripling survival from sudden cardiac arrest via early defibrillation without traditional education in cardiopulmonary resuscitation. *Circulation* 2002; **106**: 1065–1070.
18. Cummins RO, Chapman PJ, Chamberlain DA, Schubach JA, Litwin PE. In-flight deaths during commercial air travel. How big is the problem? *J Am Med Assoc* 1988; **259**: 1983–1988.
19. Crewdson J. Code blue: survival in the sky. *Chicago Tribune*. Special Report 1996, June 30.
20. Final rule, April 12, 2001. Washington, DC: Federal Aviation Administration, 2001. Accessed November 22, 2004, at http://dmses.dot.gov/docimages/pdf62/126161_web.pdf
21. O'Rourke MS, Donaldson E, Geddes JS. An airline cardiac arrest program. *Circulation* 1997; **96**: 2849–2853.
22. Page RL, Joglar JA, Kowal RC *et al.* Use of automated external defibrillators by a U.S. airline. *N Engl J Med* 2000; **343**: 1210–1216.
23. Goodwin A. In-flight medical emergencies: an overview. *Brit Med J* 2000; **321**: 1338–1341.
24. Alves PM, de Freitas EJ, Mathias HA *et al.* Use of automated external defibrillators in a Brazilian airline. A 1-year experience. *Arq Bras Cardiol* 2001; **76**: 310–314.
25. Szmajer M, Rodriguez P, Sauval P, Charetteur M-P, Derossi A, Carli P. Medical assistance during commercial airline flights: analysis of 11 years experience of the Paris emergency medical service (SAMU) between 1989 and 1999. *Resuscitation* 2001; **50**: 147–151.
26. Aviation Medical Assistance Act of 1998, Pub. L. No. 105–170, H.R. 2843, 105th Cong. (1998). Accessed November 22, 2004, at http://dmses.dot.gov/docimages/pdf48/84064_web.pdf
27. Emergency Telemedicine Centre. http://www.medaire.com/comm_air.html. Accessed June 18, 2004.
28. Valenzuela TD, Roe DJ, Nichol G, Clark LL, Spaite DW, Hardman RG. Outcomes of rapid defibrillation by security officers after cardiac arrest in casinos. *N Engl J Med* 2000; **343**: 1206–1209.
29. Fedoruk JC, Paterson D, Hlynka M, Fung KY, Gobet M, Currie W. Rapid on-site defibrillation versus community program. *Prehospital Disaster Med* 2002; **17**: 102–106.
30. Caffrey SL, Willoughby PA, Pepe PE, Becker LB. Public use of automated external defibrillators. *New Engl J Med* 2002; **347**: 1242–1247.
31. Davies CS, Colquhoun M, Boyle R, Chamberlain D. A national programme for on-site defibrillation by lay persons in selected high-risk areas: initial results. *Heart* (under review).
32. Wassertheil J, Keane G, Fisher N, Leditschke JF. Cardiac outcomes at the Melbourne Cricket Ground and Shrine of Remembrance using a tiered response strategy – a forerunner to public access defibrillation. *Resuscitation* 2000; **44**: 97–104.
33. The Public Access Defibrillation Trial Investigators. Public access defibrillation trial. *N Engl J Med* 2004; **351**: 1–10.

34. Becker L, Eisenberg M, Fahrenbruch C, Cobb L. Public locations of cardiac arrest: implications for public access defibrillation. *Circulation* 1998; **97**: 2106–2109.
35. Pell JP, Sirel JM, Marsden AK, Ford I, Walker NL, Cobbe SM. Potential impact of public access out of hospital cardiopulmonary arrest: retrospective cohort study. *Br Med J* 2002; **325**: 515.
36. Samson R, Berg R, Bingham R. Use of automated external defibrillators for children: an advisory statement from the Pediatric Advanced Life Support Task Force, International Liaison Committee on Resuscitation. *Resuscitation* 2003; **57**: 237–243.
37. Stiell IG, Wells GA, Field BJ III *et al.* Improved out-of-hospital cardiac arrest survival through the inexpensive optimization of an existing defibrillation program. OPALS study phase II. Ontario Prehospital Advanced Life Support. *J Am Med Assoc* 1999; **281**: 1175–1181.
38. Forrer CS, Swor RA, Jackson RE, Pascual RG, Scott C, McEachin C. Estimated cost effectiveness of a police automated external defibrillator program in a suburban community: 7 years experience. *Resuscitation* 2002; **52**: 23–29.
39. Groeneveld PW, Kwong JL, Liu Y *et al.* Cost-effectiveness of automated external defibrillators on airlines. *J Am Med Assoc* 2001; **286**:1482–1489.
40. Nichol G, Hallstrom AP, Ornato JP *et al.* Potental cost-effectiveness of public access defibrillation in the United States. *Circulation* 1998; **97**: 1315–1320.
41. Nichol G, Valenzuela T, Roe D, Clark L, Huszti E, Wells GA. Cost effectiveness of defibrillation by targeted responders in public settings. *Circulation* 2003; **108**: 697–703.
42. Paradis NA, Martin GB, Rivers EP, *et al.* Coronary perfusion pressure and the return of spontaneous circulation in human cardiopulmonary resuscitation. *J Am Med Assoc* 1990; **263**: 1106–1113.
43. Steen S, Liao Q, Pierre L, Paskevicius A, Sjöberg T. The critical importance of minimal delay between chest compressions and subsequent defibrillation: a haemodynamic explanation. *Resuscitation* 2003; **58**: 249–258.
44. Eftestøl T, Sunde K, Aase SO, Husøy JH, Steen PA. Predicting outcome of defibrillation by spectral characterization and nonparametric classification of ventricular fibrillation in patients with out-of-hospital cardiac arrest. *Circulation* 2000; **102**: 1523–1529.

CHAPTER 18

Cost-effectiveness of implantable cardioverter-defibrillators

Giuseppe Boriani and Greg Larsen

Introduction: relevance of the cost-effectiveness issue

The field of cardiology occupies a special place in the highly topical healthcare cost-containment issue. In a major survey on healthcare costs in the United States, heart disease turned out to be the most costly medical condition, with 57 506 million US dollars being spent in 1997, for providing health care to affected patients, with a mean expense of 3379 US dollars for each patient requiring treatment [1]. Clearly, one of the most relevant problems of current cardiologic practice must be appropriate deployment (in patients appropriately selected according to consensus guidelines) of a series of treatments whose proven efficacy is accompanied by relatively high costs [2]. Such options include implantable cardioverter-defibrillator (ICDs), devices for cardiac resynchronization therapy, drug-eluting stents and devices for left ventricular assistance. In the particular setting of sudden-death prevention, the high costs of ICDs represent a major financial hurdle.

Advantages of an economics-based approach

Despite the mounting costs that healthcare systems have had to face in recent years, the balancing of benefits against costs has yet to become a primary criterion for deciding whether a medical treatment should be covered by public services. Instead, both policymakers and healthcare providers have largely focused on cost projections, with a consequent tendency to limit or even reject costly new treatments, despite proven clinical efficacy. In other words, consideration of the effects of adopting a new treatment has mainly been based on strictly financial concerns rather than on in-depth economic analysis [3]. Even today, in the United States the Food and Drug Administration and Medicare do not take advantage of cost-effectiveness analysis as a valuable tool for deciding resource allocation [4]. The same applies for the vast majority of public decision-makers in Europe.

Cost-effectiveness and cost–benefit analysis have been proposed in various fields of medicine to determine which alternative treatment is most likely to provide maximum health benefits for a given level of financial resources, or which treatment provides a given level of health benefits at the lowest cost. Cost-effectiveness estimates express clinical outcome in terms of "years of added life" or "quality-adjusted life years gained"; on the other hand, cost–benefit analysis directly assigns a monetary value to therapeutic benefits [3–7]. Both these analytical approaches are designed to weigh up the benefits and costs of given medical treatments in order to provide a formal basis for implementation decisions.

Cost-effectiveness ratios

Cost-effectiveness analysis is designed to evaluate the cost of any therapeutic intervention with respect to its predictable outcome benefits [3,5,6,8]. The *cost* of a therapy includes both the direct costs (initial cost of therapy, costs to maintain therapy, and costs caused by any adverse effects) and the indirect costs paid by patients, their families, and/or the community. Effectiveness is measured as the mean extra number of years survived as a result of a treatment. Incremental cost-effectiveness analysis involves comparison of alternative therapeutic strategies. The cost-effectiveness ratio is commonly expressed as dollars per year of life saved ($/YLS). In the literature [8], a treatment is considered very attractive if the cost-effectiveness ratio ranges between 0 and 20 000 $/YLS; attractive between 20 000 and 40 000 $/YLS; borderline between 40 000 and 60 000 $/YLS; unfavorable between 60 000 and 100 000 $/YLS; and absolutely unfavorable above 100 000 $/YLS.

Cost-effectiveness ratios of various cardiovascular and noncardiovascular treatments are listed in Table 18.1. It is evident that cost-effectiveness ratios can vary considerably depending on the type of population in treatment. Identification of high-risk patients ("patient targeting") [8] seems to be the single most important issue in order to reach a favorable cost-effectiveness ratio.

An important general observation regards some prolonged treatments without particularly high up-front costs; in the absence of major long-term benefits in terms of survival the ultimate cost-effectiveness ratios of such strategies may turn out to be surprisingly unfavorable. Examples include lipid lowering treatments in patients at relatively low risk, as well as antihypertensives and antithrombotic treatment with clopidogrel [8–12].

The ICD: a treatment with a high up-front cost but proven efficacy

The ICD has traditionally been seen as an expensive form of treatment, with high up-front costs due to the device itself and the implant (followed over time by maintenance costs for device replacement). Since the ICD first appeared in

Table 18.1 Cost-effectiveness of various treatments.

Treatment Strategy	Substrate	Patient Characteristics	$/YLS or $/QALY Gained
Very favorable cost-effectiveness (<20 000 $/YLS)			
Pacemaker	Complete AV block		1400
Beta-blockers	Post-MI	High risk	3600
Anticoagulant drugs	Mitral stenosis	AF, f, age 35	4200
Lovastatin	Hyperlipidemia	Sec prev, chol ≥250 mg/dl, f, age 45–54	4700
Simvastatin	Hypercholesterolemia in CAD	Age 59, cholesterol 309 mg/dl	1200 (m) 3200 (f)
Simvastatin	Hypercholesterolemia in CAD	Age 59, cholesterol 213 mg/dl	2100 (m) 8600 (f)
Simvastatin	Hypercholesterolemia in CAD	Age 70, cholesterol 309 mg/dl	3800 (m) 6200 (f)
Simvastatin	Hypercholesterolemia in CAD	Age 70, cholesterol 213 mg/dl	6 200 (m) 13 300 (f)
PTCA	Ischemic heart disease	Severe angina, age 55, m, normal EF, 1-vessel disease	8700
CABG	Ischemic heart disease	Severe angina, main left main coronary stenosis	9200
Aspirin	Ischemic heart disease	Sec prev	11 000
PTCA	Ischemic heart disease	Severe angina , age 55, m, low EF, 1-vessel disease	11 600
Captopril	Post-MI	LVEF ≤0.40, age 60	10 200
Enalapril	Heart failure		10 300
Endocardial ICD without EPS	VT/VF	LVEF ≥0.25	14 200
CABG	Ischemic heart disease	Nonsevere angina, 3-vessel disease	18 500

(Continued)

Table 18.1 (Continued).

Treatment Strategy	Substrate	Patient Characteristics	$/YLS or $/QALY Gained
Favorable cost-effectiveness (20–40 000 $/YLS)			
Beta-blockers	Post-MI	Low risk	20 200
Anti-hypertensive therapy	Hypertension	Diastolic AP ≥ 105 mm Hg	20 600
Lovastatin	Hyperlipidemia	Sec prev, chol < 250 mg/dl, m, age 55–64	20 200
Catheter ablation	VT in structural heart disease patients with ICD	Patients with frequent VT episodes	20 923
Endocardial ICD with EPS	VT/VF	Age ≥75	25 700
Streptokinase	Acute myocardial infarction		27 700
Screening with exercise testing after myocardial infarction[a]	Ischemic heart disease	Previous uncomplicated myocardial infarction	21 700–36 166
Primary stent in PTCA	Ischemic heart disease	Angina, age 55, m, 1-vessel disease	26 800
Endocardial ICD with EPS	Ischemic heart disease	Low EF, nSVT, high risk	27 000
Clopidogrel	Ischemic heart disease	Sec prev in patients ineligible to aspirin	31 000
Endocardial ICD	Heart failure	NYHA class II–III, LVEF ≤ 35%	33 192
Borderline cost-effectiveness (40–60 000 $/YLS)			
Anti-hypertensive therapy	Hypertension	Diastolic AP 95–104 mm Hg	41 900
CABG	Ischemic heart disease	Severe angina, 2-vessel disease	42 500
Cardiac transplant	Severe heart failure		44 300
Lovastatin	Hyperlipidemia	Sec prev, chol < 250 mg/dl, f, age 55–64	48 600
Ambulatory peritoneal dialysis			57 300
Radio frequency ablation	WPW	Without symptoms, age 40	57 100
Hospital hemodialysis			59 500

Unfavorable cost-effectiveness (60–100 000 $/YLS)

CABG	Ischemic heart disease	Nonsevere angina, 2-vessel disease	72 900
Lovastatin	Hyperlipidemia	Prim prev, chol ≥300 mg/dl, no risk factors (RF), m, age 55–64	78 300
Coronary care unit admission	Suspected acute MI	Patients with 20% probability of acute myocardial infarction	78 000
Heart transplantation	Terminal heart disease	Patients aged 55 or younger	100 000

Very unfavorable cost-effectiveness (>100 000 $/YLS)

PTCA	Ischemic heart disease	Nonsevere angina, age 55, normal LVEF, 1-vessel disease (left anterior descending)	109 000
Clopidogrel	Ischemic heart disease	Sec prev with clopidogrel alone in all patients or in combination with aspirin	130 000
Neurosurgery	Malignant intracranial tumor		325 000
Coronary care unit admission	Suspected acute MI	Patients with 5% probability of acute myocardial infarction	328 500
CABG	Ischemic heart disease	Nonsevere angina, 1-vessel disease	1 142 000
Lovastatin	Hyperlipidemia	Prim prev, chol≥300 mg/dl, no risk factors (RF), f, age 45–54	2 024 800

Notes: AF = atrial fibrillation; AP = arterial pressure; CAD = coronary artery disease; CABG = coronary artery by-pass graft; Chol = cholesterolemia; EPS = electrophysiological study; f = female; ICD = implantable cardioverter-defibrillator; LVEF = left ventricular ejection fraction; m = male; MI = myocardial infarction; nSVT = nonsustained ventricular tachycardia; Prim prev = primary prevention; Proph = prophylaxis; PTCA = percutaneous transluminal coronary angioplasty; RF = coronary risk factors; Sec prev = secondary prevention; VF = ventricular fibrillation; VT = ventricular tachycardia; WPW = Wolff–Parkinson–White syndrome; $/YLS = dollars per year of saved life; $/QALY = dollars per quality-adjusted year of life gained.

Source: Modified from: Kupersmith [8], Tengs *et al.* [9], Johannesson *et al.* [10], Boriani *et al.* [11], and Gaspoz *et al.* [12].

[a] Assuming discounted life expectancy of 6–10 years with coronary revascularization.

clinical practice, the indications for use of ICDs have broadened dramatically from a few selected patients with previous cardiac arrest to a large cohort of patients with heterogeneous underlying heart diseases, identified as subjects at high risk of sudden death [13–16]. Transvenous implantation has markedly decreased the hospitalization costs and contributed to widespread use of ICD systems [13,17,18]. Despite marked price reductions in the last decade, the cost issue continues to limit full acceptance and application of ICD therapy, especially as regards increased use for primary prevention of sudden death [11,19–22].

The clinical efficacy of ICDs has been clearly demonstrated in specific subsets of patients. Table 18.2 summarizes the results of main randomized controlled trials [23–31] – regarding both primary and secondary prevention of sudden cardiac death – in terms of ability to improve overall survival. It is noteworthy that ICD efficacy was generally associated with favorable values for "number needed to treat" to save a life, much lower than those reported for a series of widely used pharmacological treatments (Figure 18.1). Analysis of the results of randomized controlled trials involving over 6000 patients [7] have prompted definition of consensus guidelines for ICD use [14–16]. Indications for devices with cardioversion-defibrillation capabilities are also expected to increase in view of the increasing evidence emerging from the Comparison of Medical Therapy, Pacing, and Defibrillation in Heart Failure (COMPANION) study [30] that cardiac resynchronization therapy in patients with severe heart failure may improve overall survival, in addition to providing favorable effects in terms of quality of life, exercise capacity, and reductions in hospitalization due to heart failure [32–37].

Implementation of ICD use in clinical practice

Even when the information derived from randomized controlled trials has been incorporated into consensus guidelines, barriers to widespread implementation still exist [38]. Although it is difficult to assess the degree of compliance to consensus guidelines in daily practice, indirect evidence suggests that even in the United States the actual rate of ICD implantation is lower than projections based on the current guidelines [39]. Such a gap could be of major relevance for public health, considering the evidence of ICDs' efficacy in primary prevention of sudden death in patients with severe left ventricular dysfunction/heart failure provided by the Multicenter Automatic Defibrillattor Implantation Trial (MADIT II) and Sudden Cardiac Death in Heart Failure Trial (SCD-HeFT) trials [21,22,29,31].

Marked discrepancies clearly exist in the implementation of clinical indications to ICD implantation based on randomized studies (MADIT II, SCD-HeFT) testing the impact of device therapy on primary prevention of sudden death. For instance, there are still major differences between the implant rates in the United States and Europe [2]. This heterogeneity reflects variations between different countries regarding general economic status, type of

Table 18.2 Main prospective controlled trials on treatment with ICD versus control in primary and secondary prevention of sudden death.

	Number of Patients	Mean Age (Years)	Women (%)	NYHA Class >II(%)	Mean LVEF (%)	Follow-up (Months)	Annual Control Group Mortality (%)	Relative Risk Reduction in Total Mortality with ICD (%)	p-value in the Comparison of ICD Versus Control for Overall Survival
Secondary prevention trials									
AVID (1997)	1016	65	21	9	32	18 ± 12	12	31	<.02
CIDS (2000)	659	64	15	11	34	36	10	20	.142
CASH (2000)	288	58	20	17	45	57 ± 34	9	23	.081
Metaanalysis (2000)	1866	63	18	11	34	28	—	28	.0006
Primary prevention trials									
MADIT (1996)	196	63	8	—	26	27	17	54	.009
MUSTT (1999)	704	67	10	24	30	39	14	51	<.001
MADIT II (2002)	1232	65	15	29	23	20	10	31	.016
COMPANION (2004)	1634	66	23	86	22	16	19	43	.002
SCD-HeFT (2004)	2521	60	23	30	25	45.5	7.2	23	.007

Notes: ICD = implantable cardioverter-defibrillator; LVEF = left ventricular ejection fraction.

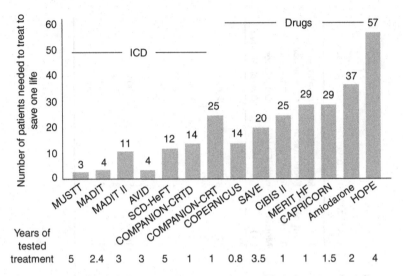

Figure 18.1 Number needed to treat (NNT) to save one life in a series of studies related to ICD treatment or various pharmacological treatments. CRT = cardiac resynchronization therapy; CRTD = cardiac resynchronization therapy + defibrillation capabilities.

healthcare system, and arrangements for reimbursement of device costs [2,40]. Moreover, a decision not to implant an ICD in a patient with a MADIT II or SCD-HeFT indication can entail very different potential medicolegal implications in different countries [41]. Such considerations may help explain why ICD implant rates can vary considerably even among European countries sharing broadly similar economic status.

Available ICD cost-effectiveness estimates

Table 18.3 provides an overview of cost-effectiveness estimates of ICD treatment generated by observational data, projections based on decision models (retrospective analysis), and – more recently – randomized trials [11,42–50]. Use of ICDs in selected patients (or subgroups of patients) at high risk of sudden death has often generated cost-effectiveness estimates that are comparable with or lower than other accepted treatments, including renal dialysis, which costs about 50 000–60 000 $/YLS [8,9,11,21]. Nevertheless, a broad range of cost-effectiveness ratios have emerged, ranging from economically attractive to very expensive values. In general, the recent randomized trials have provided less attractive ratios than those derived from the initial modeling studies [51]. A further source of variability is the time horizon within which cost-effectiveness is estimated. When Hlatky and Bigger [52] projected the results of all the trials published until 2001, to gauge the full gain in life expectancy, they obtained a cost-effectiveness ratio of 31 500 $/YLS, in line with what is currently considered fully acceptable in developed countries.

Another important variable regards the ICD setting (primary/secondary prevention of sudden death). For primary prevention of sudden death, cost-effectiveness has been evaluated prospectively in the context of MADIT I [27], which enrolled patients with coronary artery disease, low left ventricular ejection fraction (≤0.35), nonsustained ventricular tachycardia, and inducibility of ventricular tachycardia resistant to procainamide at electrophysiological study. Cost-effectiveness analysis of MADIT I [42] generated an economically attractive figure of 27 000 $/YLS for use of ICD versus amiodarone; however, this did not substantially affect implementation of ICD in clinical practice in some European countries (11,15,21). A similar analysis of SCD-HeFT recently estimated 33 192 $/YLS for the ICD [50], indicating that its use in primary prevention may be justifiable from the standpoint of cost-effectiveness [53]. Two secondary prevention studies – AVID [47] and CIDS [44,45] – revealed higher cost-effectiveness ratios for the ICD with respect to alternative treatments. An analysis of Antiarrhythmic Versus Implantable Defibrillator (AVID) [47], which considered hospital charges in all enrolled patients and overall health care costs in a subgroup of patients, concluded that ICD is moderately cost-effective (Table 18.3). In the context of CIDS, calculation of the cost-effectiveness ratio in the sickest patients (those with at least two risk factors for sudden death) led to a much more affordable cost-effectiveness ratio [45]. Indeed, even in studies [11,21,43,45] showing an economically unattractive cost-effectiveness estimate for the ICD overall, it was possible to identify subgroups of patients for whom this option appeared much more favorable or attractive. One type of risk stratification analysis that could be crucial for proper estimates of cost-effectiveness in specific subgroups of patients would be assessment of the risk of sudden cardiac death set against the competing risk of nonsudden cardiac [46] (Table 18.2). Therefore, better patient targeting based on improved risk stratification might be helpful for attempts to maximize health outcomes in a context of limited economic resources.

All the available studies agree that use of ICDs is associated with a "favorable" cost-effectiveness profile (i.e. <50 000 $/YLS) in patients with lower left ventricular ejection fraction, who have the highest risk of sudden cardiac death. Further data – especially as regards long-term follow-up – are required for patients with higher left ventricular ejection fraction.

Current limitations of ICD cost-effectiveness analysis

An important limitation of currently available ICD cost-effectiveness estimates regards the lack of data on long-term benefits. This is largely because rapid demonstration of efficacy is especially prized in prospective trials involving ICDs. So far, these trials have generally been stopped as soon as efficacy has been statistically demonstrated in terms of reduced mortality. Therefore, the follow-up of the patients enrolled has tended to be far shorter than the life expectancy of many patients implanted with an ICD in everyday practice. This

Table 18.3 Cost-effectiveness of ICDs.

Author, Year	Type of Study	$/YLS or $/QALY Gained
Kuppermann, 1990	Secondary prevention (decision-model study on data from Medicare)	17 100
Larsen, 1992	Secondary prevention (decision-model study): ICD versus amiodarone	21 000
Kupersmith, 1995	Secondary prevention (decision-model study) ICD versus EPS-guided therapy ICD without EPS, with LVEF $\geq$ 40%	25 700 14 200
Kupersmith, 1995	Secondary prevention (decision-model study) With LVEF < 25% With LVEF $\geq$ 25%	44 000 27 200
Wever, 1996	Secondary prevention: ICD versus class III antiarrhythmic drugs	11 315
Owens, 1997	Secondary prevention: ICD versus amiodarone With mortality reduction of 40% With mortality reduction of 20%	27 300 54 000
Mushlin, 1998	Primary prevention (MADIT study) If transvenous ICD If life of ICD >4 years	27 000 22 800 12 500
Sanders, 2001	Primary prevention (decision-model study based on a registry of 2924 patients): ICD versus no treatment If 60% reduction in sudden cardiac death With LVEF $\leq$ 30% With LVEF 31–40% With LVEF $\geq$ 40% If 80% reduction in sudden cardiac death With LVEF $\leq$ 30% With LVEF 31–40% With LVEF $\geq$ 40%	59 800 116 800 258 800 46 100 85 900 178 600
O'Brien, 2001	Secondary prevention (CIDS study): ICD versus amiodarone	138 803
Sheldon, 2001	Secondary prevention (CIDS study): ICD versus amiodarone With <2 risk factors With $\geq$2 risk factors	595 828 42 377
Owens, 2002	Primary and secondary prevention: ICD versus amiodarone assuming 25% reduction in overall mortality by the ICD At 12% annual mortality rate If sudden death/nonsudden death ratio = 4 If sudden death/nonsudden death ratio = 1 If sudden death/nonsudden death ratio = 0.25	36 000 55 400 116 000

(Continued).

Table 18.3 (Continued).

Author, Year	Type of Study	$/YLS or $/QALY Gained
Larsen, 2002	Secondary prevention (AVID study): ICD versus amiodarone or sotalol	66 677
Weiss, 2002	Secondary prevention (observational study: matched pair analysis of Medicare patients)	78 400
Chen, 2004	Primary prevention in heart failure patients, NYHA class II and III (decision-model study)	97 861
Mark, 2004	Primary prevention in heart failure patients, NYHA class II and III (SCD-HeFT study)	33 192

Notes: EPS = electrophysiological study; ICD = implantable cardioverter-defibrillator; LVEF = left ventricular ejection fraction; $/YLS = cost per year of life saved; $/QALY gained = cost per quality-adjusted year of life gained.
Source: Modified from Boriani *et al.* [11] and updated [42–50].

bias is highly relevant since the high initial cost of the device can markedly affect cost-effectiveness estimates, particularly when the follow-up is not long enough to assess the full benefits of ICD treatment [52,54]. Some cost-effectiveness studies extended the time horizon by means of data extrapolation [43–45,47], although this may obviously introduce further biases. Ultimately, such biases can only be avoided by longer-term follow-up or registry studies. At present, there is only one available study assessing the efficacy of ICDs in the long-term [55]. This secondary prevention study performed on a sub-set of CIDS patients from a single center indicated that ICD use in patients followed for up to 11 years (mean, 5.9 years) was associated with a much higher relative risk reduction (43%) than at earlier time points (20% at 3 years) [25, 55]. Although derived from a relatively small patient population, this finding suggests that midterm analyses can lead to underestimates of the long-term efficacy of ICDs, implying overly pessimistic cost-effectiveness ratios [56].

A further limitation of the available cost-effectiveness estimates is that patients' preferences and health-related quality of life associated with ICD use have yet to be systematically taken into account. This deserves to become a topical area of study, especially in the setting of primary prevention of sudden death in patients with a long expected survival, such as those with arrhythmogenic genetic cardiac diseases [15] or with hypertrophic cardiomyopathy [57].

Finally, it should be underlined that none of the randomized controlled trials was specifically conceived for assessing cost-effectiveness as one of the primary endpoints. Prospective studies specifically designed to evaluate cost-effectiveness over time could be extremely valuable for healthcare systems.

Possible solutions to the ICD cost issue

The high cost of ICDs raises the question of how to facilitate implementation of indications derived from studies regarding primary prevention of sudden death such as MADIT II and SCD-HeFT [19–22]. Several approaches to the problem have been suggested. The major obstacle seems to regard the financial resources needed to cover the expected steep rise in ICD implants. The authors of MADIT II expressed the hope that market forces would drive down the price of ICDs, and this may provide one of the potential answers to the economic problems raised by this trial. An additional approach was outlined by JT Bigger [20] in an editorial commenting MADIT II. He proposed that more careful screening of candidates, with selection criteria based on analysis of the characteristics of patients within the MADIT-II population who gained the greatest benefits, could help improve cost-effectiveness. A subgroup analysis [58] of MADIT II showing that those patients with a wide QRS complex at baseline (>120 ms) had a greater reduction in total mortality suggesting a criterion to maximize survival benefits from ICD implantation. Despite the methodological biases inherent in this *post hoc* analysis, financial coverage by Medicare was established in June 2003, only for MADIT II patients with a QRS interval >120 ms. Reevaluation of this criterion, as strongly advocated by the Heart Rhythm Society and leading experts in the field [22], has been done recently in the light of the results of SCD-HeFT.

Continued price reductions will clearly be important to stimulate wider use of ICDs, and the importance of this factor is likely to be greater in Europe than in the United States. One cost-cutting strategy could involve provision of simpler and less sophisticated devices ("shock-only devices with a total capability of 8–10 shocks") at lower prices [19]. The idea of using a "Volkswagen instead of a Rolls-Royce" [19] is certainly an attractive proposition. In our view, however, particular care would need to be dedicated to patient selection in order to avert a series of clinical pitfalls (device exhaustion due to arrhythmic storms, loss of full protection after delivery of some shocks owing to limited shock capabilities, etc.).

Reduced implantation costs could provide another way of making ICD therapy more economically feasible. The possibility of implanting a single-chamber ICD on an outpatient basis was explored in the SCD-HeFT trial [31]; it is noteworthy that this approach was associated with a favorable cost-effectiveness value of 33 192 $/YLS [50]. Further evaluations are required to assess, in which patients this approach for ICD implant is safe and appropriate in current practice.

What has to be stressed is that ICD price cuts can markedly improve cost-effectiveness, making ICD therapy a more economically viable proposition [43]. Further long-term evaluation of the cost-effectiveness and cost-utility of ICDs could provide a basis identification of subsets of patients for whom the implant can be considered affordable for primary prevention of sudden death within the context of current prices and prevailing economic constraints.

Such evaluations could readily be reviewed to take advantage of any price cuts.

A further economic issue regards the use of ICDs providing cardiac resynchronization therapy in the heart failure setting [21,30,36,37,59]. The problem is particularly thorny because of the current high cost of these sophisticated models which, however, are of proven efficacy in terms of quality of life, morbidity and mortality, as validated by prospective controlled studies [30,32–37].

Conclusions

Despite continuing price reductions, cost is likely to remain a major determinant for fuller acceptance and implementation of ICD therapy." Therefore, the problem of how broadened evidence-based indications to implantation can be translated into routine clinical practice will have to be addressed in the light of available economic resources. Cost-effectiveness analysis provides the most appropriate tool for weighing ICD costs against likely eventual outcome benefits. Since great emphasis has been traditionally placed on the relatively high up-front device costs, this approach appears appropriate for assessing (for specific subsets of patients) whether implantation will eventually be more or less economically valid with respect to alternative treatments characterized by continuing costs rather than a high initial burden. Analysis of randomized controlled trials indicates that use of ICDs in patients with lower left ventricular ejection fraction (who run the highest risk of sudden cardiac death) is associated with cost-effectiveness ratios similar to, or better than, other accepted treatments, such as renal dialysis. Improvement in risk stratification for sudden death and assessment of ICD cost-effectiveness in specific subgroups of patients appears mandatory for any attempt to maximize health outcomes in a context of limited economic resources.

Within this complex scenario, the cardiologist responsible for decisions regarding the well-being of individual patients may often be confronted by "societal" limitations (limited economical funding) or by "individual" imperatives (offering the best to each patient). Specific suggestions based on long-term cost-effectiveness (which can also be generated by international registry studies) are urgently required to help translate the results of controlled trials into daily clinical practice, offering appropriate care to individual patients even in an era of economic constraints.

Acknowledgment

We are grateful to Robin M.T. Cooke for writing assistance.

References

1. Cohen JW, Krauss NA. Spending and service use among people with the fifteen most costly medical conditions, 1997. *Health Affairs* 2003; **22**: 129–138.

2. Ryden L, Stokoe G, Breithardt G *et al.* Patient access to medical technology across Europe. *Eur Heart J* 2004; **25**: 611–616.
3. Meltzer MI. Introduction to health economics for physicians. *Lancet* 2001; **358**: 993–998.
4. Tunis SR. Why Medicare has not established criteria for coverage decisions. *N Engl J Med* 2004; **350**: 2196–2198.
5. Mark DB, Hlatky MA. Medical economics and the assessment of value in cardiovascular medicine: part I. *Circulation* 2002; **106**: 516–520.
6. Mark DB, Hlatky MA. Medical economics and the assessment of value in cardiovascular medicine: part II. *Circulation* 2002; **106**: 626–630.
7. Hlatky MA. Evidence-based use of cardiac procedures and devices. *N Engl J Med* 2004; **350**: 2126–2128.
8. Kupersmith J. Cost-effective strategies in cardiology. In: Hurst JW, *et al.*, eds. *The Heart, Arteries and Veins*, 9th edn. McGraw-Hill, New York, 1998: 2557–2578.
9. Tengs TO, Adams ME, Pliskin JS *et al.* Five-hundred life-saving interventions and their cost-effectiveness. *Risk Analysis* 1995; **15**: 369–390.
10. Johannesson M, Jonsson B, Kjekshus J *et al.* Cost effectiveness of simvastatin treatment to lower cholesterol levels in patients with coronary heart disease. *N Engl J Med* 1997; **336**: 332–336.
11. Boriani G, Biffi M, Martignani C *et al.* Cost-effectiveness of implantable cardioverter-defibrillators. *Eur Heart J* 2001; **22**: 990–996.
12. Gaspoz JM, Coxson PG, Goldman PA *et al.* Cost effectiveness of aspirin, clopidogrel, or both for secondary prevention of coronary heart disease. *N Engl J Med* 2002; **346**: 1800–1806.
13. Zipes DP, Wellens HJJ. What have we learned about cardiac arrhythmias? *Circulation* 2000; **102**: IV52–IV57.
14. Gregoratos G, Abrams J, Epstein AE *et al.* ACC/AHA/NASPE 2002 guideline update for implantation of cardiac pacemakers and antiarrhythmia devices: a report of the American College of Cardiology/American Heart Association task force on practice guidelines (ACC/AHA/NASPE committee to update the 1998 pacemaker guidelines). *J Am Coll Cardiol* 2002; **40**: 1703–1719.
15. Priori SG, Aliot E, Blomstrom-Lundqvist C *et al.* Task force on sudden cardiac death of the European Society of Cardiology. *Eur Heart J* 2001; **16**: 1374–1450.
16. Priori SG, Aliot E, Blomstrom-Lundqvist C *et al.* Update of the guidelines on sudden cardiac death of the European Society of Cardiology. *Eur Heart J* 2003; **24**: 13–15.
17. Boriani G, Frabetti L, Biffi M *et al.* Clinical experience with downsized lower energy output implantable cardioverter-defibrillators. *Int J Cardiol* 1998; **66**: 261–266.
18. DiMarco JP. Implantable cardioverter-defibrillators. *N Engl J Med* 2003; **349**: 1836–1847.
19. Zipes DP. Implantable cardioverter-defibrillator: a Volkswagen or a Rolls Royce – how much will we pay to save a life? *Circulation* 2001; **103**: 1372–1374.
20. Bigger JT. Expanding indications for implantable cardiac defibrillators. *N Engl J Med* 2002; **346**: 931–933.
21. Boriani G, Biffi M, Martignani C, *et al.* Cardioverter-defibrillators after MADIT-II: the balance between weight of evidence and treatment costs. *Eur J Heart Failure* 2003; **5**: 419–425.
22. Reynolds MR, Josephson ME. MADIT II (second Multicenter Automated Defibrillator Implantation Trial) debate: risk stratification, costs, and public policy. *Circulation* 2003; **108**: 1779–1783.

23. The Antiarrhythmic Versus Implantable Defibrillator (AVID) Investigators. A comparison of antiarrhythmic drug therapy with implantable defibrillators in patients resuscitated from near-fatal ventricular arrhythmias. *N Engl J Med* 1997; **337**: 1576–1583.

24. Kuck KH, Cappato R, Siebels J *et al.* Randomized comparison of antiarrhythmic drug therapy with implantable defibrillators in patients resuscitated from cardiac arrest: the Cardiac Arrest Study Hamburg (CASH). *Circulation* 2000; **102**: 748–754.

25. Connolly SJ, Gent M, Roberts RS *et al.* Canadian implantable defibrillator study (CIDS): a randomized trial of the implantable cardioverter defibrillator against amiodarone. *Circulation* 2000; **101**: 1297–1302.

26. Connolly SJ, Hallstrom AP, Cappato R *et al.* Meta-analysis of the implantable cardioverter-defibrillator secondary prevention trials. AVID, CASH and CIDS studies. Antiarrhythmics Versus Implantable Defibrillator study. Cardiac Arrest Study Hamburg. Canadian Implantable Defibrillator Study. *Eur Heart J* 2000; **21**: 2071–2078.

27. Moss AJ, Hall J, Cannom DS *et al.* Improved survival with an implantable defibrillator in patients with coronary disease at high risk for ventricular arrhythmia. Multicenter Automatic Defibrillator Implantation Trial Investigators. *N Engl J Med* 1996; **335**: 1933–1940.

28. Buxton AE, Lee KL, Fisher JD *et al.* A randomized study of the prevention of sudden death in patients with coronary artery disease. Multicenter Unsustained Tachycardia Trial investigators. *N Engl J Med* 1999; **341**: 1882–1890.

29. Moss AJ, Zareba W, Hall WJ *et al.* Prophylactic implantation of a defibrillator in patients with myocardial infarction and reduced ejection fraction. *N Engl J Med* 2002; **346**: 877–883.

30. Bristow MR, Saxon LA, Boehmer J *et al.* Cardiac resynchronization therapy with or without an implantable defibrillator in advanced chronic heart failure. *N Engl J Med* 2004; **350**: 2140–2150.

31. Bardy GH, Lee KL, Mark DB *et al.* Amiodarone or an implantable cardioverter-defibrillator for congestive heart failure. *N Engl J Med* 2005; **352**: 225–237.

32. Cazeau S, Leclercq C, Lavergne T *et al.* Effects of multisite biventricular pacing in patients with heart failure and intraventricular conduction delay. *N Engl J Med* 2001; **344**: 873–880.

33. Abraham WT, Fisher WG, Smith AL *et al.* Cardiac resynchronization in chronic heart failure. *N Engl J Med* 2002; **346**: 1845–1853.

34. Bradley DJ, Bradley EA, Baughman KL *et al.* Cardiac resynchronization and death from progressive heart failure. A meta-analysis of randomized controlled trials. *JAMA* 2003; **289**: 730–740.

35. McAlister FA, Ezekowitz JA, Wiebe N *et al.* Systematic review: cardiac resynchronization in patients with symptomatic heart failure. *Ann Intern Med* 2004; **141**: 381–390.

36. Boriani G, Biffi M, Martignani C *et al.* Cardiac resynchronization by pacing: an electrical treatment of heart failure. *Int J Cardiol* 2004; **94**: 151–161.

37. Auricchio A, Abraham WT. Cardiac resynchronization therapy: current state of the art: cost versus benefit. *Circulation* 2004; **109**: 300–307.

38. Zipes DP. Guidelines: tools for building better patient care. *J Am Coll Cardiol* 2001; **38**: 2088–2090.

39. Ruskin JN, Camm AJ, Zipes DP, *et al*. Implantable cardioverter defibrillator utilization based on discharge diagnoses from Medicare and managed care patients. *J Cardiovasc Electrophysiol* 2002; **13**: 38–43.

40. Simoons ML. Cardiovascular diseases in Europe: challenges for the medical profession. *Eur Heart J* 2003; **24**: 8–12.

41. Schwartz PJ, Breithardt G, Howard J, *et al*. The legal implications of medical guidelines. A task force of the European Society of Cardiology. *Eur Heart J* 1999; **20**: 1152–1157.

42. Mushlin AI, Hall J, Zwanziger J, Gajang E, *et al*. The cost-effectiveness of implantable cardiac defibrillators: results from MADIT. Multicentre Automatic Defibrillator Trial. *Circulation* 1998; **97**: 2129–2135.

43. Sanders GD, Hlatky MA, Every NR, *et al*. Potential cost-effectiveness of prophylactic use of the implantable cardioverter-defibrillator or amiodarone after myocardial infarction. *Ann Intern Med* 2001; **135**: 870–883.

44. O'Brien BJ, Connolly SJ, Goeree R, *et al*. Cost-effectiveness of the implantable cardioverter-defibrillator. Results from the Canadian Implantable Defibrillator Study (CIDS). *Circulation* 2001; **103**: 1416–1421.

45. Sheldon R, O'Brien BJ, Blackhouse G, *et al*. Effect of clinical risk stratification on cost-effectiveness of the implantable cardioverter-defibrillator: the Canadian implantable defibrillator study. *Circulation* 2001; **104**: 1622–1626.

46. Owens DK, Sanders GD, Heidenreich PA, *et al*. Effect of risk stratification on cost-effectiveness of the implantable cardioverter-defibrillator. *Am Heart J* 2002; **144**: 440–448.

47. Larsen G, Hallstrom A, McAnulty J, *et al*. Cost-effectiveness of the implantable cardioverter-defibrillator versus antiarrhythmic drugs in survivors of serious ventricular tachyarrhythmias. *Circulation* 2002; **105**: 2049–2057.

48. Weiss JP, Saynina O, McDonald KM, *et al*. Effectiveness and cost-effectiveness of implantable cardioverter-defibrillators in the treatment of ventricular arrhythmias among Medicare beneficiaries. *Am J Med* 2002; **112**: 519–527.

49. Chen L, Hay JW. Cost-effectiveness of primary implantable cardioverter-defibrillator for sudden death prevention in congestive heart failure. *Cardiovasc Drug Ther* 2004; **18**: 161–170.

50. Mark DB. Cost-effectiveness of ICD therapy in the Sudden Cardiac Death in Heart Failure Trial (SCD-HeFT). Presented at the Late Breaking Trials session of the Annual Meeting of the American Heart Association, New Orleans, November 10, 2004.

51. Lynd LD, O'Brien BJ. Cost-effectiveness of the implantable cardioverter-defibrillator: a review of current evidence. *J Cardiovasc Electrophysiol* 2003; **14**: S99–S103.

52. Hlatky MA, Bigger JT. Cost-effectiveness of the implantable cardioverter defibrillator. *Lancet* 2001; **357**: 1817–1818.

53. Jauhar S, Slotwiner DJ. The economics of ICDs. *N Engl J Med* 2004; **351**: 2542–2544.

54. Salukhe TV, Dimopoulos K, Sutton R, *et al*. Life-years gained from defibrillator implantation: markedly nonlinear increase during 3 years of follow-up and its implications. *Circulation* 2004; **109**: 1848–1853.

55. Bokhari F, Newman D, Greene M, *et al*. Long-term comparison of the implantable cardioverter defibrillator versus amiodarone: eleven-year follow-up of a subset of patients in the Canadian Implantable Defibrillator Study (CIDS). *Circulation* 2004; **110**: 112–116.

56. Boriani G, Biffi M, Martignani C. Letter regarding article by Bokhari, *et al.* "Long-term comparison of the implantable cardioverter defibrillator versus amiodarone: eleven-year follow-up of a subset of patients in the Canadian Implantable Defibrillator Study (CIDS)." *Circulation* 2005; **111**: e26.
57. Boriani G, Maron B, Shen WK, *et al.* Prevention of sudden death in hypertrophic cardiomyopathy: but which defibrillator for which patient? *Circulation* 2004; **110**: e438–e442.
58. Moss AJ. Findings in MADIT II substudies. *Eur Heart J Suppl* 2003; **5**: I34–I38.
59. Nicol G, Kaul P, Huszti E, *et al.* Cost-effectiveness of cardiac resynchronization therapy in patients with symptomatic heart failure. *Ann Intern Med* 2004; **141**: 343–351.

Index

Page numbers in *italics* refer to figures and those in **bold** to tables, but note that figures and tables are only indicated when they are separated from their text references.